"*The Sambo Encyclopedia: Comprehensive Throws, Holds, and Submission Techniques* is a great book and Steve Scott is a great coach! If you want to know what sambo is all about, this is the book to read."

—Jan Trussell
World, Pan American, and US Nationals sambo champion

"I have been lucky to have spent my entire career training under Steve Scott. He has taken me from a 27-year-old recreational grappling enthusiast to the highest levels of competition in less than ten years. Because of Steve's guidance and tutelage, I have won silver at the Sambo Masters World Championships, medaled twice at the Pan American Sambo Championships and most recently a silver in 2019. I won the Sambo National Championship and trained over the world with world-class athletes and coaches. I owe this all to Steve Scott and a healthy respect for hard work.

"In addition to training under Steve, I have the honor of being his *uke* during seminars, photo shoots, and video tutorials. This role has allowed me to witness the impact he has had on the grappling community through his books, videos, and teaching. Through it all, he has remained dedicated to maintaining the spirit and ethos of sambo while pushing the boundaries of what we train and how we train it. Steve is a true innovator and has done more for the teaching and theory of sambo than anyone I know.

"While his coaching credentials are exemplary (he has coached multiple world champions), it is his writing that I believe will be his greatest legacy to the grappling community. In particular, his work in bringing sambo instruction and theory to an English speaking/reading audience will truly set him apart from his contemporaries. Steve has the ability to breakdown complex physical technique and action into simple chains of physics and body mechanics. He rarely speaks above his audience, instead consistently striving to communicate the theory and application in an approachable manner.

"I train with Steve Scott on a daily basis and yet I still look forward to each and every book, knowing that I will be better for reading it."

—Derrick Darling
Sando judo, silver medalist Sambo Masters World Championship
Silver and bronze medalist, Pan American Sambo Championship
National Sambo Championship

"Steve Scott is a world-class coach of sambo, judo, and jujitsu. Steve's own competitive background includes winning two national sambo championships as well as many high-level judo tournaments. As a coach he has produced three world sambo champions and a world medalist. Steve has been coach of the US World and Pan American Sambo Teams, the US Jr. World and Pan Am Judo Teams, and many others. I first met Steve at the US Olympic Committee Coach's College in the 1980s where we were selected to represent judo. As I got to know Steve, I was impressed by the depth of his knowledge in all aspects of judo, sambo, and other grappling arts. Even more impressive is his ability to impart his knowledge to others. I highly recommend *The Sambo Encyclopedia: Comprehensive Throws, Holds, and Submission Techniques* by Steve Scott. Now, for the price of a book you can tap into Steve's vast experience and learn how to take your game to the next level."

—John Saylor
Three-time US national judo champion, Pan American medalist
Head Coach US Olympic Training Center judo team (1983-1991)
Author of *Strength and Conditioning Secrets of the World's Greatest Fighters*
Director Shingitai Jujitsu Association

"Steve Scott's impressive tome is exactly what the title declares: *The Sambo Encyclopedia: Comprehensive Throws, Holds, and Submission Techniques*. This comprehensive book really is an encyclopedia of the Russian martial art of sambo. It pragmatically guides you through throws, takedowns, transitions, armlocks, leg locks, hold-downs, and breakdowns from this Russian martial sport. This incredible resource belongs in every sambo practitioner's library, and it's a book that will help anyone who desires to up their grappling skills through sambo's techniques and training methods."

—Alain Burrese, JD
5th dan Hapkido, former army sniper
Author of *Survive a Shooting, Hard-Won Wisdom From The School of Hard Knocks, How to Protect Yourself by Developing a Fighter's Mindset, 101 Safety and Self-Defense Tops, 101 More Safety and Self-Defense Tips, Lost Conscience, Tough Guy Wisdom Vols. 1-3* and DVD *Hapkido Hoshinsul*

"*The Sambo Encyclopedia* by master grappler Steve Scott offers an excellent opportunity to explore the major aspects of sport sambo! This book presents an interesting perspective on many grappling moves. Practical lessons can be learned even by seasoned grapplers who are not very knowledgeable about sambo's methods. Scott displays a lot of winning moves and the numerous clear photos in his book are well described with detailed captions. If you had to own only one book on sambo, this would be it. Highly recommended for anyone interested in effective grappling!"

—Andrew Zerling
Martial arts veteran, multi-award winning author
Author of *Sumo for Mixed Martial Arts: Winning Clinches, Takedowns, and Tactics*

The Sambo Encyclopedia

Comprehensive Throws, Holds, and Submission Techniques

by

Steve Scott

YMAA Publication Center

Wolfeboro, New Hampshire

YMAA Publication Center, Inc.
PO Box 480
Wolfeboro, New Hampshire, 03894
United States of America
1-800-669-8892 • info@ymaa.com • www.ymaa.com

ISBN: 9781594396557 (print) • ISBN: 9781594396564 (ebook) • ISBN: 9781594399008 (hardcover)
Copyright © 2019 by Steve Scott
All rights reserved including the right of reproduction in whole or in part in any form.
Copy editor: Doran Hunter
Cover design: Axie Breen
This book typeset in Adobe Caslon and Franklin Gothic

Illustrations courtesy of the author, unless otherwise noted.

20220924

Publisher's Cataloging in Publication

Names: Scott, Steve, 1952- author.

Title: The sambo encyclopedia : comprehensive throws, holds, and submission techniques / by Steve Scott.

Description: Revised and corrected edition. | Wolfeboro, New Hampshire : YMAA Publication Center, [2019] | "For all grappling styles"--Cover. | Originally published in 2015 by Turtle Press. | Includes bibliographical references.

Identifiers: ISBN: 9781594396557 (print) | 9781594396564 (ebook) | 9781594399008 (hardcover) | LCCN: 2019949656

Subjects: LCSH: Sambo wrestling--Handbooks, manuals, etc. | Sambo wrestling--Training. | Wrestling--Training. | Wrestling holds--Training. | Hand-to-hand fighting, Oriental--Training. | Hand-to-hand fighting--Training. | Judo--Training. | Mixed martial arts--Training. | Martial arts-- Holding--Training. | BISAC: SPORTS & RECREATION / Martial Arts & Self-Defense. | SPORTS & RECREATION / Wrestling.

Classification: LCC: GV1197.5 .S36 2019 | DDC: 796.8120947--dc23

Editor's Notes: Throughout this book, readers will see mention of US Judo, judo's national governing body. This organization is also known as US Judo, Inc. and USA Judo. For our purposes, the terms are synonymous.

SAMBO is a portmanteau of the Russian words *samozashchita bez oruzhiya*, which literally translates as "self-defense without weapons." Sambo is sometimes spelled sombo in English. For our purposes, the terms are synonymous.

Printed in USA.

Contents

Chapter One: The Essentials of Sambo   15

Chapter Two: The Throwing Techniques of Sambo   34

Chapter Three: The Leglocks, Ankle Locks, and Hip Locks of Sambo 118

Chapter Four: The Armlocks of Sambo   182

Chapter Five: The Holds and Breakdowns of Sambo   276

Chapter Six: Epilogue   327

This book is dedicated to Dr. Ivan Olsen, the father of American Sambo.

INTRODUCTION

Almost every culture on this planet has its own system of wrestling or fighting, and it was the culture of the people who made up what was then the Soviet Union that gave birth to the rugged sport of sambo. There have been few books written in the English language on this subject, and with sambo's recent surge in popularity, it is a good time to offer a serious, technical look at the Russian martial sport that has changed the way the martial arts world looks at grappling.

On the pages of this book, you will find the nuts and bolts of sambo: what makes it unique and what makes it work. It is my intention to provide to you a reliable resource that you can use for many years to come. Sambo is a perfect example of the famous architect Louis Sullivan's adage, "Form ever follows function." Sambo's overarching philosophy emphasizes efficiency over aesthetics and victory over defeat. In keeping with the pragmatic approach of sambo, this book will present a wide variety of throws, takedowns, transitions, armlocks, leglocks, hold-downs, and breakdowns. All presented in the functional, efficient, and no-nonsense manner that makes sambo what it is.

Sambo was born in the old Soviet Union, and its roots are steeped in the social fabric of the diverse people who lived during that time. It's a demanding fighting sport that either makes the best out of you or takes the best from you. This author sincerely believes that sambo is the most demanding grappling sport that has ever been devised.

Sambo's early technical theories were based largely on Kodokan judo, but theories and techniques from other martial arts and fighting styles, both native to the Soviet republics and from outside the Soviet Union, were also included. Vasili Oshchepkov, one of the men who initially developed what later became known as sambo, trained in Japan under judo's founder Jigoro Kano. Oshchepkov didn't hide the fact that judo was the basis for the new form of grappling combat he developed, and he lost his life for it. A victim of Stalin's purges in the late 1930s, Oshchepkov died in a Soviet prison accused of being a Japanese sympathizer and spy, but it is believed he was arrested because of the credit he gave judo for sambo's early technical development instead of claiming it was purely a Soviet invention. But, Oshchepkov (as well as Viktor Spiridonov and others) put into motion the philosophical and technical foundation that remains to this day. While judo was the initial martial discipline that Oshchepkov studied, he, Viktor Spiridonov and their collaborators and students traveled across the Soviet Union taking the best they could find from the many regional wrestling styles they encountered. As a result of this research and development, the fighting discipline that had no formal name other than being called "judo" or "freestyle wrestling" by Oshpechkov and "samoz" by Spiridonov (until the Soviet government officially named the sport sambo) evolved and took on a form and personality all its own. It was Anatoli Kharlampiev, the man recognized as the "father of sambo" and a student of Oshchepkov and Spiridonov (as well as other early pioneers) who gave this form of personal combat a name and gained for it formal recognition by the Soviet government on Nov. 16, 1938.

Eventually, sambo was the primary style of wrestling a promising youngster would take up in the Soviet Union. As the child grew and developed, he might be able to train in the Olympic sports of judo, freestyle wrestling, or Greco-Roman wrestling. He might also have stayed in the primary sport, sambo, and pursued his athletic career in this native wrestling style of the Soviet Union. Whichever was chosen, it was sambo that was his primary wrestling and grappling education.

This book is the result of years of training and coaching and comes from my perspective as a coach, sambo wrestler, and mat official from the United States.

SAMBO ENCYCLOPEDIA

Sambo's history in the United States is a colorful one, and I was around for many of its early years. I've met a lot of people and been to a lot of places, and it is hoped that this experience is reflected on the pages of this book in a positive way. There have been a number of books and videos produced about the sport of sambo, and it's my hope that this book provides a helpful contribution to the existing body of knowledge on the subject and provides a reliable resource for anyone who is interested in sambo.

From a technical perspective, it's probably obvious to say, but I'll say it anyway; not every technique in the sport of sambo is included in this book. What you will see are a lot of realistic, functional, and effective technical skills presented from this author's perspective and based on sambo's eclectic technical and theoretical foundation. The photographs used in this book were, in large part, taken during actual workouts at our Welcome Mat Training Centers. I've made every attempt to include on these pages the technical skills that form the basis of what sambo is as well as provide analysis of many of the distinctive moves that make sambo the unique and effective fighting sport it is.

To the trained observer, sambo techniques (especially the throwing techniques of sambo) have a distinctive "look" to them. Years ago, my good friend John Saylor, who was a US National Judo Champion and Pan American Judo Championships medal winner as well as the head coach of the US Olympic Training Center's judo squad, commented to me that he spotted (as he put it) "a distinct sambo flair" to how I performed and taught throwing techniques. This led to an interesting technical discussion about (on the surface level) stylistic differences (and on the substantive level) biomechanical differences (and similarities) between sambo's approach to technical acquisition and application in contrast to judo's approach. John and I were coaching at one of his yearly Shingitai training camps (John is the director of the Shingitai Jujitsu Association) when he observed how the athletes from my club (with our strong sambo background) were using both gripping and body space to control and unbalance opponents when throwing them. In essence, the sambo-trained athletes generally were in closer proximity to their opponents than the judo-trained athletes, and the sambo-trained athletes tended to use their gripping to control their opponents more at the shoulder than at the arm. Pulling an opponent at the elbow wasn't (and isn't) the only way

to disturb an opponent's balance, and in many cases the sambo-trained athletes jammed the opponent's arms in rather than out. Basically, the sambo-trained athletes "broke the balance" of opponents in a different way than the judo-trained athletes did, and the resulting throw had a different look to it. A trained observer (like John Saylor) will immediately recognize the differences. Both approaches work. But, from a perspective based on sambo's utilitarian and functional approach, both should be learned and practiced, and it's up to the athlete to determine which works best for him (or her). This pragmatic approach is seen in all aspects of technical and tactical skill in sambo. If the idea is to beat an opponent and beat him decisively, then use any skill or tactic that is permitted by the rules of the sport.

I would like to thank Becky Scott, who, besides being my wife and best friend, is one of America's all-time great sambo champions and is the first woman from the United States to win a World Sambo Championship (in 1983 at the first World Sambo Championships for women in Madrid, Spain). Her advice during the writing of this book is appreciated. My sincere thanks to David Ripianzi and his team at YMAA Publications, especially to this book's patient and hard-working editor, Doran Hunter,

Many thanks to Derrick Darling, Gregg Humphreys, Mike Pennington, Ken Brink, Kelvin Knisely, Sandi Harrelson, Ben Goehrung, Jeff Suchman, Jake Pursley, Jarrod Fobes, John Zabel, Aric Weaver, Chico Hernandez, Anthony Ishmael, JT Thayne, Dre Glover, Julie Patton, Eric McIntosh, Andre Coleman, Eric Millsap, Chris Heckadon, Bob Rittman, Kyle Meredith, Will Cook, Kyle Elliott, Greg Fetters, Slava Nozhnik, and Jeff Owens for their help. These people are gifted athletes, coaches, and technicians, and their skill is what you see on the pages of this book.

My gratitude and respect go to Maurice Allan, MBE, the Scotsman who was my first sambo coach, and to Ken Regennitter, my judo and jujitsu coach and the person who suggested to me that I give sambo a try. I'm glad I listened to Ken's advice.

Finally, I want to dedicate this book to Dr. Ivan Olsen, the father of American sambo. Ivan was my mentor, and the mentor to many sambo wrestlers and coaches in the United States. He was the Chairman of the AAU (Amateur Athletic Union) Sambo Committee for many years and responsible for the early growth of the sport in the United States. Ivan was a great wrestling coach and leader, but an even greater human being. Many of us owe him a lot.

The skills presented in this book have all passed the tests of both time and competition. There is no filler or fluff here. Everything presented has been used successfully in all levels of competitive sambo. I am a firm believer that fundamentally sound skills performed by a motivated and well-conditioned athlete who has molded what he knows to work for him with a high rate of success is hard to beat. This is the approach I have taken as an athlete and as a coach, and I hope to convey that as an author in this book as well. Sambo is a real test of fitness, skill, and courage. It is my goal to provide a text that can be used by anyone who wants to put on a red jacket or a blue jacket and test his or her character in the rugged sport of sambo.

Steve Scott

AUTHOR'S NOTE

The scope of this book is to present sambo's unique technical approach in throwing techniques, submission, and holding techniques and the other supporting skills that make sambo what it is. The emphasis will be on presenting a variety of skills based on their function and utility in actual sport combat. There are some skills that are, if not identical, at least similar in appearance to skills in judo or wrestling. Some of these skills will be presented on these pages, but more emphasis will be placed on the skills that are characteristic and distinctive to sambo.

In some of the photographs in this book, the athletes demonstrating the skills are not wearing sambo jackets or uniforms, while in others, they are. This is done so that in the photo series where a submission technique is presented, you get a better view of what each appendage or part of the body is doing. Showing a photo where you, the reader, can get a better view of what each arm, leg, or other part of the body is doing will provide a better picture of how to do the move. Be assured that what is being presented in a photo where the athletes are not wearing sambo jackets is something they would also be doing when wearing sambo jackets. In some cases, such as in throwing techniques, the athletes in the photos wear a jacket (kurtka) because the actual application of the technique may rely on the use of the jacket or belt.

As in all combat sports or fighting arts, safety is paramount and the author, editors, and publisher of this book wish to stress that anyone practicing the skills presented in this book do so under the guidance of a competent, qualified coach or instructor. Practice safely and respect your training partners, and when someone taps out or signals submission verbally, respect it and stop applying the technique. Remember the old sambo adage when working out: "When in doubt, tap out."

The use of Russian names for the techniques and skills presented in this book will not generally be used. Unlike judo, where it is common to learn the names of techniques in Japanese, Russian terminology, at least from this author's experience, has not been widely used in sambo. As a result, the names of the various techniques presented in this book will be descriptive in nature and reflect the specific function of the particular technique.

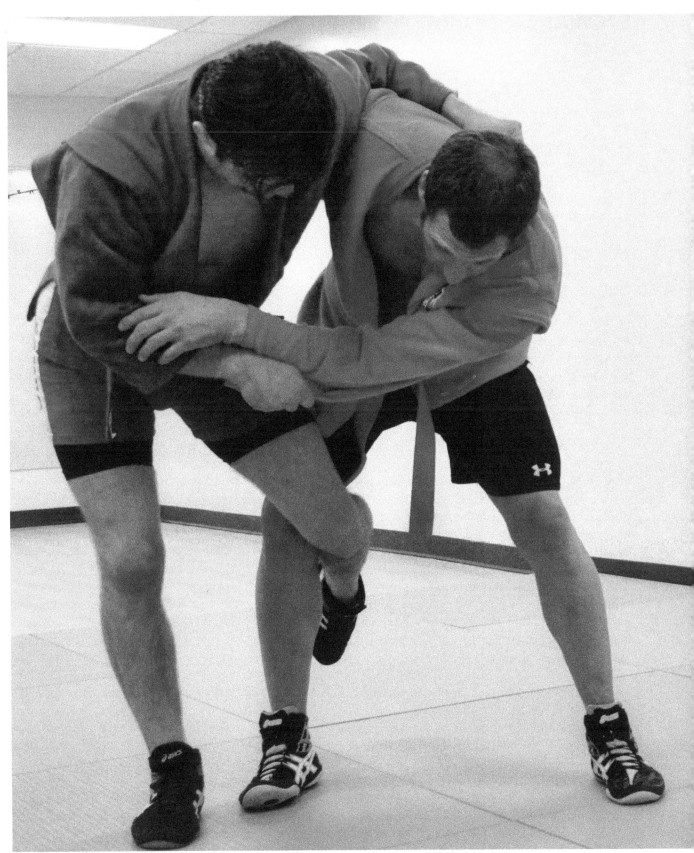

Chapter One: The Essentials of Sambo

"Sambo is not for the faint of heart."

SAMBO: NOT FOR THE FAINT OF HEART

The young newspaper reporter was looking for an angle for his story about the national sambo tournament I was hosting sometime back around 1985 or so in Kansas City, Missouri. I had given him the necessary background information on the sport; the rules, history, who was competing that day, and the other bits of information that would give the reporter more than enough information to provide an interesting story to his readers. As it turned out, he was fascinated with what took place on the mat and stayed for most of the tournament. Since this was sambo and not the far more popular (and known) sports of baseball, basketball, or football (and I imagine the reporter wasn't too high up on the food chain in the newsroom at the time), the local newspaper ran a small, perfunctory article in the back of the sports section in the morning edition the next day. But the opening sentence of that reporter's brief story has stayed with me ever since. He wrote, "Sambo is not for the faint of heart."

He was right. Sambo isn't for the faint of heart, or for the faint of body for that matter. It's one of the most technically rich and diverse as well as physically demanding sports ever devised. Sambo is a tough sport practiced by tough men and women. It isn't hyperbole when I write this statement. It's simply true. It's my sincere belief that, in any given year, the men and women who win the World Sambo Championships are some of the best, if not the best, grapplers on the planet. No offense is intended or meant to any other grappling or wrestling sport or the people who do them, but sambo requires the very best, and then expects more, from anyone who does it.

Coming out of Stalin's regime in the old Soviet Union, sambo has stood the test of time, world events, and the evolution of combat sports to make a huge and lasting impact. Sambo has altered how many people in judo, jujitsu, mixed martial arts, and other fighting sports have looked at these martial arts and has been a catalyst for innovative technical change in just about every fighting sport or art that has come in contact with it. I know that my first sport, judo, has been changed forever (and for the better in my opinion) because of sambo's influences.

When Soviet athletes appeared on the international scene in the late 1950s and early 1960s, they changed the way sport was done—any sport. Their training methods were considered the best in the world at that time. The Soviet Union was, among other things, a sports machine that cranked out world-class athletes every year, seemingly getting better every year until the wall came crumbling down...both literally and figuratively. The Soviet Union wanted to make a political statement and one of the ways they made it was through their athletes in the world of international sport. Where better than on the world stage of the Olympic Games? The Soviet sports machine, born after the ruins of World War II, was introduced to the world in the 1950s and early 1960s; and since sambo wasn't an Olympic sport, the next best things were judo and wrestling.

The 1964 Olympics in Tokyo, Japan, served as the stage for the world's first look at sambo when a team of sambo/judo men from the Soviet Union competed in the Olympic judo event. The Soviets entered four athletes and won four bronze medals, placing second as a team behind Japan. The initial exposure of this strange form of grappling certainly changed the way everyone did any form of wrestling or grappling ever since those sambo men walked onto that judo mat in Tokyo.

The unusual, yet effective, throws that the sambo men in the 1960s were doing in international judo tournaments had not ever been seen on the world stage before. In addition, these sambo grapplers seemed to have a sixth sense on how to get an opponent, almost any opponent, into some kind of armlock. These Soviet sambo men meant business. They didn't care about the aesthetics of any given throw, hold, or submission technique. They simply cared about the functional aspect of how to go about beating any and every opponent they faced. And, not only that, these guys were in shape. Their fitness levels were superb; and because they were so physically dominating, they made their technical execution of their unusual skills even more effective and impressive.

These Soviet sambo wrestlers didn't approach judo the way the Japanese did. The sambo men didn't train to perfect a technique, as was the accepted Japanese (and world) view of judo. Instead, these sambo men trained to become proficient with techniques in a variety of situations. Emphasizing utility over aesthetics, they molded the technique to work for them and had no qualms about changing a move to make it work for their own body type or weight class. In the seclusion and isolation of the Soviet regime, the sport of sambo developed into a mature and efficient combat sport parallel to the development of the sport of judo: rooted in the technical concepts of Kodokan judo with influences of wrestling styles from throughout the Soviet empire. In reality, sambo was the Soviet Union's counterpart to judo during that period of history.

Essentially, sambo places emphasis on fast-paced, powerful, and functional throwing techniques and equally fast-paced, powerful, and functional groundfighting techniques. Fitness is a key component in a sambo wrestler's arsenal and serves as the foundation for technical and tactical superiority.

There are two basic versions of sambo. One is combat sambo that emphasizes self-defense and resembles mixed martial arts in sambo jackets. The other, presented on the pages of this book, is called borba sambo, or grappling-based sambo. This author's interest has usually been on the grappling side of sambo, but I have found that the self-defense techniques used in sambo are efficient, to the point, and applicable in any situation. While there is much to be learned from the self-defense aspect of sambo, this book will present the sport approach and look at some of the skills that make sambo unique in the world of wrestling and grappling. One book can't possibly do justice to this fascinating sport, so I will present some of the skills that have worked for my athletes and me through our years of involvement in sambo.

Technically, the most useful way to describe borba (grappling) sambo is that it is primarily a throwing and submission sport. I say this because the focus of action is throwing an opponent to the mat and transitioning quickly into a joint lock or hold-down. The groundfighting that takes place in sambo has the ultimate goal of making the opponent submit. Hold-downs are seen as a way of controlling or immobilizing an opponent on the mat and picking up some points in the score until you are able to secure a submission technique. Presently, the rules of sambo allow for throws, takedowns, holds, elbow submissions, and leg submissions. Choking an opponent is not permitted in the grappling sport of sambo, but this may be changed in the future. (However, "freestyle sambo," initially developed by Steve Koepfer of New York, is a popular and innovative adaptation of the sambo rules that allows

choking techniques.) The combat version of sambo allows for everything done in grappling sambo, but also including chokes, punching, and kicking. I was always fascinated by sambo's attitude of accepting anything that works and the philosophy of molding the technique to make it work for the person doing it, whether it's in combat sambo or borba sambo.

To the Soviets who invented sambo, and to the exponents all over the world who practice the sport, sambo is considered one of many styles of wrestling or grappling or fighting available. The sports of judo, freestyle wrestling, Greco-Roman wrestling, or any of the traditional folk styles of wrestling found anywhere in the world are, to the sambo exponent's way of thinking, fundamentally similar. The major differences are simply in the rules of the sport and the emphasis each sport may place on specific techniques or tactics. A good throw is a good throw no matter what sport it's done in, who does it, or what type of garment is worn. The same thing can be said about an armlock, hold, or any other technical skill. The emphasis, in every case, is that the skill is done in a functionally efficient and effective manner.

For many years following the Second World War, sambo was the primary wrestling style in the Soviet Union, and the other styles of international wrestling and judo were secondary to their native sport of sambo. This is why sambo so greatly influenced the way the Soviets did judo, freestyle wrestling, and Greco-Roman wrestling for many years and why sambo has made such a lasting impression on anyone who participates in wrestling, judo, or grappling today. Sambo wrestlers who participate in the many mixed martial arts events popular today prove that sambo places emphasis on both skill and fighting ability. Again, as said in the opening paragraph, sambo isn't for the faint of heart.

When sambo wasn't selected as a demonstration sport in the 1980 Moscow Olympics or the 1984 Los Angeles Olympics, the sport began to decline in popularity. However, there has been a real resurgence in the last few years, and many new people are training in sambo today. Sambo's new-found popularity is (to a great degree) the result of sambo men who have done well in the various mixed martial arts events held all over the world in recent years. Much like its initial rise in popularity back in the 1960s when the Soviet sambo men took the judo world by storm, a younger generation of sambo athletes is winning in the new international sporting event of mixed martial arts.

SAMBO ENCYCLOPEDIA

Sambo, by its very nature, is an eclectic and wide-open approach to mat combat. Embracing a philosophy of effectiveness over beauty, it is no wonder that grapplers, fighters, and wrestlers all over the world have discovered that sambo is worth learning.

A BRIEF HISTORY OF SAMBO

In 1918, the Soviet ruler Vladimir Lenin created a program of military training for the newly formed Soviet Army. Part of that new program was the development of a hand-to-hand fighting program. In 1923, the Soviet government opened a new physical training center called the Dynamo Sports Society and hired a military combat veteran of World War One named Viktor Spiridonov. Spiridonov had conducted extensive research into the various styles of wrestling and fighting that comprised the Soviet Union as well as research on wrestling and fighting styles from other countries as well.

Working independently of Spiridonov was Vasili Oshpechkov, who, in 1911, as a young man of 19 traveled from his native Vladivostok to Tokyo to become one of the first non-Japanese to be admitted to the Kodokan Judo Institute in Japan. In 1913, Oshpechkov was promoted to Shodan (first-degree black belt) and returned to Vladivostok to teach judo in his hometown. In 1917, Oshpechkov returned to the Kodokan in Japan and was promoted to Nidan (second-degree black belt). When Oshpechkov again returned to his native Russia after spending several years in China, he combined his knowledge of Kodokan judo with a myriad of other fighting systems ranging from wushu of China to the various grappling and fighting styles of the republics of the Soviet Union and even to the more western styles of wrestling and boxing. At that point in time, Oshpechkov called his fighting system the generic name of "judo" and also sometimes called it "freestyle wrestling." In 1929, Oshpechkov joined Spiridonov at the Dynamo Sports Society, and working with a team of other experts and students, endeavored to develop a comprehensive and practical form of hand-to-hand combat for the Soviet military. One of those students was Anatoli Kharlampiev, who would a few years later be recognized as the official founder of what was to become known as sambo.

Tragically, Vasili Oshpechkov was a victim of the Soviet dictator Josef Stalin's purges and in 1937 was arrested and executed as a spy for Japan. Up to this time, Oshpechkov was one of the driving forces behind the eclectic fighting system that was forming in the Soviet Union, and with his death Anatoli Kharlampiev took the reins of leadership in what was to become known as sambo. For the sake of clarity, it is important to point out that Oshpechkov never used the name "sambo" when describing what he taught. Oshpechkov called what he did "judo," "freestyle wrestling," or similar descriptive terms, and it was Kharlampiev who eventually managed to get the Soviet government to use the name sambo.

To best understand sambo both historically and technically, it's a good idea to get some basic background about its primary underpinning: Kodokan judo. Prof. Jigoro Kano formed Kodokan judo in 1882 in Tokyo, Japan. Drawing directly on Prof. Kano's writings and what many judo exponents since have written is that Kodokan judo is (first and foremost) a method of physical education and character development. The sporting aspect of judo was of secondary importance to Prof. Kano. As a judoman (as well as a sambo man) myself, this author sincerely believes Jigoro Kano was a brilliant man and that his gift of Kodokan Judo to the world is certainly appreciated. From what can be ascertained, Vasili Oshpechkov believed this as well and wanted to bring judo to his native Russia; and in the process, adapt it to meet the needs of his countrymen. All of the early pioneers of what was to become known as sambo agreed that this eclectic method of personal combat was primarily a fighting art and a fighting sport. So, it is fair to say that sambo was formed as a method of fighting and, more specifically, fighting as a competitive activity. Historically, Viktor Spiridonov (the other primary innovator of what was to be later called sambo) had less interest in sambo as a competitive activity than Oshpechkov did. Oshpechkov believed that skill in actual combat could be best developed by skill in competitive fighting. Sambo's doctrines and traditions are less concerned with physical education or character development than with developing fighters. That's not to say sambo cannot be used as a vehicle to teach good sportsmanship or other positive values; it most certainly can. But like boxing and wrestling, sambo's primary purpose is that of a fighting sport and not a method of physical education as Kodokan judo is.

Sambo is the acronym for the Russian name that means "self-defense without weapons" (SAMozashchita Bez Oruzhiya). Initially called "samozashchita" and shortened to "samoz" by Viktor Spiridonov as early as around 1923, it was primarily through the work of Anatoli Kharlampiev that "judo freestyle wrestling" (later to be officially called "sambo" in 1948) was recognized as an official sport of the Soviet Union's "All Union Sports Committee" on Nov. 16, 1938. For this reason, Anatoli Kharlampiev is considered to be the official founder of sambo, but credit should also be given to Oshpechkov, Spiridonov, and others who came before him. However, it was the hard work of Kharlampiev that prevented sambo from disappearing from history in this tumultuous time in both world and Russian history.

In 1939, first National Sambo Championships were held in the Soviet Union, and held again 1940. World War II forced the suspension of this tournament, but in 1947 the tournament was started again. By the early 1950s, the military-style combat sambo and the competitive borba (wrestling) sambo were officially made distinct of each other, with the combat sambo practiced by the military and police and the borba sambo practiced by everyone else. (Author's note: this book concerns itself with borba sambo only.)

Sambo became an international sport in 1966 when the International Amateur Wrestling Federation (FILA) recognized sambo as an international style of wrestling (along with freestyle and Greco-Roman). The first European Sambo Championships were held in Riga, Latvia, in 1972. The first World Sambo Championships were held in 1973 in Tehran, Iran. The first World Sambo Championships for women were held in 1983 in Madrid, Spain. The first U.S. National AAU (Amateur Athletic Union) Sambo Championships were held in 1975 in Mesa, Arizona, for men and in 1980 in Kansas City, Missouri, for women. The first U.S. AAU National Youth Sambo Championships were held in 1980 in Kansas City, Missouri. In 1984, FILA dropped sambo from its program and the International Amateur Sambo Federation (FIAS) was formally organized.

In 2001, combat sambo was expanded from military and police use to become a separate sport and the Combat Sambo Federation of Russia was formed. Combat sambo has become a popular international sport and a good many professional mixed martial arts fighters come from a combat sambo background.

Sambo was a recognized sport in the 1983 Pan American Games in Caracas, Venezuela, with the hopes (at least in the sambo community) of gaining acceptance in the 1984 Olympics in Los Angeles. This was sambo's first and only (up to the present time) appearance in the quadrennial Pan American Games sanctioned by the International Olympic Committee.

When sambo wasn't selected as a demonstration sport in the 1980 Moscow Olympics or the 1984 Los Angeles Olympics, the sport began to decline in popularity both internationally and in the United States. However, there has been a real resurgence in the last few years, and many new people are training in sambo today. Sambo's new-found popularity is the result of sambo men who have done well in the various mixed martial arts events held all over the world in recent years. Much like its initial rise in popularity back in the 1960s when the Soviet sambo men took the judo world by storm, a younger generation of sambo athletes is winning in the new international sporting event of mixed martial arts.

Sambo is also spelled "sombo," which was the spelling first used, to my knowledge, in the early 1980s here in the United States. The "o" spelling was implemented to have Americans use the "ah" sound rather than the "aa" sound in the name. The phonetic spelling helped, and most Americans now pronounce the name of the sport correctly. I remember back in the 1970s when I became involved in sambo, most people pronounced it wrong. Additionally, the word "sambo" had rather negative racial connotations in the past and replacing the "a" with an "o" served as a way of disassociating a great grappling sport from any negative associations. However, times have changed for the better in that regard and most people today use the "sambo" spelling and that is what is used in this book.

References

- Adams, Andy. "Russia Prepares to Export Sambo." *Black Belt Magazine*, February 1967.
- Adams, Andy. "Sambo, the Russian Self-Defense Sport." *Black Belt Magazine*, July 1967.
- Anderson, Scott. "Is This Eclectic Martial Art What America Needs For Self-Defense?" *Black Belt Magazine*. February 1998.
- Green, Thomas and Joseph R. Svinth, eds. *Martial Arts of the World*, Santa Barbara, CA: ABC-CLIO, 210.
- Gulevitch, Dimitri. *Judo Times Magazine*, May 1974.
- Porter, Major Phil. "Judo in the Olympics." *Black Belt Magazine*, February 1965.
- Sonnen, Scott. "The History of Hidden Sambo." USADojo.com.

A TECHNICAL ANALYSIS OF SAMBO

Sambo is a grappling sport that places primary emphasis on throwing and submission techniques with secondary emphasis on holding (or pinning) techniques. Sambo matches start with both grapplers in a standing position directly in front of each other. The sambo uniform, consisting of a jacket with belt, shorts, and shoes, provides the primary means of contact for the sambo grapplers or wrestlers. A sambo wrestler's goal is to throw his (or her) opponent to the mat and finish the opponent off with a submission technique. If, in the process, the sambo wrestler is able to (by opportunity or by choice) hold his opponent to the mat to control him, the sambo wrestler will use that hold-down to score points and ultimately attempt to finish the opponent off with a submission technique.

Fundamentally, sambo techniques consist of armlocks, leglocks, throws, and hold-downs. There are also supplementary technical skills that make the armlocks, leglocks, throws, and hold-downs happen. An analogy is a solid brick house. The throws, armlocks, leglocks, and hold-downs are the bricks and the supplementary skills such as transitions, breakdowns, gripping, and other ancillary skills serve as the cement that holds the bricks together to form a solid structure.

TECHNICAL CATEGORIES FOR SAMBO

There are thousands of techniques and moves in the sport of sambo, and it would be impossible to list or categorize every one of them. In this regard, sambo is an open-ended activity with a continually expanding technical base. Since sambo is such a dynamic and fluid activity, some of these categories blend or blur into one another. So, in an effort to provide a general analysis of the technical skills of sambo as well as to provide a general guide for the purposes of teaching and learning, the following curriculum is presented.

THROWING TECHNIQUES

The throws of sambo are designed to take an opponent to the mat or ground with control and force in order to score a "total victory" or maximum points. A secondary purpose of a throw is to immediately follow up after the throw to a submission technique or hold-down.

The maximum score of total victory is awarded for throwing an opponent to the mat with control and largely onto his back with the thrower remaining standing and in control of his posture.

Four Points: A throw that could be scored as a total victory except the thrower lands on his opponent or in some other way finishes the throw without remaining standing.

Two Points: A throw where the person being thrown lands primarily on his side or back side.

One Point: A throw where the person being thrown lands on his buttocks, hip, or entirely on his side or on his front on his chest and stomach area.

A secondary purpose of a throw is to immediately follow up after the throw to a submission technique or hold-down.

In some throwing techniques, high amplitude or lifting an opponent high into the air is achieved and in other throws, it is not.

Wheel Throws

In these throwing techniques, the attacker throws his opponent forward and over his body. Imagine a wheel, with the thrower standing upright and in the middle of the wheel; another example is the action of a windmill turning. The thrower "wheels" his opponent forward and over the thrower's body at a fairly constant rate of speed.

There are three basic variations of wheel throws.

1. Wheel Throw with Both Feet on the Mat

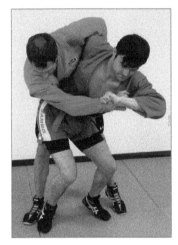

Both of the attacker's feet are on the mat as he throws his opponent.

2. Wheel Throw with One Foot on the Mat

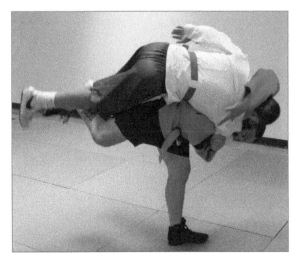

The attacker supports himself with one foot on the mat as he throws his opponent.

3. Wheel Throw with Attacker on One or Both Knees

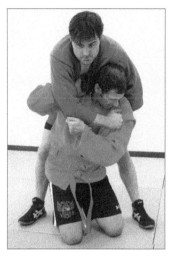

The attacker drops under the center of gravity of his opponent as he throws him.

Rotation Throws

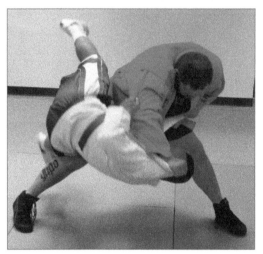

In these throwing techniques, the attacker throws his opponent forward and over his body in a rotational manner. An analogy is the action of a tornado with the strong rotation in a horizontal or semi-horizontal direction. Rotation throws are similar to wheel throws except that in a rotation throw, the person being thrown spins or turns in a forward or backward direction over the thrower's body or part of his body.

Momentum Throws

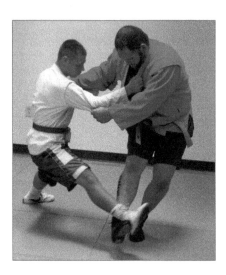

These are foot sweeps, leg hooks, or other throws where the person being thrown has one part of his body move at a faster speed and in a different direction than the opposing end of his body.

Body Weight Throws

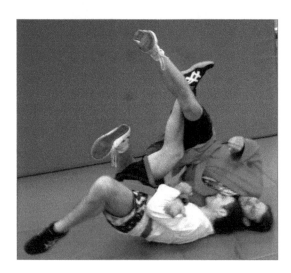

In these throws, the attacker commits his body and "sacrifices" it to go to the mat or ground in order to throw his opponent.

Lifting and Pick-Up Throws

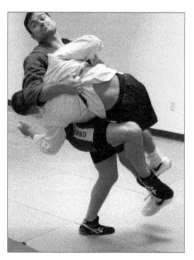

These are high amplitude throws where the attacker picks his opponent up or uses any part of his body, legs, arms, or hips to lift his opponent up and off the mat.

A Comment on Takedowns

The term "takedown" is used in all styles of wrestling and combat sports, from freestyle wrestling to mixed martial arts. It is commonly used as a generic term for any throw or transition from a standing position to the mat.

Specifically, takedowns are moves designed to start from a standing position with the goal of taking the opponent to the mat or ground in order to control him there. The secondary goal of a takedown is to score points in the process.

A takedown is not entirely a throw and not entirely a transition. A takedown is a move where the attacker takes his opponent from his feet in a standing position to the mat or ground with the purpose of simply gaining further control when on the mat and not necessarily a specific submission technique or hold. Sometimes, a takedown is applied with such skill and force that a total victory or points are scored as in a throw. Just as often, a takedown can immediately lead into a submission technique or hold-down; but the important factor is that the attacker simply wants to take his opponent to the mat with the singular intent of gaining further control once there. For this reason, takedowns are considered to be a form of transition from standing to the mat or ground.

TRANSITIONS

In transitions, the attacker uses any move with a specific goal of securing a submission or finishing technique against his opponent. A transition is unlike a throw, where the attacker's primary purpose is to gain total victory or maximum points and follow through to the mat or ground with a hold-down or submission technique as a secondary purpose. A transition takes place when one sambo wrestler moves from one position to another in an attempt to secure a specific submission technique, throw, or hold-down. There are four primary categories of transition techniques.

Standing to Groundfighting Transition

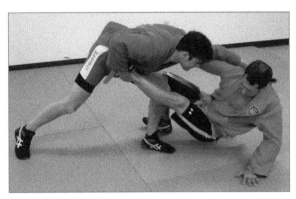

This transition takes place when the attacker takes his opponent to the mat with a specific finishing hold or technique in mind and immediately applies it. This photo shows a classic example of the attacker using an ankle pick that takes his opponent to the mat so that the attacker can immediately apply an ankle lock or another finishing hold.

Standing to Standing Transition

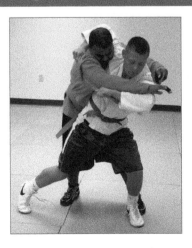

This transition takes place when one grappler attacks his opponent with a throw and switches to another throwing technique that ultimately throws the defender. These are the "combination attacks" or "continuation attacks" used in sambo (sometimes called "linked attacks"). They are as follows:

1. The attacker has every intention of throwing his opponent with the initial attack, but the defender's actions force the attacker to immediately follow up with another throwing attack, and he scores with it.
2. The attacker fakes or feigns an initial attack, forcing his opponent to react in a specific way, and the attacker immediately follows up with a second throwing attack and scores with it.

Groundfighting to Standing Transition

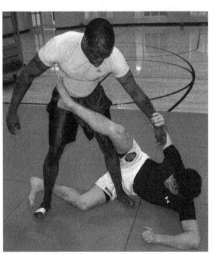

The attacker is on the mat or ground, and his opponent is standing. In this transition, the attacker works from the bottom and can apply a throw or finishing hold by taking his standing opponent to the mat. This photo shows the attacker positioned on the mat and using a scissors throw against his standing opponent.

Groundfighting to Groundfighting Transition

This type of transition takes place when the attacker moves from one groundfighting position into another groundfighting position. There are two basic types:

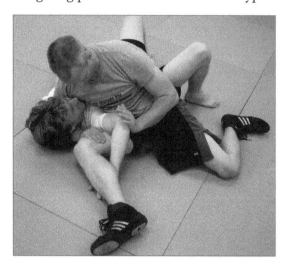

The first transition occurs when one sambo wrestler moves from a specific technique to another technique. This is a common transition. When one sambo wrestler holds his opponent for twenty seconds and scores four points, the mat official will instruct the sambo wrestler to "go for the submission." The sambo wrestler who holds his opponent will immediately attempt a submission technique as shown in this photo.

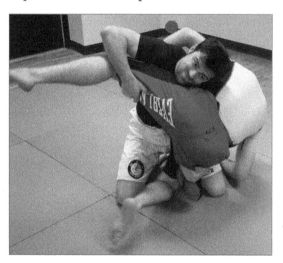

The second type of transition in a groundfighting-to-groundfighting situation is what is called a "breakdown." In a breakdown, the attacker takes his opponent from a stable to an unstable position. The attacker follows up with a finishing hold or submission technique.

UPPER BODY SUBMISSIONS

These techniques are the armlocks of sambo. The primary target of an armlock is the opponent's elbow joint but, realistically, a great deal of stress and pain is applied to the opponent's shoulder as well. There are three primary applications of armlocks in sambo: the cross-body armlock, the bent armlock, and the straight armlock. Sambo has many functional and effective armlocks, and sambo exponents take great pride in the many innovative armlocks that are used in both borba (grappling) sambo and combat sambo.

Cross-Body Armlock

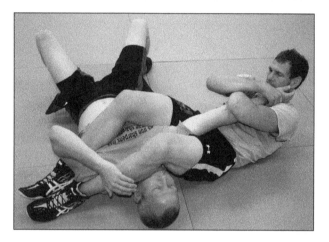

Sambo has many effective and functional applications and variations of the cross-body armlock. Basically, a cross-body armlock is a straight armlock with the defender's arm being levered over the attacker's crotch (serving as the fulcrum). Many sambo wrestlers have exceptional skill in the cross-body armlock. For more information on cross-body armlocks, get the book *Juji Gatame Encyclopedia* by this author and published by YMAA Publication Center.

Bent Armlock

There are two basic applications of the bent armlock. The first is with the defender's hand pointing upward and the second is with the defender's hand pointing downward.

1. Upward Bent Armlock

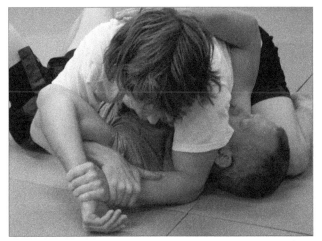

There are many bent armlock variations, but the defining characteristic of this armlock is that the defender's arm is bent in an upward direction with his hand pointing the same direction as his head.

2. Downward Bent Armlock

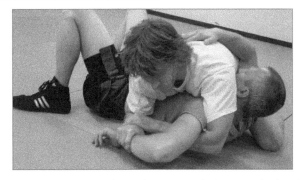

As with the upward application of this armlock, the bent armlock in the downward direction has many functional variations but the primary characteristic is that the defender's arm is bent and his hand is pointed in the same direction as his feet. A variation of the bent armlock, the compression bent armlock (also called a "slicer"), is often applied from a downward position.

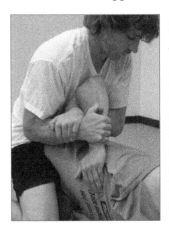

3. Compression Bent Armlock

In a compression variation of the bent armlock, the attacker taps and isolates his opponent's arm either above or below the elbow, and the attacker wedges his arm between the top and bottom portions of the defender's arm. The attacker bends the arm in, applying pressure. This is also known as a "slicer" armlock.

Straight Armlock

The straight armlock has a large number of variations and applications, but the fundamental principle that applies to every straight armlock is that the attacker straightens out his opponent's arm and applies pressure.

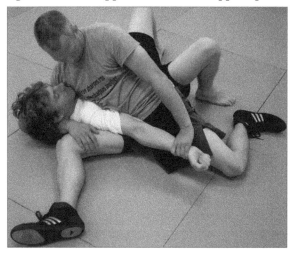

This basic variation of the straight armlock is a classic example of a lever and fulcrum in action. The attacker controls his opponent's right arm and stretches it out straight over the attacker's right upper leg.

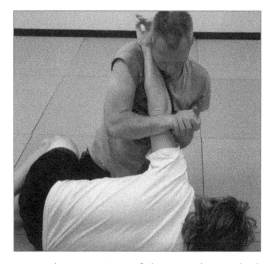

Here is another variation of the straight armlock with the attacker trapping his opponent's left arm against the attacker's shoulder and head as the attacker uses a square grip to pry inward and add pressure to the elbow joint. There are several other variations of the straight armlock that are functional and effective in addition to what has been shown.

LOWER BODY SUBMISSIONS

The lower body submissions in sambo attack any joint from the waist down. Sambo is recognized for its many innovative, effective, and downright nasty lower-body submissions. A lower-body submission is a joint lock directed against the opponent's knee, hip, or ankle joints. Knee locks where the attacker bends his opponent's knee and causes pain in the joint are legal when the lower leg is in line with the upper leg. In other words, no twisting of the joint is permitted. A knee lock with the knee straight is often called a knee bar, and this is permitted as long as there is no cranking or side bending movement at the knee joint. A hip lock is permitted as long as there is no lower back pressure and the pressure is directly aimed at the hip joint. An ankle lock must be applied with the joint in a straight line. In other words, heel hooks, twisting ankle locks, and toeholds are not permitted in the rules of sambo. A total victory can be scored from the application of a lower-body submission when the grappler having the joint lock applied on him taps the mat, makes a gesture of surrender, or verbally submits or yells out.

Straight Knee Locks

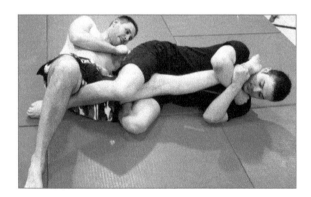

These are also called "knee bars" because the attacker "bars" his opponent's knee joint against a fulcrum, forcing it to straighten and cause pain.

Bent Knee Locks

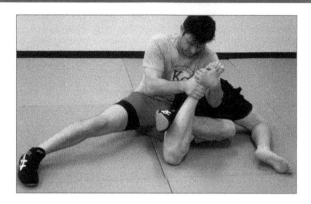

The attacker applies pressure on his opponent's knee by bending it and wedging his foot or leg (or simply bending it) and applying pressure on the joint. When applying a bent knee lock in the sport of sambo, the attacker must make sure his opponent's lower leg is parallel to his upper leg and not crank or twist the knee joint.

Ankle Locks

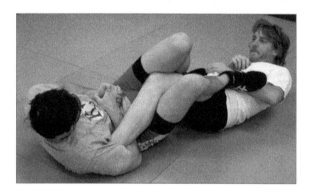

In the sport of sambo, ankle locks where the ankle is stressed in a straight line with the leg are legal. Twisting or turning the ankle is not permitted. This means that, in sport sambo, heel hooks, toeholds, and twisting ankle locks are not permitted. However, these holds are used in combat sambo, and it's highly recommended that every sambo wrestler study and know a variety of ankle locks, whether they are permitted in the rules of sambo or not. Since most sambo wrestlers also participate in a variety of other fighting and grappling sports, it's important to be well-versed in all phases of submission holds.

Compression Locks

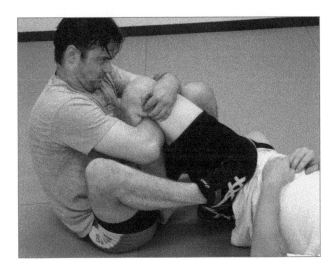

A compression lock creates pressure on a ligament, tendon, or muscle, causing pain. More often than not, most compression leglocks also accompany a bent leglock or a straight ankle lock, making the submission technique all the more uncomfortable for an opponent.

Hip Locks

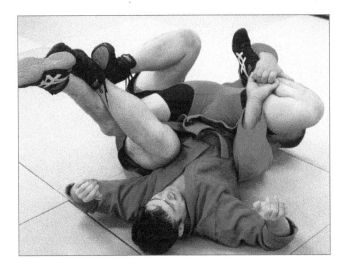

What are called hip locks are often painful holds where the attacker will pry or lever open his opponent's hips or will apply pressure to the hip joint itself.

HOLD-DOWNS

The hold-downs of sambo are not pins. They are immobilizations where the attacker holds his opponent to the mat for a specified period of time with torso-to-torso contact. If torso-to-torso contact is broken, the hold is broken. Pinning an opponent's shoulders to the mat is not the object of a hold-down in sambo. A sambo match cannot be won with a hold-down as in the sport of judo. Often, a sambo wrestler will use a hold-down to score points and then transition to a submission technique.

A hold-down occurs when the attacker's torso (front, side, or back) is in contact with the defender's front or side torso. Total victory cannot be achieved with a hold-down. A hold-down must be in effect for twenty seconds for the maximum score of four points to be awarded by the mat official. A hold-down of at least ten to nineteen seconds will score two points. The maximum amount of points for hold-downs allowed in a sambo match is four. Often, a sambo wrestler will attempt to hold his opponent for twenty seconds (to get the maximum score of four points) and then transition from the hold-down to a submission technique. A hold-down in sambo should be viewed as a "time hold" (a phrase first used by Gene LeBell to the best of the author's recollection) with two primary purposes. First, the attacker holds his opponent to the mat for a long enough period of time in order to give the attacker sufficient time to secure a finishing or submission technique. The second purpose is for the attacker to immobilize or control his opponent to secure maximum points (four points). So, a hold-down is not a "pin" in the wrestling sense of the word, where the goal of a pin is to force an opponent's shoulders to the mat for a touch fall or specified period of seconds. Because of this, the term "hold-down" will be used in this book while the word "pin" will not be used to any great extent.

Hold-Down outside Opponent's Leg or Legs

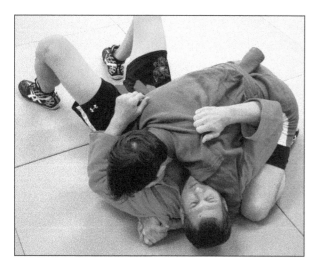

The emphasis of a hold-down in sambo is to maintain torso-to-torso contact with the attacker's front, side, or back torso in contact with his opponent's front side. Often, the most advantageous position is to control an opponent in a hold-down from the side or upper body areas so that the opponent does not have a chance to grapevine or entwine the attacker's legs.

Hold-Down between Opponent's Leg or Legs

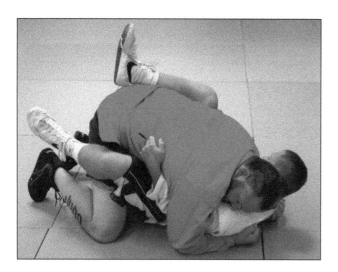

Unlike judo, where the attacker must be free of his opponent's legs to secure a hold-down, the rules of sambo allow the attacker to be positioned between his opponent's legs or have a leg scissored (as in a half-guard from jujitsu).

CONTROLLING WITH THE LEGS

Before we leave the subject of technical skills, let's analyze one of the most identifiable aspects of sambo: how sambo wrestlers use their legs to control and manipulate each other in the application of many throwing techniques, transition techniques, and groundfighting techniques. The "leg entwining" or "leg wrapping" as it is called in throwing techniques, the "leg lacing" as it is called when doing lower body submissions, and the "grapevine" as it is called when using hold-downs or controlling and opponent to perform an upper body submission, are all methods used in sambo to control an opponent's legs.

Leg Entwining

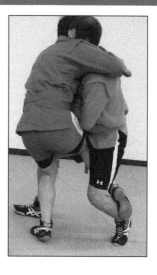

The grappler on the left is using his right leg to entwine his opponent's left leg. A sambo wrestler will use either leg to entwine either one of his opponent's legs, depending on the situation. As in many European and Central Asian styles of wrestling, sambo uses this method of controlling with the legs in a large number of throwing techniques. Also called "leg wrapping," this is an effective way for a sambo wrestler to trap and control his opponent's leg as both a way of setting up an opponent for a throw or in the actual execution of a throwing technique. Called "kawazu gake" in judo, this maneuver is not permitted in the contest rules of judo. Be careful, as leg entwining can be dangerous and serious knee injuries can result if it is applied wrong. This photo shows one of the many ways a sambo grappler will entwine his opponent's leg.

Leg Lacing

There are many varieties of leg lacing, but these two are commonly used.

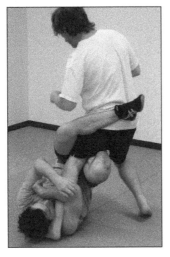

In this application of leg lacing, it's handy to visualize someone lacing his boot strings all the way up the boot so that it fits tightly on the foot and leg. The grappler standing is "wearing" a boot (the grappler on the mat) and the grappler on the mat is using his feet and legs (as well as his hands and arms) to "lace" himself tightly on his opponent's leg. Doing this traps and controls an opponent's leg so that the attacker can better apply a lower-body submission or take his opponent to the mat to transition to a finishing hold. Generally, the term "leg lacing" refers to the attacker wrapping his legs around his opponent's leg from the bottom up (from the foot area up the length of the leg); however, this isn't always the case.

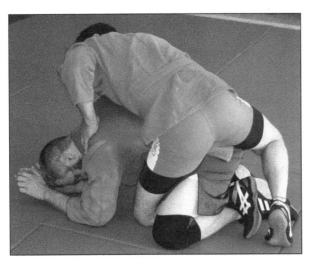

The grappler on top is using his left leg to lace or entwine his opponent's left leg as a method of control to apply a bent leglock. Some people call this a near leg

ride, grapevine, or a leg lace (or other name), so it really doesn't matter what terminology you use; the important thing is to use it so that it works for you.

Grapevines

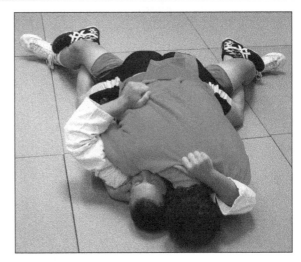

When a sambo wrestler uses both of his legs to wrap (entwine) both of his opponent's legs, that is often called a grapevine. Actually, "grapevine" is a pretty generic term, but it's used often when specifying this particular situation.

LEARNING AND APPLYING SAMBO SKILLS

It goes without saying that there are many technical skills that make up the sport of sambo; some skills are the big things that are obvious while other skills are the small things that aren't so obvious but that make the big things happen. As the great basketball coach John Wooden said, "Small things make big things happen."

Sambo is pragmatism applied to combat sports. A defining feature of sambo is the functional way it is taught from the very beginning. Let's briefly examine how the technical skills of sambo are taught.

One of the major attractions I had to sambo as a young man was how Maurice Allan taught it to me. I didn't realize it at the time, but how Maurice presented what sambo was and how it could be best applied was a major turning point in my life, both as an athlete and as a coach. From my all too brief time training with Maurice, I spent the rest of my life delving into the functional approach to skill development that sambo was (and is) known for. First of all, Maurice was (and is) an excellent coach with a tremendous amount of knowledge. But the functional, performance-based approach to the teaching, learning, practice, and application of sambo (or any fighting sport for that matter) is one of the major reasons sambo is effective as a combat sport. So what follows is a good blueprint for approaching the subject of skill development—not just for sambo, but for any skilled activity.

A RATIONAL APPROACH TO SKILL DEVELOPMENT

First of all, let's define "skill." Skill is the application of a movement (a technique) that achieves a predetermined goal with a consistently high rate of success in relation to the circumstances or situation. It's the practical application of a technique. When someone says (about another athlete), "He has good technique," that actually implies that the person has good skill at performing the technique, often under stressful conditions.

Now, let's define "technique." Technique is a distinct, specific, and identifiable movement pattern, in and of itself. It's the generally accepted way of performing a throw, hold, armlock, or leglock.

> TECHNICAL TIP: A technique is a specific, unique, and identifiable movement. Skill is the actual application of that movement.

Sambo is pragmatic and quite direct when it comes to the teaching, learning, practicing, and mastering of technical skill. More will be said in following chapters, but make no mistake about it, sambo's emphasis is on results. To achieve the best results, it is imperative that any athlete wishing to achieve mastery of his or her sport must be as efficient as possible in the learning, development, and application of the skills that make up the sport (in this case, sambo).

The goal of both the coach and athlete must be to ensure that personal application and performance of every technique is as successful as possible. A technique is only as good as how it is applied. A technique is a tool. How well the technique is applied is called skill.

Because of this, every technique has to be modified to fit the needs of every human being who does it. The coach's role is to adapt the technique so that it is efficient for the person doing it.

For an improvement in skill to take place, it must be learned and practiced in the way it is to be performed. In other words, it is essential that the athlete practice the way he or she intends to use it in a realistic or competitive situation. Skill development takes place at the same time both technically and tactically. It is important to make your opponent fight your kind of fight, from both a technical and tactical point of view. To do this, it is fundamentally important to develop the skills, both technically and tactically, that emphasize the best use of your movement and the best use of nullifying your opponent's movement; then, make his movement work to your advantage.

As World Sambo Champion Maurice Allan once told me, "Make your technique work for you." From the very start of learning a fundamental skill, the coach must take great care to mold the technique so that its essential fundamental movement is best exploited and applied by the athlete or student learning the movement. This differs from the approach used traditionally in judo (as an example) where the student or athlete must fit his body to meet the preconceived structure, parameters, and limitations of the technique. There is no doubt that the novice (or any) athlete must learn the fundamentally sound application of any and every technique. However, it is incumbent on the coach to (as quickly as possible) make that technique fit the needs of the athlete learning it. Not every technique is for every athlete. Everyone is different, and some moves simply don't work for some people. This is why it is important for a coach to assess every student or athlete as well as possible and see if a technique "fits." If it doesn't, the coach may modify it so that it does, or the coach may choose to work with the athlete on another move that better suits the athlete. Some techniques may not work initially, but may be effective after a period of time or with physical or emotional development on the part of the athlete. In any event, it's the coach's job to help guide his or her protégé in a direction that is most successful for the athlete.

Sambo is a tough physical sport, but it's also a highly technical sport that requires every athlete who participates in it to have a high degree of functional technical skill. The basis of functional and efficient technical skill is physical fitness. A sambo wrestler must be physically fit enough to not only apply highly functional and refined technical skill, he must also be fit enough to dominate his opponent and beat him. As I have told my athletes for years, "Show up in shape." But this means more than simply showing up in shape. It most definitely means that if you want to win, you have to be physically dominant; not simply to beat an opponent, but to beat him with skill.

This philosophy has very real ramifications. The object of competing in sambo (or any sport, especially a fighting sport) is to win. This may sound harsh to some people, but it is objectively true. If you enter into a fight and your goal is not winning, you are in serious trouble. With this in mind, every athlete must have the best level of fitness humanly possible. A primary objective of every athlete should be to dominate his opponent and control him with a high degree of physical contact. An athlete should strive to apply constant pressure to an opponent so that the opponent will (1) break down and fatigue physically, which leads to (2) the opponent breaking down and fatiguing mentally, which leads to (3) the opponent breaking down and making a technical or tactical mistake, making it possible to beat him.

STRUCTURED TRAINING

Structured training is not only necessary, it is essential and central to success. You have to train hard, but just as important, you have to train smart. Continuing with our rational approach to skill development, there is a planned follow-up approach to the actual training so that the technical and tactical skills that have been developed will be put to effective use. Just like using a road map to best arrive where you want to go and avoid getting lost along the way, an athlete needs a similar "map" in his or her development. What follows is a viable and effective "road map" that can be used by coaches and athletes to best arrive at their competitive destinations and avoid getting lost along the way.

From my experience and training as a coach, there are three primary factors or parts that comprise the overall, effective development of athletes. When it comes down to the nitty-gritty of "training smart," the three parts that follow have proven to form a solid foundation in the development of athletes at all levels, from novices to world-class sambo wrestlers. These three parts are (1) Structured Learning and Drill Training, (2) Free Practice or Sparring, and (3) Competition. The first two parts should take place at every workout or practice. The third part is the actual tournament or competition that is necessary to measure all aspects of a particular athlete's development and level of ability.

Structured Learning and Drill Training

An athlete doesn't get good simply by showing up and rolling on the mat with his buddies for a couple of hours, even if he does it on a regular basis. Learning and retaining what is learned requires structured training. Remember, education is learning; training is applying that learning to actual situations. We previously discussed using a rational approach to the teaching of skills, so let's analyze how to effectively see to it that athletes retain these skills and know how to apply them in realistic and competitive situations.

The first part of an effective workout is planned and structured drill training. There are drills for just about every aspect of what takes place in a real situation or in a match. There are drills for fitness and conditioning, drills for skill learning and development, drills for specific situations that take place in a match both technically and tactically, and drills for everything else that actually happens.

Drill training eliminates, to a great extent, the goofing off that can take place in a practice session. Through intelligent drill training, the athletes can learn skills more easily and the coach can regulate time better. Drills can prevent a team from going stale because drill training provides a variety of situations in training. Really, just about any situation in sambo can be drilled on (and should be, for that matter). Drills can be used to teach new skills or reinforce already-learned technical or tactical skills. Drill training is the most effective method of teaching learned, automatic, or efficient spontaneous behavior in sambo (or any sport). Drill training is efficient because the drills themselves can vary so much in content and context.

Drill training is effective if a coach uses it wisely. Drilling, like anything else, can be overdone. Often, a coach can teach an underlying movement, skill, or tactic by using a well-planned drill or game. This is where a drill can have more than one use, even though it has a specific purpose. An example is teaching a throw using a crash pad. This not only teaches the mechanics of the throw, it also teaches the student to follow through with more force since the person being thrown and taking the fall is landing on about eight inches of foam. Learning how to throw an opponent with control and force is a good skill, and using crash pads is handy for this purpose.

A coach can better dictate the tempo or pace of the workout so that the actual training session will be as hard or as light as the coach desires. A coach should constantly vary the drills so that they don't become boring or lose effectiveness. A coach should also coordinate the drills to suit the skill level of the group or team. Drills that are too easy or too difficult are ineffective and could do more harm than good.

Drill training can develop technical and tactical skill, fitness, coordination, confidence, or whatever the coach wants for his athletes and team.

Drills can be classified into two basic groups.

Skill Drills

Skill drills emphasize teaching or reinforcing already-learned technical or tactical skills. When discussing skill drills, there are two varieties that are used. (1) Closed-ended drills, which teach or reinforce specific technical or tactical behavior. This is also called a "fixed drill." The student must work on a specific skill or exercise repeatedly to develop that particular skill in a specific, automated, or learned reaction. (2) Open-ended drills, which are drills where a student is often presented a basic or specific situation and he must adapt or react to it using his own initiative or already-learned skills. Often, what are called "situational drills" are good examples of an open-ended drill. The coach places his athletes in a situation and the athletes must react using already-learned behavior as well as their own initiative. A coach can develop realistic, effective drills by carefully observing situations that actually take place in a sambo match. Situational drills effectively reinforce successful behavior in athletes so that they practice the technical or tactical skills actually used in a competitive situation.

Fitness Drills

Fitness drills emphasize physical development and coordination. Often, the value of drills overlaps so that a drill that is primarily a skill drill will often have fitness value too. When doing fitness drills, it is important that they are not boring. I often like to say that I "fool my athletes into having a hard workout" because they enjoy themselves so much. This is where using a variety of games that can be played on the mat are useful, even for adults. Games aren't just for kids; adults like to enjoy practice as well. A coach will do well to remember that unless he is working with a group of professional athletes who get paid for what they do, the people on his mat are there because they want to be there. This may make some coaches cringe, but it is okay for an athlete to actually enjoy himself or herself during a workout.

There are several good books on mat drills and games on the market, but I recommend the one I wrote, *Drills for Grapplers*, published by Turtle Press. Also, John Saylor and I coauthored an excellent book, *Conditioning for Combat Sports*, also published by Turtle Press. If you get these books, you will have an extensive amount of information that is useful for the purpose of drilling for fitness.

TECHNICAL TIP: Education is learning. Training is applying that learning to actual situations.

Free Practice

The second part of successful training is what the Japanese call "randori" or "free practice." Call it "going live," "rolling," or any name you wish, the premise of this aspect of training is to provide an organized and structured time for the athletes to use their own initiative and experiment with the technical and tactical skills they know.

Free practice is what the name implies. It's practice (first and foremost) and it's not a competition. Every coach should carefully monitor free practice. As a coach, set specific goals for every round of free practice that your athletes engage in. Likewise, as an athlete, set goals for yourself and be sure to discuss them beforehand with your coach and teammates. I like to compare it to sparring in boxing. There is always a reason for a sparring session in boxing. Fighters don't just get in the ring and beat the snot out of each other; they get in the ring for specific reasons, and those reasons are whatever the coach or trainer has in mind for them. It's the same for free practice in sambo or any of the grappling sports; every session of free practice must have a purpose. Just showing up and beating up on each other simply creates too many injuries and turns the training session into a time when the stronger, more experienced (and tougher) grapplers often tend to pick on the newer and weaker athletes on the mat and beat them up. This type of training simply creates predators, and predators (no matter what species, human or animal) tend to pick on the weak rather than seek out those who will actually challenge them. I've been a coach for a long time and I was an athlete before that, and it's been my experience that the guys who are predators in the gym are almost always the guys that can't be relied on in a tournament or in a real competitive situation. This is just my personal advice to coaches, but if you have someone in your gym who views free practice as a time to keep a record of "wins" and "losses," then he's a detriment to your team and to the welfare of your students and athletes, and he should either change his attitude or change the place where he works out. I've had guys who "collect scalps" or keep a record of "wins" and "losses" in free practice, and they have always been shown the door.

To sum it up: free practice should always have a purpose and should always be monitored by the coach. It should be considered as a time to prepare for the real thing, a competition.

TECHNICAL TIP: Free practice is not a tournament. Nobody wins or loses in free practice. It's practice, period.

Competition

This is the actual test for an athlete. There are a lot of tests in life and competing against another human being who is fit, motivated, and skilled is about as honest a test as anyone can find. I've often told my athletes, "It's a fight, not a game." It's important to remember that what we do isn't a game. It's the real thing. You have every intention of throwing your opponent to the mat or crank his (or her) arm or leg to the point that it forces him to surrender to you. That's not playing, that's fighting.

But, it's a fight with a set of ethics that are enforced by the rules of the fight. This is what separates war from sport. A fighting sports is simply personal combat with a mutually agreed set of rules and governed by ethical behavior. What our society calls "sportsmanship" is (fundamentally) ethical and moral behavior applied to sporting or competitive situations; in our case, competitive fighting. For this reason, sportsmanship isn't simply an old-fashioned notion of being a gentleman or lady. It's a vital part of the competitive process, and without it, sports (especially fighting sports) would not be possible. Through the accepted rules and mores of sportsmanship, athletes, coaches, and anyone connected with the activity have a certain standard of behavior to exhibit. Without good ethical training developed by honest, sincere effort and an adherence to the rules of the sport, athletes (especially those athletes in combat sports where aggressive behavior is required for success) become predators. Sport (in this case, sambo) would be impossible to continue from one generation to the next without a definite set of ethics and sportsmanship.

The concepts of competition and sportsmanship force the athlete to take risks. If someone is only willing to compete when he is assured of winning, he will never amount to much as an athlete (or anything else in life). Winning is more fun than losing but that's only true if an athlete has accepted the risk of losing. If a sport (or anything else in life) isn't worth the risk, it's not worth the reward.

Okay, let's turn our attention to the throwing techniques of sambo.

References

DeMars, Dr. AnnMaria and James Pedro, Sr. *Winning on the Ground*. Valencia, CA: Black Belt Books, 2013.
Gleeson, Geof. *All about Judo*, Wakefield: EP Publishing, 1975.
Gleeson, Geof. *Judo Inside Out*. Wakefield: Lepus Books, 1983.
Scott, Steve. *Winning on the Mat*, Santa Fe, NM: Turtle Press, 2011.

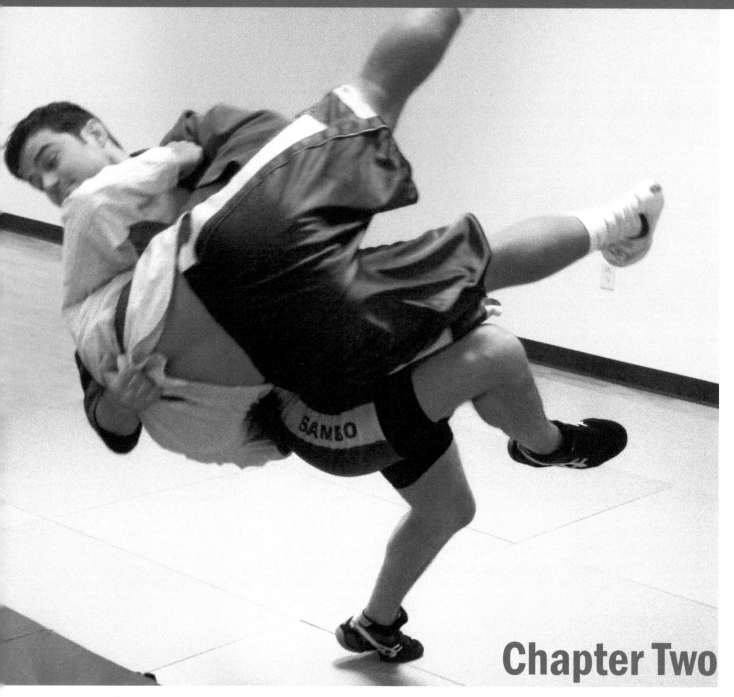

Chapter Two
The Throwing Techniques of Sambo
"Make the technique work for you."

THE CORE CONCEPTS OF THROWING TECHNIQUES

The purpose of a successful throwing technique in sambo is to get an opponent to the mat or ground as effectively as possible with control. A sambo grappler can win a match outright by a total victory by throwing his opponent to the mat with control (largely on the back or backside, or if the opponent lands in a bridge) with the thrower remaining standing at the conclusion of the throw. To some mat officials, amplitude and force, or impetus, also counts in the equation, but not always. Sambo is actually a throwing and submission sport, with a throwing technique serving as a means to the end the match, and if that doesn't happen, the throw can result in the attacker following through to the mat or ground and forcing an opponent to submit. And sambo matches start with both athletes standing and facing each other. Knowing how to skillfully and effectively throw an opponent to the mat is a vital part of sambo.

The development of sambo's many technical skills, especially in throwing techniques, comes from a variety of sources, with the emphasis primarily coming from Kodokan judo of Japan, chida-oba of Georgia and kurash of Uzbekistan as well as other wrestling styles. More specifically, the biomechanical concepts of what makes a throwing technique work and work with a high rate of success in a functional way come directly from Vasili Oshpechkov's study of judo in the early 1900s and the subsequent additions from the wrestling styles gleaned from the various Soviet republics as well as the innovative ideas and practices by later generations of sambo exponents. These core mechanical skills apply to every throwing technique used in sambo, and while in many cases these specific skills blend in together in a rapid and explosive application, they are, indeed, all part of the total picture of how to effectively throw an opponent to the mat or ground.

It's also important to remember that it requires two sambo wrestlers for a throw (or any technique) to happen. The attacker must control his opponent's body, but he also must control his body as well. With this in mind, let's analyze the core movements of what makes a throwing technique in sambo work. These are the sum parts that make the whole of a throwing technique. To start, let's look at the core root of sambo's throwing mechanics that come from Kodokan judo.

The three parts of every throw in Kodokan judo are: (1) kuzushi—controlling and unbalancing the opponent; (2) tsukuri—fitting into and building the technique; and (3) kake—executing the throw. Sambo's approach to the analysis and synthesis of a throwing technique comes directly from Kodokan judo and is pretty much the same; however, there are other areas of emphasis taught at the core level that are important to point out.

So with this in mind, let's analyze the parts of a throwing technique. If you've read my book on judo, *Winning on the Mat*, you will recognize the following underlying and foundational principles of a functional approach to throwing techniques.

It's useful to consider a throwing technique as a weapon. The action of throwing another human being down to the ground or mat is a ballistic movement based on fundamentally sound principles of biomechanics. You can use it, and it can be used against you. It's much like a gun in that sense. Like any other tool or weapon, it has no personality or life of its own and how you use it is up to you. If you go into a gunfight with a .22 caliber handgun and your opponent has a .44 Magnum, you may be in trouble. But, if you're more willing to shoot and know how to shoot that .22 straighter, faster, and more accurately than your opponent does his .44 Magnum, you might come out the winner in that gunfight.

I compare the caliber of a gun's bullet to the training you put into your throw. The more powerful the bullet combined with a rifled barrel on the gun means that gun will shoot with its full ballistic effect. If you've done your speed/strength training so that you have tremendous plyometric strength when performing the throw, then you have a .44 Magnum bullet. But if you haven't put in the physical effort, then you're only shooting a .22 caliber bullet. If you've gone to the shooting range and practiced both smart and hard, and know how to handle that handgun in realistic situations, then you're most likely going to shoot both accurately and fast when in a real gunfight. But if you've only shot the gun a few times and not under realistic situations, then you'll most likely not shoot very straight or fast enough when you need to. I think you get the analogy by now. It takes a combination of physical fitness training along with lots of serious training on the mat to have the explosive power and technical ability to throw an opponent in a real situation.

The following formula is one that I favor when describing what happens in every successful throw: P + M = C. P (position) combined with M (mobility or movement) results in C (control of your opponent). This is true for any phase of grappling or fighting but is especially true when it comes to throwing an opponent. You're fighting someone who is on his feet and can move, and as a result can either attack you or defend against your attack. Your position and the position your opponent is in are vital to the execution of a successful throw or takedown. Often, how you move and how you make your opponent move dictate both your position and his position. You have controlled the situation and can effectively throw your opponent when you've been able to control both your opponent's position and movement as well as your own. Now, how you go about doing that takes some study and a lot of hard work on the mat. That's what I'll cover on the following pages.

All the techniques of sambo (and specific to this chapter, the throwing techniques) are performance-based skills. In other words, the efficiency of the performance of any given technique is the primary judgment of success. "Style" points are not given, so the aesthetics of the throw are secondary to its effect. In essence, the effectiveness of the throw determines its aesthetic value. As former U.S. National Sambo Champion Shawn Watson remarked, "It's only pretty if it works." What this means, from a coaching point of view, is that the functional purpose of the technique is taken into account when any biomechanical skill is initially taught to an athlete. As the athlete increases his or her skill in the application of the fundamental technique, his or her coach quickly guides the athlete into making the move more efficient for that athlete personally. Right from the start, the core and fundamental application of a move (again, specific to this chapter, a throwing technique, but it is true for any move in sambo) is taught so that it best works for the athlete doing it. The fundamental move is not altered so much that it fails to retain its purpose and effectiveness, but for example, a tall, slender athlete will learn a basic throw in a slightly different way than a short, stocky athlete will. While the specific fundamental throwing technique is the same, the people doing it are not, and a good coach (whether a sambo coach, or a coach of any sport) will make alterations and adjustments so that the technique being worked on best suits the purposes of the athlete doing it. For instance, a basic hip throw looks pretty much the same no matter who does it, but for that hip throw to work best for a tall athlete, specific accommodations will have to be made. If the athlete learning the hip throw is short, the technique will be presented to him so that it works best for his specific physical attributes. In other words, the technique is altered to best work for the athlete doing it as opposed to a more "cookie cutter" approach. Not everyone is the same, so it makes more sense to teach (from a coaching point of view), learn (from an athlete's point of view), and train in the most efficient way possible so the most effective results can be gained from the performance of the technique. Rather than an athlete fitting a throw, the throw fits the athlete. To the sambo exponents who developed the technical basis of the sport, the end result was the primary object. In other words, the form of the technical movement must be (first and foremost) functional, efficient and, taking it a step further, efficient with a high rate of success particular to the person doing it. While the original basis of sambo's technical development, especially in throwing techniques, is based on Kodokan judo, heavy influences from (especially) chida-oba and kurash have formed the mechanical processes of sambo to a significant degree. Kodokan judo teaches the building blocks of kuzushi (unbalancing the opponent), tsukuri (building or fitting into the technique), and kake (execution of the technique). In some cases, a fourth element is taught: kime (finishing or following through with the technique) as separate but integrated elements of a throwing technique. Sambo does the same, but because of its technical background in other grappling sports in addition to judo, the building blocks often seem to blend together and in some cases may even be done at the same time so that the end result looks like a technique based on brute strength rather than what it is: a combination of physical fitness and efficient biomechanical application of movement, balance, speed, and control.

Another important thing to consider is that some techniques seem more natural to some people than others. We're all different, and in many cases a particular throw or type of throw seems more "natural" to you than others. If this is the case, go with it and try to develop that throw so that it works for you in real situations. Give it a while and take the time to see if that throw is a good one for you. In the end, it may or may not be something you can use now, but you may keep it on the back burner and use it later in your career.

TECHNICAL TIP: Elite and world-class skills are fundamental skills that have been developed to their full potential. As he is learning the fundamental or core skills of a throwing technique (or for that matter, any technique, whether it's a throw, submission technique, or hold-down), the sambo grappler will develop and adapt that move so that it fits him like a glove. As World Sambo Champion Maurice Allan once said, "Make the technique work for you."

FITNESS IS ESSENTIAL

Without exception, the performance of effective and efficient throwing skills (or any technical skill) is based on the fitness level of the person doing it. In other words, if you want to perform the skills of sambo (or anything for that matter) with efficiency and a high rate of success, you must be physically capable of doing it. Remember, when you train for a sambo match, you're training for a fight, not a game. Sure, it may be a fight with a set of rules but it's still a fight, and if you don't show up in shape, you'll not only lose, you'll take a beating. The idea is to show up and give the other guy the beating, so if you want to win and win with skill, it is essential that you take your physical fitness seriously.

As the well-respected strength and fitness coach Louie Simmons said about training athletes in football (paraphrased), "If you put a team of physically weak players up against a team of physically strong and fit players in a football game, the strong and fit players will win every time." The result would be the same in any fighting sport, especially sambo. This is in line with my friend John Saylor's shingitai approach to training. Fitness is a fundamental and required foundation in any athlete's development. Along with fitness, the athletes' willingness to perform and compete is essential. An athlete must have the fighting heart necessary to fight and win and must have a tactical awareness so that he can win the fight. Another key element in the shingitai approach is functional technical expertise. In other words, make the move work for you and work for you on a regular basis against opponents who are motivated, fit, and skilled. I mention our shingitai approach because, while it may not be historically rooted directly to sambo by the name of shingitai, it nonetheless is exactly what

sambo is all about. For more information on fitness for sambo (or any fighting sport), refer to the book *Conditioning for Combat Sports* that John Saylor and I coauthored and published by Turtle Press.

Suffice it to say, everything that follows is dependent on physical fitness.

AN ANALYSIS OF THE FIVE MAJOR PARTS OF A THROWING TECHNIQUE

A throwing technique is like any machine, human body, or anything else that has separate and interdependent moving parts. While there are many finite motor skills that must take place for such a complex activity as taking another human being off of his feet and moving, controlling, and throwing him through the air and onto his back, these five principal components are always present in every successful throw.

1. Control your opponent with grip, posture, and stance.
2. Control and unbalance your opponent with movement and use the momentum created by that control.
3. Build the technique to fit your body so that it works for you.
4. Execute the technique: throw your opponent with control to the mat.
5. Follow through and finish your opponent.

(1) CONTROL OPPONENT WITH GRIP, POSTURE, AND STANCE

There are several interdependent functions that take place in this initial phase of a successful throwing technique, so let's take a look at them.

Gripping and Grip Fighting

What is called a "grip" in sambo is the way you grab your opponent's jacket, belt, body, or anything else in an effort to control him. Your first contact with an opponent is usually with your hands. You have to grab him (usually) before you can throw him. Gripping or grabbing an opponent's jacket and belt are the primary methods of controlling him with your hands and arms used in all jacket-wrestling sports, including sambo. Use your hands, arms, elbows, shoulder, head, and anything else at your disposal to control the grip and control your opponent's movement. Because how a sambo wrestler grips his opponent often dictates what throw he uses, it's important to spend some time analyzing gripping and grip fighting.

Sambo has a well-earned reputation for the variety of effective methods used to grip an opponent's jacket or belt and control him with it. There are few limitations on how a sambo wrestler grabs, grips, or holds his opponent, from either a technical point of view or from the point of view of what is allowed in the rules of the sport. Any grip that works and works with a good rate of success is a good grip.

As with just about every other aspect of the sport of sambo, the skills of gripping or holding an opponent's jacket or belt come from a variety of influences. An obvious influence in the grip-fighting skills of sambo comes from judo, but a great deal of grip-fighting and controlling an opponent comes from some of the traditional folk styles of wrestling found in what was once the Soviet Union, most notably chida-oba. The Georgian sport of chida-oba has influenced modern sambo significantly. chida-oba's jacket and belt are similar to a sambo jacket except that the jacket worn in chida-oba doesn't have sleeves. As a result, gripping onto the back of the jacket as well as onto the belt is necessary in order to control an opponent to throw him. Another of these traditional styles of wrestling is kurash from Uzbekistan. Kurash can be described as "belt wrestling" where the grapplers must grab onto the opponent's belt in order to control and ultimately throw him.

A good way to think of using gripping in sambo to control an opponent is to imagine that you have a rope in both of your hands and you loop the rope over your opponent and wrap it around him, pulling it in tighter and exerting more control all the time.

If you think of the jacket and belt (or anything your opponent wears or any part of his body—or for that matter anything you wear, or any part of your body) as a tool to grab, manipulate, and use to control him, you have a good idea of sambo's approach to controlling and beating an opponent.

Your first actual point of contact with an opponent is how you grip him and how he grips you. In every throwing or takedown technique, how you grip your opponent dictates the success of the action. An important point to remember is that if you don't grip your opponent very well, you most likely won't throw him very well either. Before you can control your opponent's posture, movement, or other aspects of throwing him, you must have a grip that works for you. Your throw often flows directly from your grip, and this is why it's vital that you have good gripping skills if you want to be able to throw opponents with a high rate of success.

Each of your hands and arms, as well as shoulders and hips, work independently of each other in that they each have specific jobs to perform in the overall scheme of things. An example of this is when one hand (the "anchor hand") grips the opponent in a certain way to isolate his arm or shoulder and pull it down while the other hand (the "probing hand") and arm reaches over his shoulder to secure a back grip. The objective was to get the back grip, but one hand had to control the posture and movement of the opponent so that the other hand could get the desired grip.

Decide what you want to accomplish with your grip. What's the purpose of grabbing your opponent in the way you are grabbing him? Using the grip effectively is fundamentally important (both technically and tactically) in a sambo match. The bottom line is: Why are you gripping your opponent the way you are gripping him? What's its purpose? Here are some goals to consider when grip fighting.

1. Control your opponent's movement; shut him down and limit his posture and movement.
2. Use the grip to help control the space between you and your opponent.
3. Control or "kill" your opponent's forward or lead shoulder to limit the use of his hands, control his posture, and control his movement.
4. Use grip fighting to control the tempo or pace (in other words, how fast or slow you and your opponent move about the mat).
5. Use your grip to set up your favorite throwing attack.
6. Force your opponent to move in a specific direction.
7. Engage your opponent in grip fighting to kill time on the clock if you are ahead in the score.

8. Use the grip to neutralize your opponent's steering or anchor hand as well as his probing hand.

9. It's a simple fact that some grips work better with some throws than others. Take the time and effort in training to best match the grip to the throw that works best for you.

10. Everything is a handle. The art and science of grip fighting starts with the realization that you have to get hold of your opponent and control him in order to throw him. Use anything and everything at your disposal to grip and control your opponent. (By the way, this applies to groundfighting as well.)

TECHNICAL TIP: Any grip that works for you and works for you when you need it to work is a good grip. Experiment with using different grips for different throws in practice, and always be on the lookout for effective functional gripping methods.

Compact (Short) Grips and Extended (Long) Grips

A useful way to explain gripping an opponent in sambo is to understand what a "compact" or "short" grip is and what an "extended" or "long" grip is. A short or compact grip is one where an athlete's primary control point is his opponent's shoulders. An extended or long grip is where an athlete's primary control point is his opponent's arms. In many cases (but not all cases), a compact or short grip leads to less distance between the two athletes and may produce a slower tempo when the athlete moves about the mat. A long grip tends to lead to more space between the opponents and makes for a faster tempo when the athletes move about the mat.

Remember, how you grab or grip your opponent directly determines how close your body is in relation to his body, and more specifically to his hips, which control the center part of his body. If the attacker can control his opponent's shoulders, he can better control his opponent's hips. Controlling an opponent's hips often leads to controlling the movement of his body. A short grip is a grip where the attacker uses his hands or arms to grip and control an opponent's shoulders. This results in the bodies of the attacker and defender being in close proximity to each other. A long grip is a grip where the attacker primarily controls the defender's arms. This results in the bodies of the attacker and defender being further apart from each other.

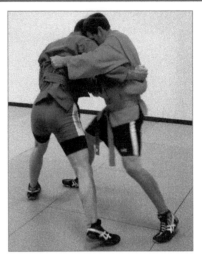

Look at how the attacker (on the right) controls his opponent's shoulders with his back grip. This results in a close proximity of the two bodies, especially at the hips.

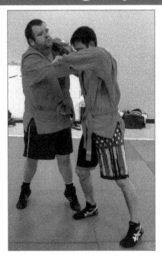

Look at how the attacker (on the right) controls his opponent's sleeve and arm with this lapel and sleeve grip. This results in a far proximity of the two bodies, especially at the hips.

IMPORTANT: While knowing how short and long grips work (and how to use them), the most important thing to remember is that everything is a handle and any grip that works for you with a high rate of success is an effective grip.

Using the Hands When Throwing

Each of the attacker's hands has a specific function, but both work together as a unit to grip, control, and ultimately throw his opponent.

The Anchor Hand and Probing Hand

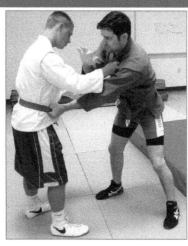

Often, a sambo wrestler wants to establish initial control of his opponent with his "anchor" hand. This photo shows the attacker (on the right) using his left hand to grab his opponent's belt. This is the attacker's anchor hand. He uses it to secure or "anchor" his opponent so that the attacker can go on to gain more control with his other hand. This photo also shows how the attacker uses his right hand as his "probing" hand. This probing hand comes into play after the attacker establishes a measure of control with his initial grip of his anchor hand. (A bit more on this later.)

The Pulling Hand

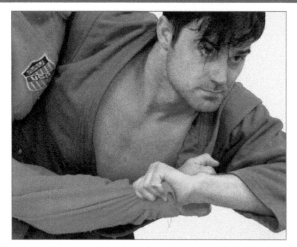

The attacker uses his left hand to pull his opponent's sleeve as he moves him and ultimately throws him.

Look at how the attacker uses his left hand to "screw up" his opponent's sleeve to tighten it. Doing this gives the attacker more control when pulling on his opponent's arm; and more control means a more effective throw.

The Steering Hand

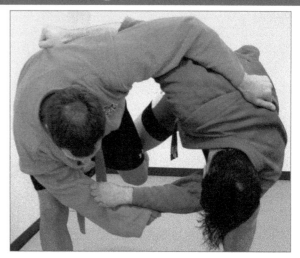

The attacker (on the left) uses his left hand to "steer" his opponent as he moves him or throws him.

A Variety of Grips

As mentioned before: any grip that works for you with a high rate of success is a good grip. In addition to Kodokan judo from Japan, the Georgian chida-oba and kurash from Uzbekistan (as well as other regional wrestling styles) have heavily influenced not only how a sambo wrestler grips his opponent, but also how he uses those grips to throw him. Chida-oba from Georgia is a wrestling style that places emphasis on throwing. Chida-oba has no groundfighting and as a result has developed sophisticated and high-flying throwing techniques over the course of its history. Many of the throws that most people recognize as "sambo throws" come directly from chida-oba. Additionally, the belt wrestling style of kurash from Uzbekistan has been influential in sambo's approach to using the belt to control and throw an opponent.

In the modern sport of sambo, pretty much any way of gripping and controlling an opponent's jacket or belt is fair game. As a result, what appear to judo or jujitsu exponents as unorthodox grips are simply the result of the eclectic history and pragmatic philosophy of the sport of sambo. Shown here are only a few of the many gripping methods used in sambo, but also take note of the grips used in the throwing techniques presented later in this chapter.

Neutral Grip: Basic Lapel and Sleeve Grip

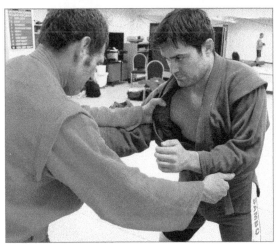

In order to practice with each other to learn and develop skill, the grapplers need a common method of gripping or holding onto each other. The lapel and sleeve grip, in the same way as used in judo, is an ideal "neutral" grip for beginners or novices (or for anyone of any skill level). With this grip, neither sambo wrestler has the advantage. It is an ideal method of taking the initial grip or hold onto an opponent particularly when practicing throws with a training partner. While this is considered a neutral grip, many sambo wrestlers use it with good results. The grappler on the left is using his left hand to grip his opponent's right lapel and using his right hand to grip his opponent's left sleeve.

Back Grip

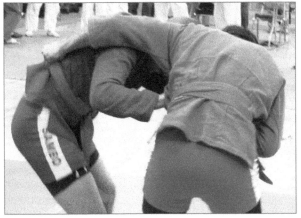

A common grip in sambo is the back grip. There are numerous variations of the basic back grip. This photo shows the athlete on the right using his left hand and arm to reach around his opponent's right shoulder and

upper arm to grab his belt. This method of using the left hand and arm to control his opponent's right shoulder and arm is the standard form of the back grip. The defender (on the left) is attempting to make distance between the two bodies by pushing with his right hand against the attacker's left hip. The attacker (on the right) could use his left hand to grab his opponent's jacket, but he has gained more control by grabbing his opponent's belt. This grip resulted in the attacker throwing his opponent for a four-point score.

Near Arm Back Grip

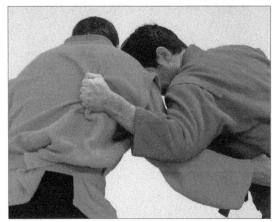

Another back grip that is useful is to use your left hand and arm (shown above) to reach around your opponent's right upper arm and grab onto his back (often gripping his jacket at his right shoulder blade area).

Georgian Grip (with Sleeve Grip)

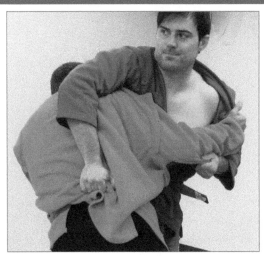

What has come to be known as the Georgian Grip (because of its derivation in Georgian chida-oba), this back-grip variation has proven to be highly effective. This photo shows the basic Georgian grip with the attacker (on right) using his right hand and arm to reach over his opponent's right shoulder. The attacker uses his left hand to grip and control his opponent's right elbow at the sleeve.

Georgian Grip (with Belt Grip)

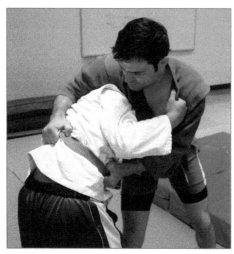

Here is the Georgian grip with the attacker using his left hand to grab and control the defender's belt and using his right hand to reach over the defender's right shoulder and grip onto the belt as shown.

Two-on-One Grip

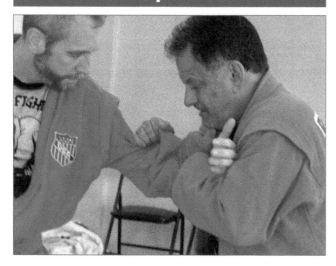

A popular and common grip used is the two on one grip as shown here. The attacker (on the right) uses his left hand to grab fairly low on his opponent's left forearm or wrist area and uses his right hand to grab his opponent's left upper arm. There are numerous variations of the two-on-one grip and this photo shows a commonly used approach to the grip.

Tightwaist Grip

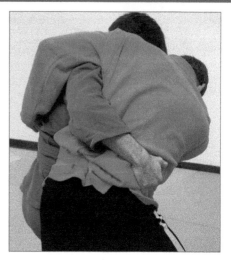

A commonly used grip that controls an opponent's hips is the tightwaist grip. Called the "tightwaist" because (as shown in this photo), the attacker uses his right hand and arm to grab tightly around his opponent's waist and hip area to control him.

Pistol Grip

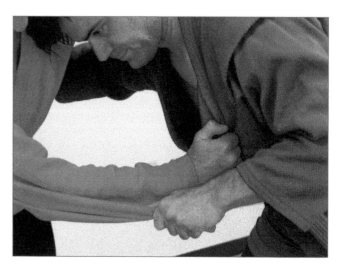

A classic example of a "long grip" is the pistol grip on the opponent's sleeve as shown here. The attacker uses his left hand to grab as low as possible on the end of his opponent's sleeve and grab it in the same way he would hold a pistol. The pistol grip is an excellent method of controlling an opponent's entire arm and controlling the distance between the two bodies.

Epaulette Grip

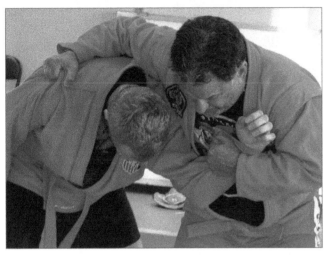

Sambo jackets have an epaulette on each shoulder for a good reason and that reason is to grip it for control of the opponent. The attacker (on the right) uses his right hand to reach over his opponent's back and grip his opponent's right epaulette. The attacker uses his left hand to grip his opponent's left arm in this example of a cross-arm grip. This is one (of many) variations of the epaulette grip.

Gripping with One Hand

Gripping an opponent with one hand and the practice of "probing," "fishing," "hunting," or "hooking" with the other hand (the non-gripping hand) is commonly seen in sambo matches. The reality of competitive sambo is that often, the kurtka (jacket) fits so tight on the opponent's body that getting only one hand on his jacket is about all a sambo wrestler can manage. In this case, grabbing the lapel of the jacket or the belt with one hand serves as an "anchor" while the other hand is used to probe or grab onto the opponent's ankle, leg, or other body part. The following three photos show how one-hand gripping is used, with the grappler on the left using his left hand to grip his opponent and using his right hand to probe and eventually use to grab his opponent's leg in an effort to throw him.

Using the Hands in One-Handed Gripping

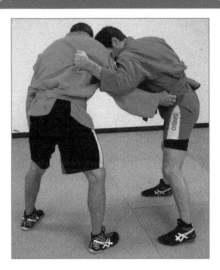

The Anchor Hand: The grappler at left uses his left hand to grip his opponent's jacket. This hand serves two primary purposes. The first use is that the attacker uses this as his "anchor" hand to initially grip and control his opponent as much as possible. The second use of the anchor hand is that the attacker uses it as his "radar" to sense how his opponent moves and then reacts accordingly.

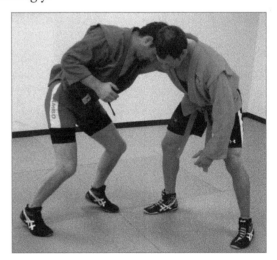

The Probing Hand: The grappler on the left has his right hand ready to "probe" or reach out as necessary to initiate his attack. This probing hand could be used to grab onto the opponent's jacket, belt, or any part of his body in an effort to see where the defender is most vulnerable. The author has called this "going fishing" or "going hunting" with the probing hand. By going fishing, you just might catch a big fish.

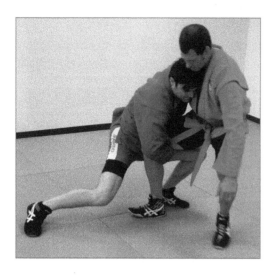

The Attack: After controlling his opponent with his left hand and probing out to find the best opportunity to attack, the attacker (on the left) uses his right hand to grab or hook his opponent's right leg in this photo. This is a typical example of how the attacker uses his hands to anchor and to probe, searching for the best moment to attack.

Posture, Body Space, and Stance

Often, the posture of your opponent (as well as your posture) dictates the type of grip you will use, which often dictates the particular attack you will choose to throw him with. How close or far your hips are in relation to your opponent's hips dictates the action of the throw. Where (and how) you stand in relation to your opponent or in relation to the mat or surrounding area is important. As will be discussed a bit later, "lead with your hips" is the best advice that can be given when talking about posture and position when engaged in standing situations. If you have your hips in good position to attack and defend with, you will be better able to control your opponent, the grip and how you throw him or defend against his throw. Good hip position in relation to your opponent stems directly from a good, upright posture.

In many cases, athletes who are physically strong tend to fight using a close distance to their opponents and use compact and short gripping, generally attempting to control the opponent's shoulders and not using longer sleeve or arm grips. That said, every athlete who is serious about sambo is physically strong, but some are stronger than others. However, as a general rule of thumb, athletes in the lighter weight classes tend to fight in a faster tempo than athletes in heavier weight classes, but that's not always the case. Again, speaking in generalities, athletes who rely less on physical strength tend to prefer a farther distance from the opponent and use grips that rely more on long levers (the arms and sleeves). This allows them more space to move freely and move in a faster tempo about the mat. Again, we have to come back to the hips. Fighting out of a more upright posture allows the athlete to move more freely in attacking and defending because his hips are closer to his opponent and he has less space to cover than if he were bent over in a crouched, defensive, or bent-over posture. Even though an athlete may use a slower tempo, it's still essential that he lead with his hips and makes it a point to keep his hips close enough to his opponent to attack and defend.

At any time in the match, an aggressive action may have to turn immediately into a defensive or neutral action. Effective sambo (or judo or any form of sport combat) relies on the concept that attack and defense are really the same thing. The situation at hand determines whether an athlete attacks, defends, or neutralizes the action. Always being in a position to attack or defend is vital to success in both standing situations and in groundfighting. Even when you have to defend yourself, always look for a chance to either neutralize his movement, turning it into your advantage, or to counter his movement and turn it into your own aggressive movement or attack.

My old friend Harry Parker was the first to tell me, "Lead with your hips." Leading with the hips is a fundamental skill. All of your attacks start with your hips. To the untrained ear, saying this makes no sense, but it's important to know why it works and know how to make it work in a real situation. By leading with your hips, you're better balanced whether you're moving or standing still and are more balanced when you move your feet. This increased balance and posture allow for better mobility and fluidity of movement. You're in better position to attack when possible and defend when necessary. This fluid movement allows you to go immediately from defending against an opponent's attack and turning it immediately into an attack of your own. Your hips are powerful and one of the primary tools you have on your body to move with skillfully in sambo and any fighting or sport.

What is called "stance" is where and how the attacker places his feet relative to his opponent. The legs and feet are extensions of the hips, and the grappler should make it a point to have his feet under his hips at all times. If a grappler has too wide or too narrow of a stance, he is often off-balance and unable to attack or defend freely. Additionally, the grappler should make it a point to have a balanced stance so that his shoulders are not too far in front of his hips. If a grappler likes to use a low, crouching-style stance and posture, he should make sure that his shoulders are in a direct line with his hips (which are in a direct line with his feet) so that he is balanced and has the ability to move quickly and effectively.

Upright Posture

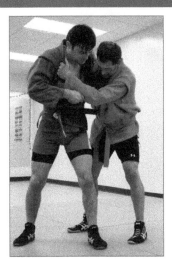

In most cases, the attacker wants to have his hips positioned no more than a hand-length away from his opponent's hips. Additionally, it's a good rule for the attacker to start with a strong, upright posture. This upright posture allows the attacker more freedom of movement and to attack and defend freely. In many cases, this upright posture lends itself to a fast-paced movement about the mat by both athletes. Just as a good boxer uses good upright posture to facilitate better movement, a sambo wrestler uses this upright posture to better allow more freedom of movement (especially with his hips) and mobility. This photo is a good example of how the hips lead the attack.

Low, Bent, or Crouched Posture

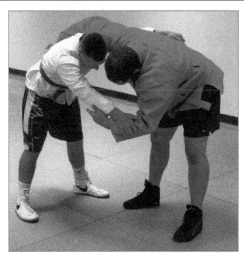

This posture is not always defensive and in many situations is anything but defensive. However, it often is used as a defensive posture. This low, bent-over posture creates the situation where there is a great deal of distance between the hips of the sambo grapplers. In many cases (but not always), this low and crouched posture results in slower movement about the mat by the athletes resulting in a slower-paced match. When using this posture, be sure to not bend over so far that your shoulders are ahead of your hips or feet. If a grappler's shoulders are forward and ahead of his hips, his balance is off and he is vulnerable to an attack.

TECHNICAL TIP: An effective posture is a well-balanced one and often the stance where the sambo wrestler's hips are in line with his feet, his shoulders are in line with his hips, and he has the ability to attack and defend freely.

Okay, from this analysis of controlling your opponent with the grip, posture, and stance, let's go on to analyze the second part of a successful throwing technique; the effective use of controlling your opponent's movement and balance.

(2) CONTROL AND UNBALANCE OPPONENT WITH MOVEMENT AND USE THE MOMENTUM CREATED BY THAT CONTROL

Controlling an opponent's balance is essential in every successful throwing attack. The key component in controlling an opponent's balance is to initially control his movement and then take advantage of it by further controlling the momentum of the action and turn it into a specific attack. By controlling the movement, the attacker will control how fast or how slow both athletes move about the mat. This is called "tempo" or "pace" and if the attacker successfully controls the pace or tempo, he will successfully control the momentum of both his body and his opponent's body. The more momentum that is developed, the more ballistic effect will be generated when the attacker actually executes the throw.

The direction of the movement that leads to the execution of the throw is also part of this phase of control. So, it's not only important that you move your opponent; it's important where and how you move your opponent. The attacker's goal is to control his opponent's direction so that his opponent's body is close enough to successfully develop and build the actual fitting in of his body into the throw.

1. Attacker Controls Grip, Posture, Body Space, and Stance

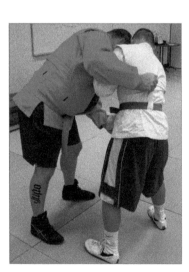

The attacker (on the left) starts the throwing process by controlling his opponent with the grip. As he does this, the attacker uses this controlling grip to determine the posture and proximity of the bodies (body space between the two wrestlers), and this all works from the stance the attacker uses.

2. Attacker Controls Balance with Movement and Momentum

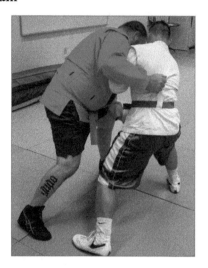

The attacker (on the left) starts to move his opponent in an effort to build the momentum.

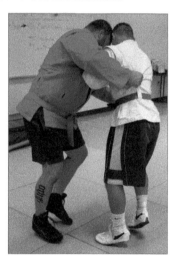

The attacker sets the tempo or pace in an effort to build the necessary momentum to increase the ballistic effect of the throw. This movement contributes to controlling and "breaking" his opponent's balance.

TECHNICAL TIP: The better you control your opponent's movement, the better you control his balance.

(3) BUILD THE TECHNIQUE TO FIT YOUR BODY SO THAT IT WORKS FOR YOU

This is the commitment of the attacker's body into the development and "construction" of the actual throwing movement. It is where and when the attacker fits his body into the throw.

3. Attacker Builds the Technique, Fitting in to Throw

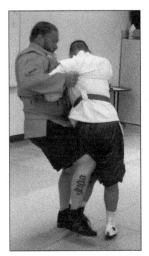

The attacker (left in photo) actually fits his body into position to throw his opponent. In this case, the attacker is using the Sliding Thigh Sweep and he uses his right leg and thigh to sweep into his opponent's left upper leg.

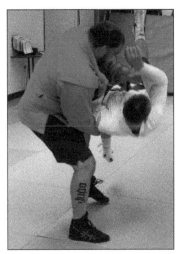

This photo shows the throw in its full effect. The attacker has successfully upended his opponent and has him in the air.

(5) FOLLOW THROUGH AND FINISH THE OPPONENT

Throwing the opponent to the mat or ground with control and force can not only win the match with a score of either total victory or four points, it also serves as a good way to take a lot of the fight out of an opponent. Throwing an opponent to the mat with force can knock the wind out of him, softening him up for a follow-up submission technique or hold-down.

5. Attacker Finishes the Throw

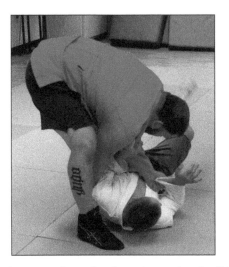

(4) EXECUTE THE TECHNIQUE: THROW YOUR OPPONENT

4. Attacker Throws His Opponent

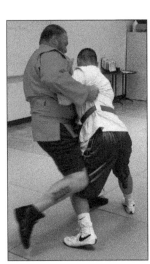

The thrower continues to use his right leg to attack his opponent as he uses the momentum built up from the movement to increase the ballistic effect of the throwing movement. As the thrower does this, you can see how all of these sequential movements blend together. The attacker is actually executing the throw at this point.

The attacker completes the throwing action by following through so that his opponent lands with control and force. The attacker should always be in position so that he can follow his opponent to the mat to secure a hold-down or submission technique if the attacker hasn't scored a total victory from the throw.

SAMBO ENCYCLOPEDIA

Total Victory from a Throw

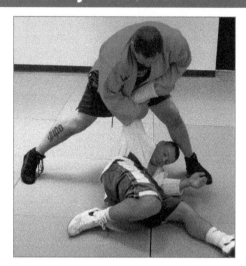

The attacker throws his opponent with control on the mat so that the attacker remains balanced and upright as he finishes the throw. In reality, it's certainly possible (and actually done) to score a total victory from a throw in sambo, but it's not common.

Four-Point Score from a Throw

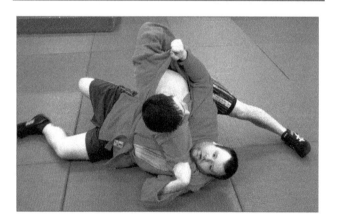

The attacker throws his opponent with good control but less than a total victory score as he follows through and lands on his opponent. Often, the momentum of the throwing attack results in the thrower landing on his opponent and making what would have been a total victory turn into a four-point score. This photo shows how the attacker is in position to follow through from a throw to a hold-down.

Finishing Hold or Technique

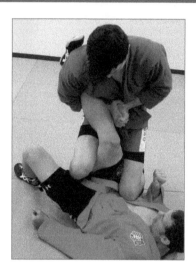

If the thrower doesn't score a total victory, his goal is to score as many points as possible from the throw and immediately apply a submission technique or hold-down. This photo shows the attacker following up from a throw with the start of a lower-body submission.

SELECTED SAMBO THROWING TECHNIQUES

What follows is a selection of throwing techniques used in sambo. Certainly not all the throwing techniques in the sport of sambo can be included in this chapter, but a variety of throws are presented that represent the wide range of diverse techniques used in the sport.

REAR THROW

This is a fundamental throwing technique in sambo, and this author introduces this throw early in a student's career.

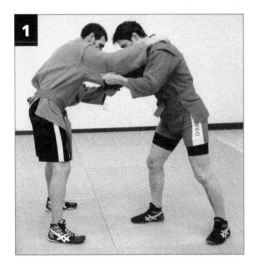

The attacker (on the right) faces his opponent.

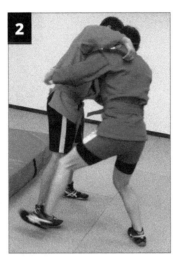

The attacker moves into the throw.

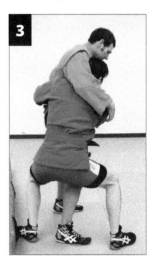

The attacker fits into the throw by moving his left foot and leg behind his opponent as shown. An important point is that the attacker must jam his head into his opponent's right front shoulder. Doing this gives the attacker a good anchor to control the opponent as the attacker throws him. At this time, the attacker uses his left hand and arm to reach around his opponent's waist and hip area. This is what is called a "tightwaist." The attacker uses his left hand to grab the defender's left hip or belt for control.

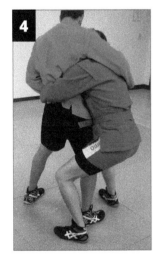

This photo shows how the attacker uses his left arm to wrap around his opponent's waist. Look at how close the attacker is to his opponent and how low the attacker bends with his knees. Also, the angle of the attack is important. The attacker's hips are lower than his opponent's hips and the attacker's front left hip area is positioned under and below the defender's right hip area.

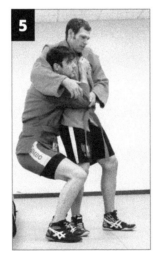

The attacker makes sure his hips are lower than the defender's hips as shown. Look at how the attacker jams his head into the defender's right front shoulder area and look at how the attacker uses his right hand to grab and control his opponent's left lapel. The attacker's feet are firmly planted on the mat with both knees bent.

REAR THROW

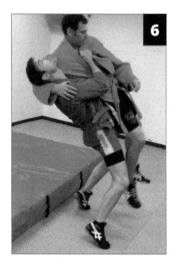

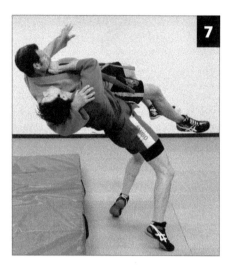

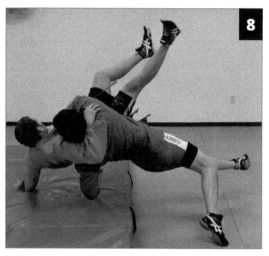

The attacker starts his lift by driving with his feet off of the mat and arching as shown. Look at how the attacker uses his right hand to control his opponent's left lapel to assist in the lifting action.

The attacker drives off both feet as he arches backward. Look at how the attacker uses his head that is wedged at his opponent's right shoulder area to "steer" his opponent as he throws him.

The attacker rotates his body to his left as he throws his opponent as shown.

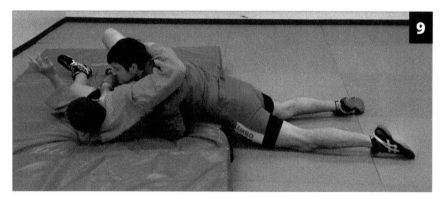

The attacker finishes the throw and follows through to the mat, making sure to land belly down and not land on his back. Doing this ensures that the referee gives the score to the attacker.

REAR THROW AS A COUNTER

Often, the rear throw is taught as a counter technique against a forward throw. This series shows the rear throw's effectiveness as a counter technique.

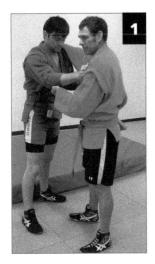

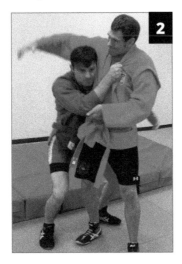

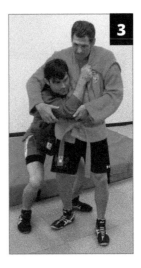

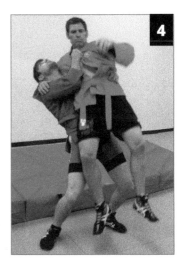

The initial attack will come from the grappler on the right and the grappler on the left will counter his forward throw.

As the attacker comes into a forward throw, the grappler on the left bends his knees so that he is below his opponent's hips and center of gravity. He also jams his head as deeply as possible into the right front shoulder and pectoral area of his opponent.

The grappler on the left is now in a solid position to throw his opponent. Look at how he uses his right hand to firmly grasp his opponent's left lapel and his left hand to start to grab around his opponent's hip to tightwaist it.

The sambo wrestler on the left lifts his opponent up. Look at how he uses his head to drive and steer his opponent and his right hand to control his opponent's body by grabbing the lapel of the jacket. The attacker springs upward with his legs to elevate his opponent.

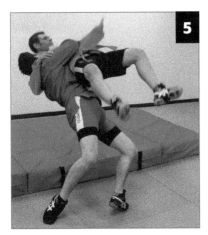

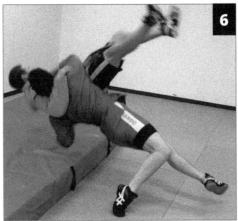

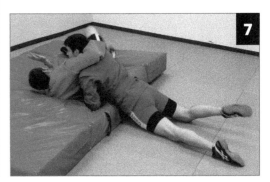

The attacker rotates his body toward his opponent as he throws him.

The attacker continues to rotate his body to his left and toward his opponent. Look at the total commitment into the throwing action.

The attacker completes the throw as shown.

SINGLE LEG THROW

There are numerous variations of this throw, but the bottom line is that if you develop a single leg throw that works for you, use it. This particular variation is one that we call the "Cuban leg grab" at our club because I first saw this variation used with great success by the Cuban team when there for a tournament in the 1980s.

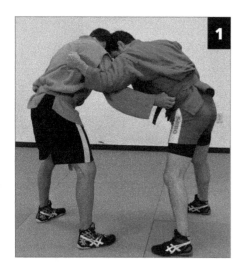
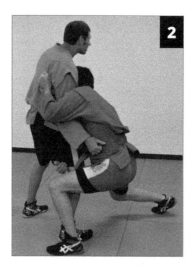
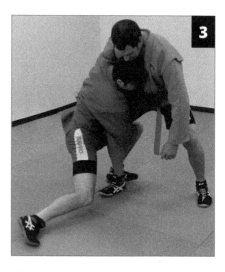

The attacker (on the right) uses his left hand to securely grip onto his opponent's jacket at the general area of the opponent's right shoulder blade. The attacker leads with his left foot.

The attacker does a lunge step with his left foot and leg as shown to get close to his opponent. As he does this, the attacker aims his left elbow down and tightens his grip with his left hand on his opponent's jacket as shown. This action traps and locks the defender's right side and controls him. As he does this, the attacker drives his head onto his opponent's right pectoral area and uses his right hand to grab deeply and around the defender's right thigh (just above the right knee).

This photo shows another view of this throw with the attacker on the left.

SINGLE LEG THROW

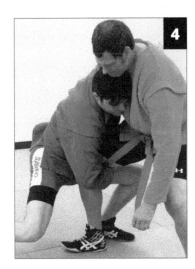

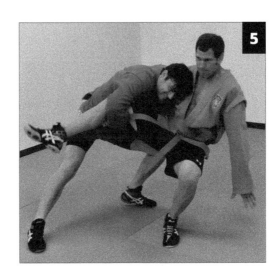

This photo shows how the attacker uses the left side of his head to push against his opponent's right pectoral and shoulder area. Look at how low the attacker is in his lunge step. However, it is important that the attacker not drop onto his right knee. If he does this, he will lose a great deal of momentum and not throw his opponent with as much ballistic effect.

The attacker uses his right hand and arm to lift the defender's right leg up and at about the height of the attacker's hips. As he is doing this, the attacker drives hard with his head and body into the defender. Doing this creates a strong throw.

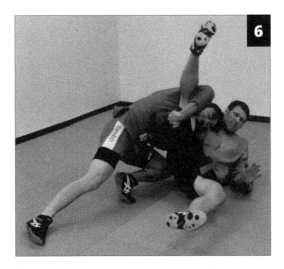

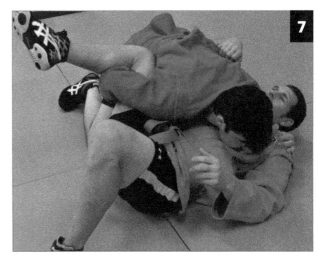

The attacker drives hard and throws his opponent onto his back with force and control to score as many points as possible and make it possible for the attacker to follow through to the mat with a finishing hold.

The attacker can immediately secure a side chest hold or other hold-down and be in a strong position to transition into securing a submission technique to win the match.

BOTH LEGS THROW

There are about as many variations of a double-leg throw as there are grapplers. This is a popular and effective throw, but make sure to use it as a throw and not simply a takedown. Sure, you can use it as a takedown to get an opponent to the mat, but go for a maximum score with a throw if you can.

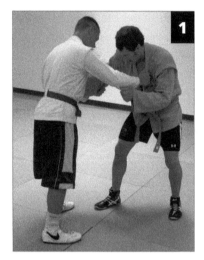

The attacker (on the right) takes a stance with his right foot slightly leading as shown.

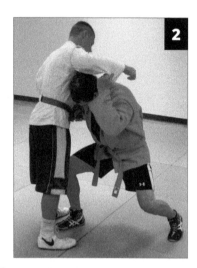

The attacker does a lunge step with his right foot and uses both hands to push his opponent's arms upward. As he does this, he starts to drive his head to his left and onto the right side of his opponent.

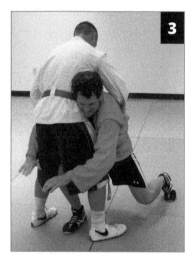

The attacker drops in low and uses both hands to start to reach and grab around his opponent's legs at the knee area.

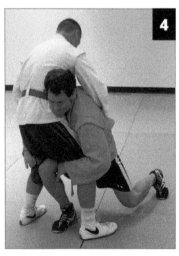

The attacker uses both hands to grab onto each of his opponent's legs just above the knee area as the attacker drives his right shoulder hard into the defender's waist at about the belt. Notice that the attacker's left knee is not resting on the mat as doing this would reduce the forward drive and momentum of the attacks; possibly lowering the score for the throw.

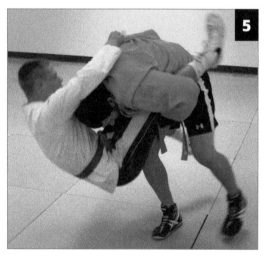

The attacker uses both hands to reap and pull onto his opponent's legs as the attacker drives forward into the throw.

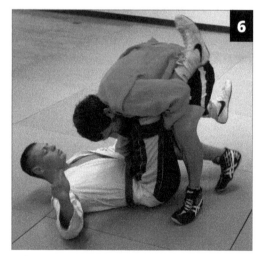

The attacker throws his opponent onto his back and can immediately transition into groundfighting.

DOUBLE LEG THIGH SWEEP THROW

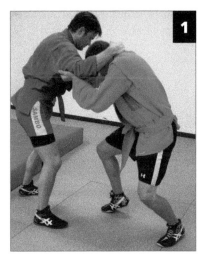

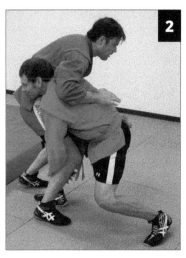

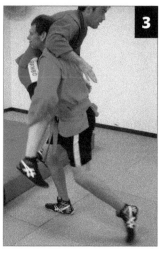

The angle of attack is important in this application of the double leg thigh sweep. The attacker (on the right) positions his body so that it is not directly facing his opponent. Instead, the attacker's body should be angled to his left and close to the defender's right leg. The attacker will shoot in, aiming for the defender's left hip. Doing this puts the attacker in a strong position to use a thigh sweep a bit later.

The attacker drops in low with his double leg throw attack as shown.

The attacker drives forward and uses both his hands and arms to pick the defender up. As he does this, the attacker makes sure to start to drive forward and to his right.

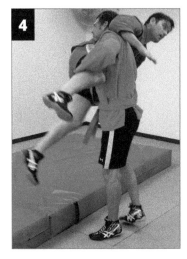

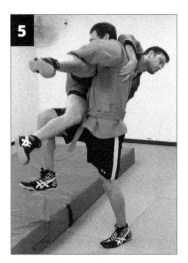

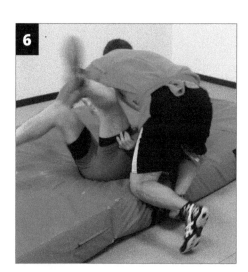

The attacker uses his hands and arms to lift his opponent and tilt the defender to the attacker's right as shown. The attacker uses his head that is placed on the defender's right hip to steer the defender's body to the attacker's right side. Look at how the attacker is now standing firmly on both feet at this point.

The attacker uses his right leg to sweep and lift the defender's left upper leg. The attacker uses his right leg to forcefully sweep and lift his opponent. Doing this adds to the amplitude of the throw. Look at how this lifting and sweeping action throws the defender to his left side.

The attacker throws his opponent to the mat.

FAR LAPEL BACK CARRY THROW

This is a standard forward throw that is a good example of a "wheel throw." Imagine a big wheel and the thrower is standing in the center of it. The attacker throws or "wheels" his opponent over his body in the same way a wheel turns.

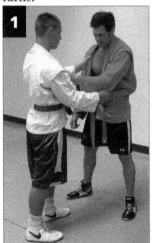

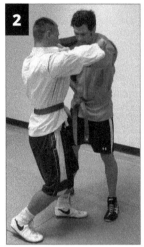

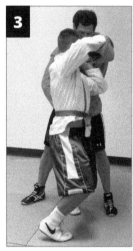

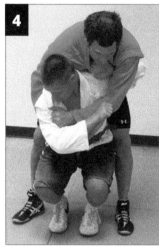

The attacker uses his left hand to grab his opponent's right lapel and uses his right hand to grip his opponent's left lower sleeve.

The attacker uses his right hand to pull and lift upward on his opponent's left sleeve as the attacker steps in with his left foot to start the throw.

The attacker continues to use his right hand to pull on his opponent's left sleeve as the attacker uses his left hand to curl up his opponent's right lapel.

The attacker turns into the throw and loads his opponent up onto the attacker's back and hip. Note how the attacker uses his left hand and arm to wrap his opponent's left lapel tightly and his left forearm to jam under his opponent's left armpit area.

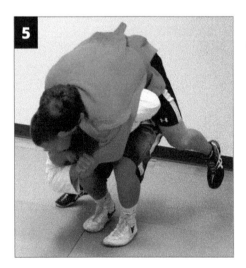

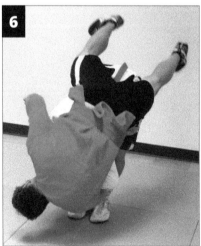

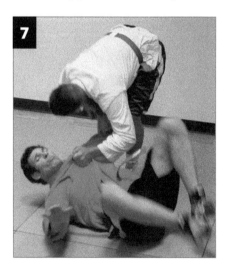

The attacker rotates to his right as he starts to throw his opponent.

The attacker throws his opponent.

The attacker throws his opponent to the mat with control and force and in this photo remains standing in order to secure a total victory score from the mat official.

HIP THROW WITH BELT GRIP

This is a standard and popular hip throw where the attacker uses a belt grip.

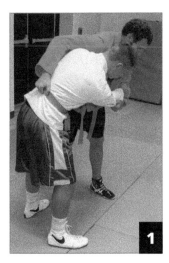

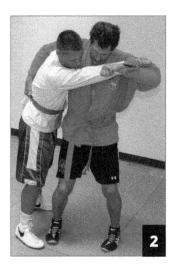

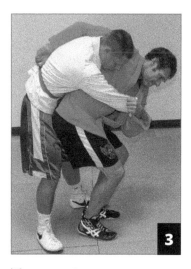

The attacker (on the right) uses his right hand to reach over his opponent's left shoulder and grips the belt as shown.

The attacker uses his left hand to pull upward and forward on the defender's right sleeve. As he does this, the attacker uses his right hand (which is holding onto his opponent's belt) to pull upward on the belt.

The attacker moves into position to throw his opponent as shown.

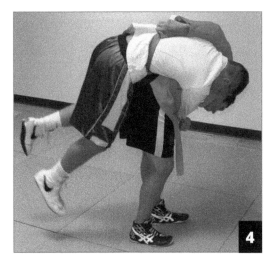

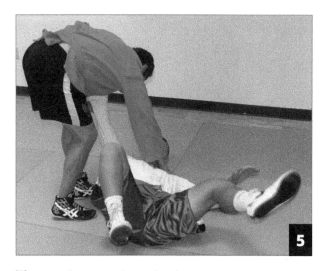

The attacker throws his opponent, making sure to pull with both his left hand (on the defender's right sleeve) and use his right hand to pull on the defender's belt.

The attacker completes the throw.

BELT GRIP

This throw is basically a variation of the hip throw with the belt where the attacker drops under his opponent onto both of his knees. This throw is effective to not only throw an opponent, but transition an opponent from standing to groundfighting.

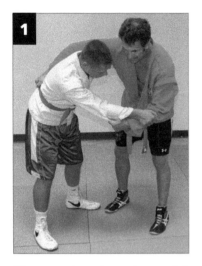

The attacker (on the right) controls the grip by using his left hand to grab low on his opponent's right sleeve and his right hand and arm to reach over the defender's left shoulder and grab his belt.

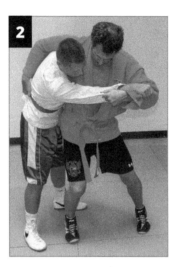

The attacker fits into the throw.

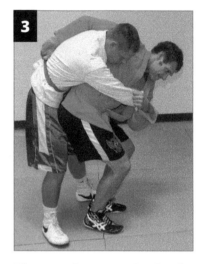

The attacker completely fits into the throw and makes sure that both of his knees are pointed to his left.

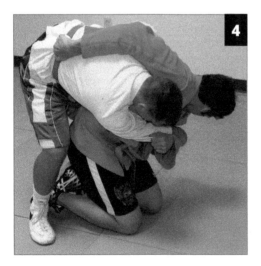

The attacker "screws himself into the mat" and onto both of his knees. Doing this causes the defender to be thrown forward and over the attacker's right hip. The attacker doesn't simply drop straight down onto his knees as doing this takes the momentum directly downward and not forward. Also, dropping straight downward onto the knees could cause injury to the knees.

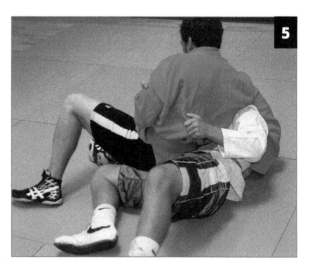

The attacker throws his opponent over his right hip and immediately secures a hold-down.

KNEE DROP ONE ARM BACK CARRY THROW

This is probably the most popular and often-used throw in a number of combat sports, including sambo.

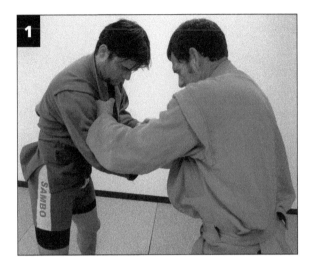

The attacker (on the right) uses his left hand to grip his opponent's right lapel. Using this short grip with the left hand helps the attacker control his opponent's right shoulder more effectively than if the attacker used his left hand to grip his opponent's right sleeve.

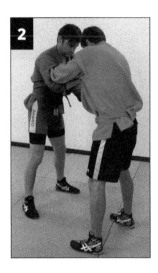

This photo shows how the attacker (on the right) stands relatively close to his opponent. The attacker uses a good, upright posture so that his hips are relatively close to his opponent's hips, allowing him to attack more quickly than if the grapplers were bent over with their hips far apart from each other.

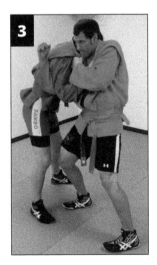

The attacker uses his left hand to pull on his opponent's right lapel as the attacker uses his right arm to hook up and under his opponent's right arm. Look at how the attacker's right arm is bent with his fist pointed straight up to the ceiling and his right elbow is pointed directly down to the mat.

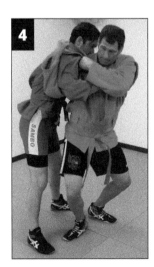

The attacker turns into the throw. It is important that the attacker uses his right arm to pinch and trap his opponent's right upper arm as shown. The attacker does not hoist his opponent up and onto his right shoulder. The attacker uses his left hand and arm to pull on the defender's right lapel as shown.

KNEE DROP ONE ARM BACK CARRY THROW

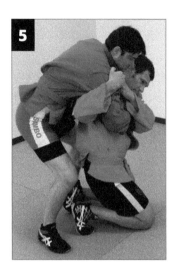

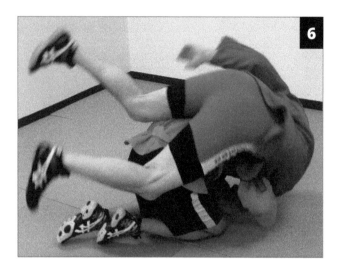

The attacker screws himself into the mat and turns downward and under the defender as shown. The attacker's right hip is pointed to his right, and the attacker's knees are together and pointed to his left. The attacker does not do a "flop and drop" where he drops straight down and onto his knees.

The attacker throws his opponent.

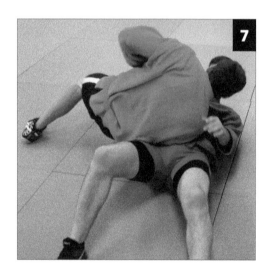

The attacker immediately transitions to a hold-down.

KNEE DROP BOTH HANDS BACK CARRY THROW

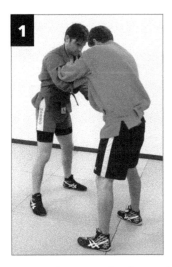

This is another popular knee-drop attack. The attacker (right) uses his left hand to grab low on his opponent's right sleeve and uses his right hand to grip onto his opponent's left lapel.

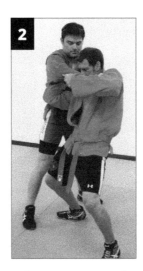

The attacker turns into the throw. As he does this, he uses his left hand to pull forward and slightly upward on his opponent's right sleeve. The attacker uses his right hand that is holding onto his opponent's left lapel to curl his right hand in, making sure not to bend his right wrist.

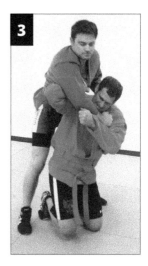

The attacker is fully committed to the throw. Look at how the attacker uses his right forearm as a wedge under his opponent's right shoulder and armpit area.

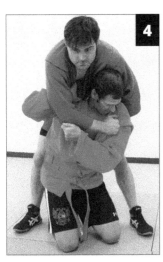

The attacker's knees are both on the mat, close together. Look at how the attacker's knees are pointed to his left and his right hip is pointed to his right. He has successfully screwed himself into the mat much like water going down a drain. The attacker does not "flop and drop" or drop straight downward on both knees.

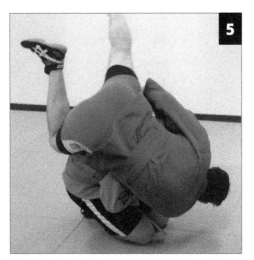

The attacker throws his opponent.

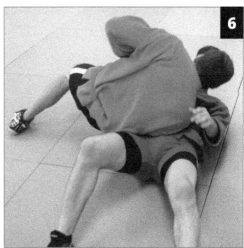

The attacker immediately follows through to a hold-down.

SIDE KNEE DROP THROW

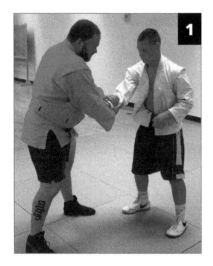

The attacker (on the left) uses both hands to grip onto his opponent's right sleeve, low on the sleeve. The attacker leads with his left foot as shown.

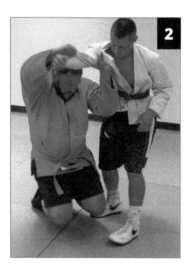

The attacker quickly swings under his opponent. As he does this, the attacker uses his right hand to pull his opponent's right sleeve and arm up and over the attacker's head. The attacker uses his left hand to grab his opponent's right lapel.

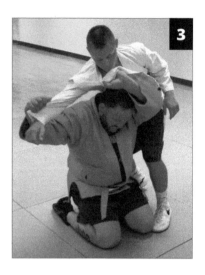

The attacker spins under his opponent and lands on both knees as shown. Look at how the attacker uses his hands and arms to control his opponent's upper body. The attacker has spun his body low and under his opponent's center of gravity.

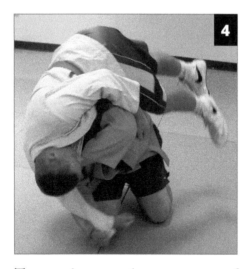

The attacker uses the momentum of his spinning action low and under his opponent's center of gravity to throw him as shown.

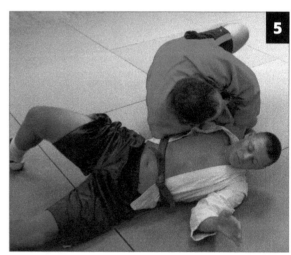

The attacker finishes the throw.

SAME SIDE LAPEL BACK CARRY THROW

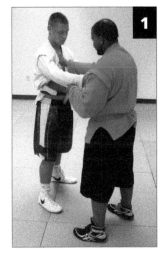

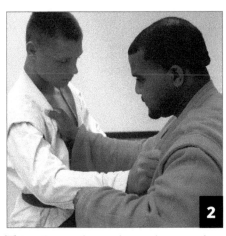

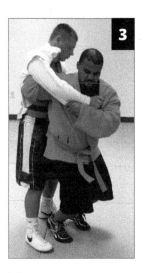

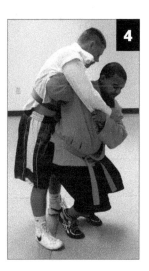

The attacker (on the right) uses his left hand to grip onto his opponent's right sleeve at about the elbow area. The attacker uses his right hand to grip his opponent's right lapel.

This photo shows how the attacker (on the right) uses his left hand to grip his opponent's right sleeve and uses his right hand to grip onto his opponent's right lapel.

The attacker uses his left hand to pull his opponent forward as he swings into the attack and curls his right hand so that it wraps tightly into his opponent's right lapel.

The attacker wedges his right forearm up and under the defender's right armpit as shown.

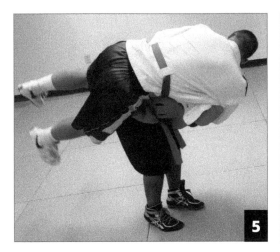

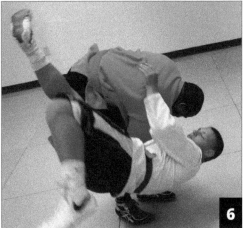

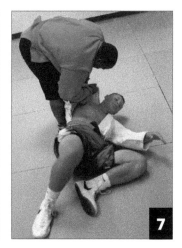

The attacker pulls with his left hand and throws his opponent over his hip.

The attacker throws his opponent.

The attacker finishes the throw. In this photo, the attacker remains standing so the mat official will most likely score the throw as a total victory.

KNEE DROP TIGHTWAIST HIP THROW

This is a useful knee-drop throw when your opponent is bent over.

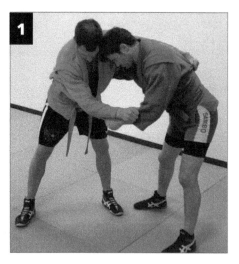

The attacker (on the right) uses his left hand to grip low on his opponent's right sleeve.

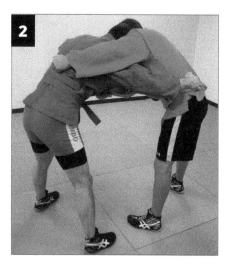

This back view shows how the attacker (now on the left in this photo) uses his right hand to grip onto his opponent's jacket or belt at the hip area. Look at how both grapplers are bent over with a lot of space between their hips. Again, this knee drop attack is ideal for this situation.

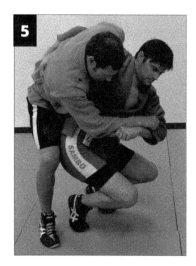

The attacker screws himself into the mat and spins under his opponent much like water going down a drain.

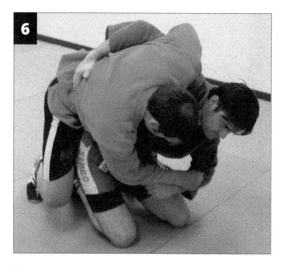

The attacker is now low and under his opponent's hips and center of gravity and is throwing him.

KNEE DROP TIGHTWAIST HIP THROW

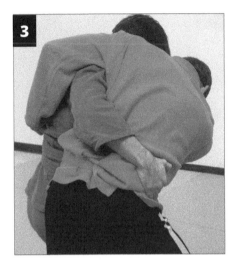

This back view shows how the attacker quickly uses his right hand to grab deeply around his opponent's waist and uses his right hand to latch onto his opponent's right hip.

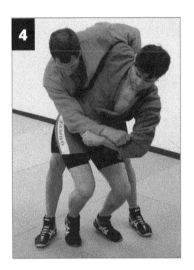

The attacker fits into position to throw his opponent as shown. Look at how the attacker's knees are pointed to his left as his right hip is pointed to his right.

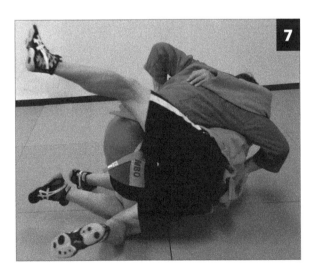

The attacker throws his opponent.

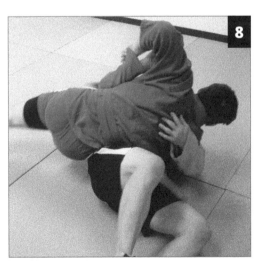

The attacker finishes the throw and immediately secures a hold-down.

CROSS GRIP TIGHTWAIST HIP THROW

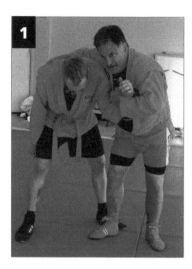

The attacker (on the right) uses his left hand to grip low on his opponent's left sleeve and arm, pulling it firmly to the attacker's chest. The attacker uses his right hand to reach behind his opponent and grips his opponent's right epaulette.

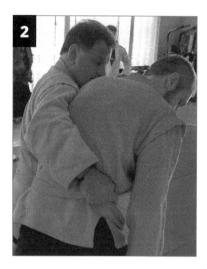

The attacker quickly uses his right hand and arm to reach around his opponent's hip area and grips his opponent's belt or right hip.

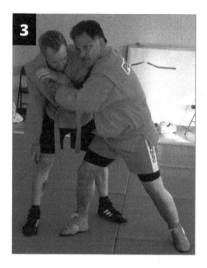

The attacker quickly uses his left hand to jam his opponent's left arm into the opponent's upper chest area. Look at how the attacker moves in very close to his opponent.

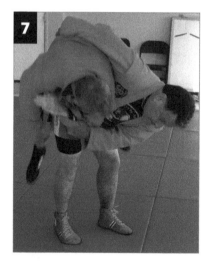

This photos shows the attack at midpoint.

CROSS GRIP TIGHTWAIST HIP THROW

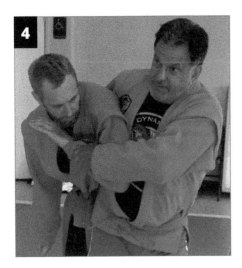

This photo shows how the attacker uses his left hand to jam his opponent's left arm into the opponent's upper body as the attacker fits into the throw.

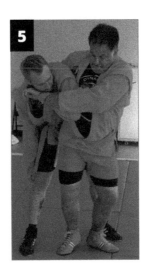

The attacker fits into the throw, moving his right hip in front on his opponent.

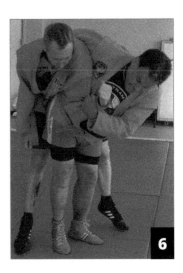

The attacker starts his throw.

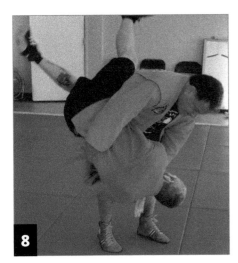

The attacker throws his opponent over his hip as shown.

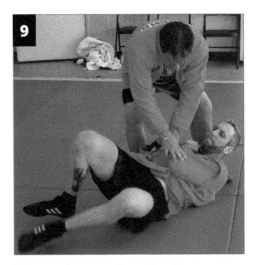

The attacker completes the throw.

SAMBO ENCYCLOPEDIA

PICK-UP HIP THROW

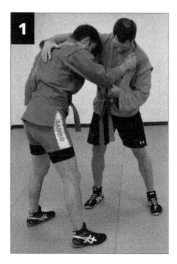

The attacker (on the left) uses his right hand to firmly grip his opponent's left lapel as shown.

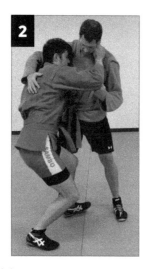

The attacker dips low and uses his left hand and arm to reach around his opponent's right side and grab high around his opponent's right leg very close to the buttocks.

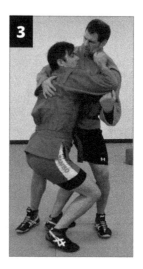

The attacker moves his feet and legs so that they are between his opponent's feet and legs. He uses his right hand that is gripping his opponent's left lapel to pull upward on the lapel.

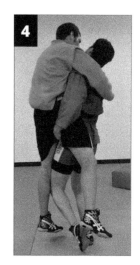

This shows how the attacker uses his left hand to grab around his opponent's right leg near the hip. Look at how he uses his left hand to hoist his opponent up and onto his left hip.

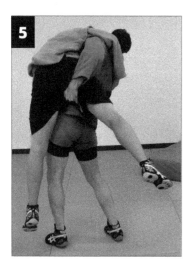

The attacker shifts his left hip in front of his opponent's body as the attacker continues to use his left hand and arm to lift up on his opponent's right leg as shown.

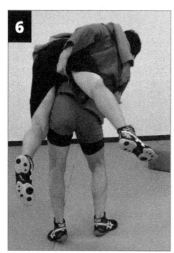

The attacker throws his opponent over his left hip as shown.

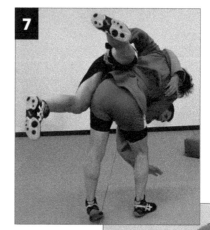

Look at how the attacker uses his left hand to control his opponent's right leg as the attacker throws him over his hip.

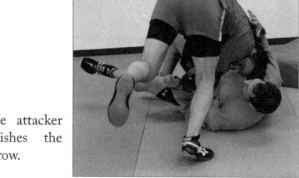

The attacker finishes the throw.

PICK-UP LEG SWEEP THROW

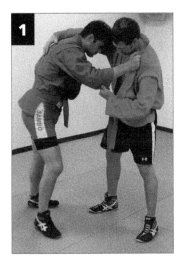

The attacker (on the left) uses his right hand to grip firmly on his opponent's left lapel.

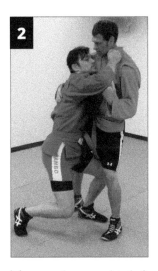

The attacker uses his left foot to step in deeply between his opponent's feet and legs. As he does this, the attacker uses his left hand to grab around his opponent's left upper leg.

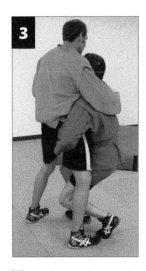

This photo shows the back view where the attacker uses his left hand to grab around his opponent's upper left leg near the buttocks.

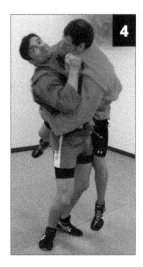

The attacker shifts his left hip in front of his opponent as he uses his right hand to lift upward on his opponent's left lapel. As he does this, he uses his left hand to lift upward on his opponent's right leg.

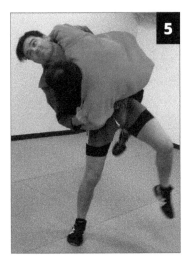

The attacker starts to sweep with his left leg. Doing this give the attacker more control of the throwing movement and allows the attacker to shift his left hip in deeper in front of his opponent.

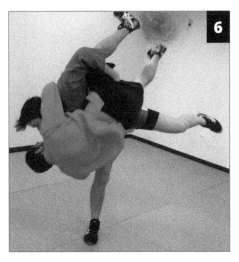

The attacker throws his opponent using a strong sweeping motion with his left leg and hip as the attacker continues to use his left hand to lift his opponent's right upper leg as shown.

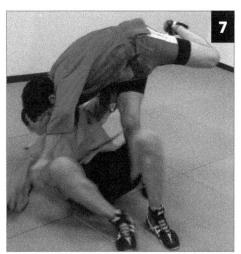

The attacker finishes the throw.

CROSS GRIP HIP SWEEP

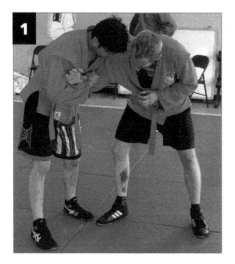

The attacker uses his right hand to grip onto his opponent's right arm and sleeve. As he does this, the attacker uses his left hand to reach around and grab his opponent's jacket or belt at the hip area.

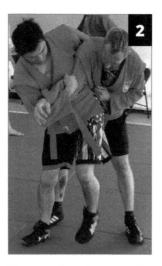

The attacker fits into the throw as shown. Look at how the attacker shifts his left hip in front of his opponent.

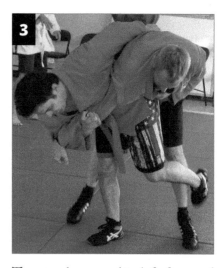

The attacker uses his left foot and leg to sweep his opponent's left leg as shown. Look at how the attacker uses his right hand to pull his opponent's right sleeve.

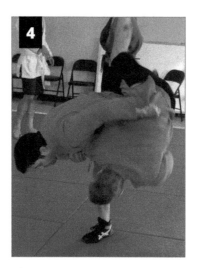

The attacker throws his opponent.

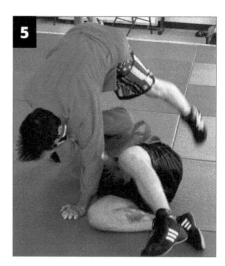

The attacker finishes the throw.

SWEEPING HIP THROW WITH GEORGIAN BELT GRIP

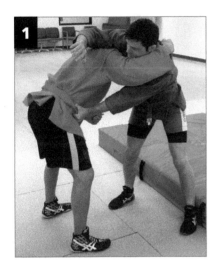

The attacker (on the right) uses his left hand to grip firmly on his opponent's belt as shown. As he does this, the attacker uses his right hand to reach over his opponent's right shoulder.

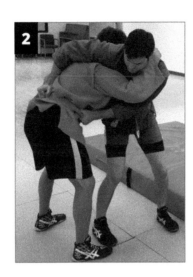

The attacker uses his right hand to reach over his opponent's right shoulder or upper arm and grips firmly onto his opponent's belt. As he does this, the attacker moves his right hip closer to his opponent.

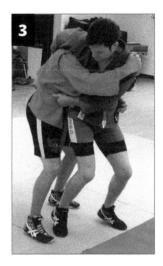

The attacker fits into the throw as shown. Look at how the attacker shifts his right hip in front of his opponent's hips.

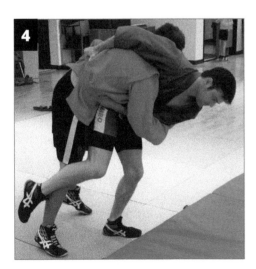

The attacker uses his right foot and leg to sweep his opponent's right upper leg as shown. Look at how the attacker uses both hands to pull on his opponent's belt as he throws him.

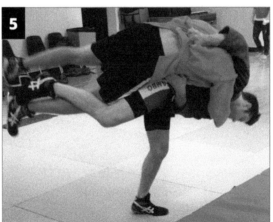

The attacker throws his opponent.

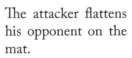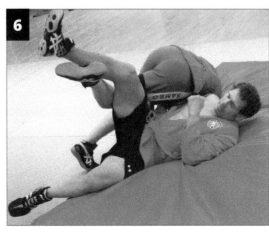

The attacker flattens his opponent on the mat.

DUCK UNDER PICK-UP HIP THROW

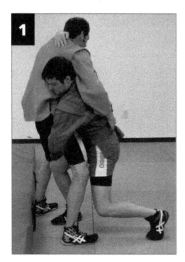

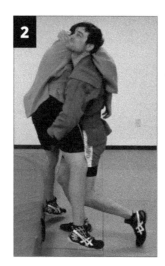

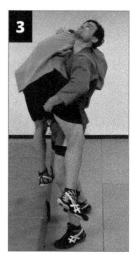

From a standard lapel and sleeve grip, the attacker (right) uses his right foot and leg to step in deeply between his opponent's legs. As he does this, he uses his right hand to grab over his opponent's left shoulder and grip onto the collar of the jacket. The attacker has now dropped low with his initial lunge step and drives his head under the defender's right arm as shown. The attacker uses his left hand and arm to grab the defender's right upper leg.

The attacker continues to step into his opponent and drives his head upward. Doing this allows the attacker to stand straight as shown. As he does this, the attacker starts to lift his opponent up and off the mat.

The attacker steps in with his left foot and has both feet firmly planted on the mat as a base. The attacker uses his right hand to pull on his opponent's collar as the attacker drives his head to his right as shown. The attacker continues to use his left hand and arm to grab around the opponent's upper leg and lift his opponent.

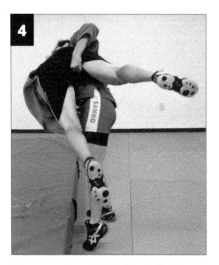

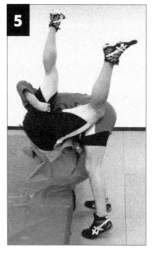

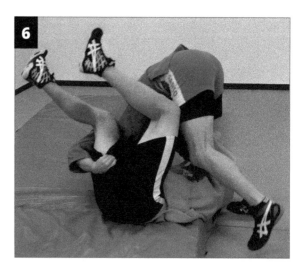

The attacker shifts his left hip so that it is in front of his opponent. Doing this helps the attacker throw his opponent over his left hip as the attacker continues to use his left hand and arm to lift his opponent.

The attacker throws his opponent over his left hip.

The attacker finishes the throw.

WINDMILL THROW

This throw has many variations and is known by various names depending on the combat sport that it is done in. This throw (in all it variations and applications) is probably one of the most popular throws, takedowns, or transitions in any grappling or fighting sport.

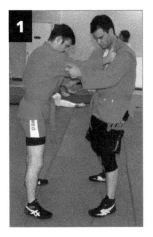
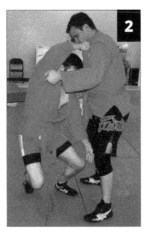
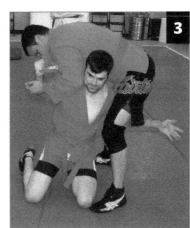

1. The attacker (on the left) uses his right hand to grip onto his opponent's left lapel.

2. The attacker turns to his right so that his left shoulder is facing his opponent. As he does this, the attacker starts to drop onto his knees and uses his right hand to pull on his opponent's left lapel.

3. The attacker drops onto both of his knees as he is positioned so that his left side is facing his opponent. The attacker uses his left hand to drive between his opponent's legs as shown.

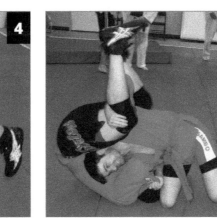
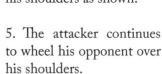

4. The attacker uses his right hand to continue to pull on his opponent's left lapel and uses his left hand and arm to hook and grab the defender's left upper leg. The attacker lifts his opponent onto the attacker's shoulders and wheels the defender over his shoulders as shown.

5. The attacker continues to wheel his opponent over his shoulders.

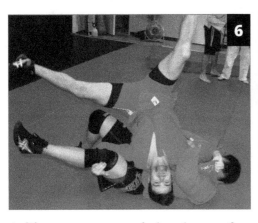
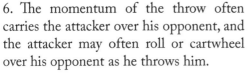

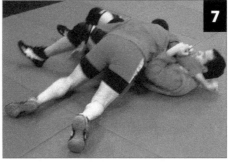

7. The attacker immediately follows through to a hold-down.

6. The momentum of the throw often carries the attacker over his opponent, and the attacker may often roll or cartwheel over his opponent as he throws him.

LEG SPLIT OR BODY DROP THROW

Here is another throw that is commonly used in every combat sport and this is because it works so well.

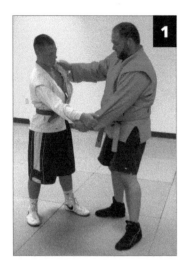

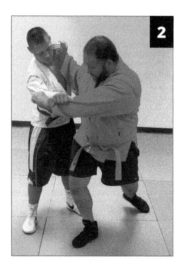

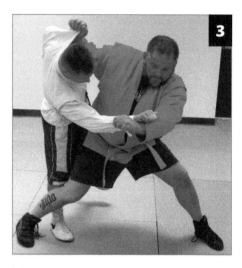

The attacker (on the right) uses his left hand to grip low on his opponent's right sleeve and uses his right hand to grip his opponent's left lapel.

The attacker uses his left hand to pull up and forward and uses his right hand and arm to jam onto his opponent's left pectoral area. As he does this, he spins backward on his right foot and swings his left foot and leg back.

The attacker splits his feet and legs wide so that the attacker's right knee is slightly bent as shown. Look at how the attacker uses his hands to control his opponent. It is important that the attacker continually pull forward with his left hand on his opponent's sleeve.

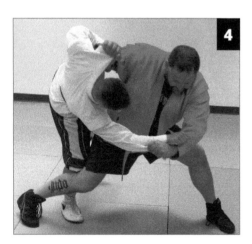

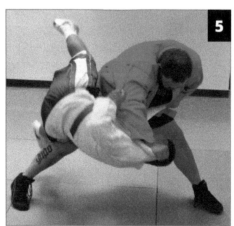

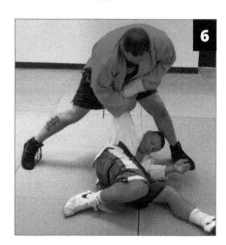

This throw catches the attacker applying the throw. Look at how the attacker's right knee is flexed.

The attacker throws his opponent. Look at how the attacker's right leg has sprung up to add more ballistic effect to the throw. Also notice how the attacker uses his hands to drive his opponent into the mat.

The attacker completes the throw.

LOW SPLIT THROW ON ONE KNEE

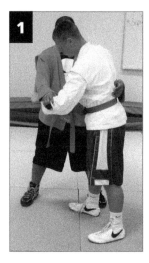

The attacker (on the right) uses his left hand to grip low on his opponent's right sleeve. Look at how the attacker leads with his right foot and has it placed slightly inside his opponent's left foot.

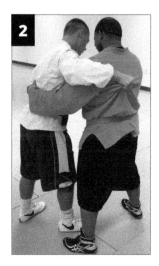

This view shows how the attacker (now on the left) uses his right hand to grip onto the back of his opponent's jacket.

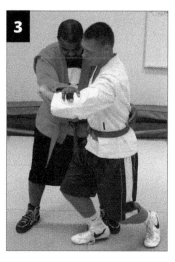

The attacker uses his left hand to pull forward as he spins on his right foot and swings his left foot backward.

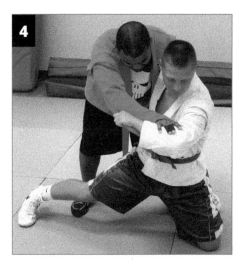

The attacker spins backward with his left foot and leg and quickly drops on his left knee as shown. As he does this, the attacker shoots his right foot and leg laterally. Look at how the attacker positions his right foot on the mat so that the foot is on the ball (and not flat). Note how the attacker's right leg is flexed with the knee pointed downward and slightly forward.

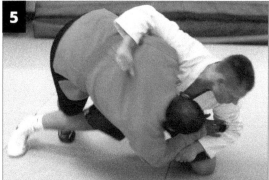

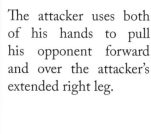

The attacker uses both of his hands to pull his opponent forward and over the attacker's extended right leg.

The attacker throws his opponent and follows through to a hold-down.

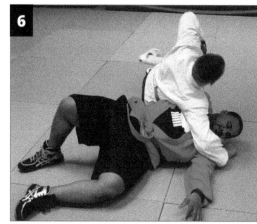

FRONT LEG-LIFT THROW

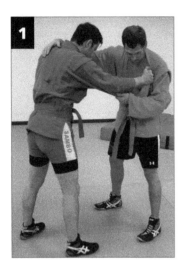

The attacker (on the left) uses his right hand to grip his opponent's left lapel.

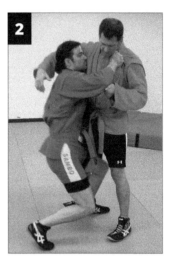

The attacker uses his left foot to step deeply between his opponent's feet and legs as shown. As he does this, the attacker uses his right hand to pull up on his opponent's left lapel and lift him. Look at how the attacker's right knee is bent and starting to drive forward. As he does this, the attacker uses his left hand and arm to grab high around the defender's right leg (at about the thigh) or upper leg.

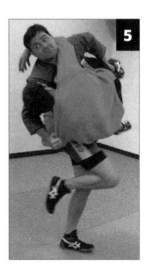

The attacker rotates to his right as he throws his opponent.

FRONT LEG LIFT THROW

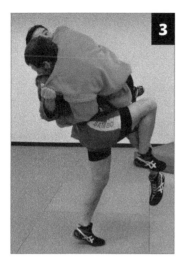

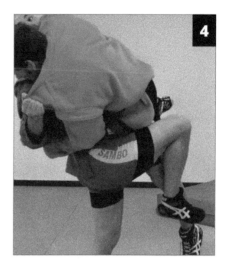

The attacker forcefully lifts and drives his right knee and leg forward and upward on the left side of his opponent's hip. As he does this, the attacker continues to use his left hand to lift upward on his opponent's right leg as the attacker uses his right hand to pull upward and back over the attacker's right side as shown. Look at how the attacker's right bent leg is lifting and sweeping the defender's body.

This photo shows how the attacker's right leg is used to lift and sweep his opponent. The attacker uses the momentum of the lifting and sweeping action of his leg to throw his opponent.

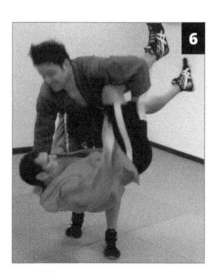

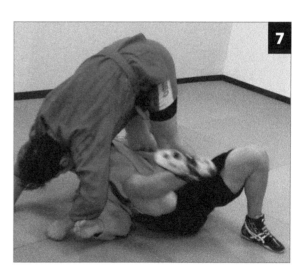

The attacker throws his opponent.

The attacker finishes the throw with the defender landing on the mat with a big boom.

FRONT LEG-LIFT THROW USING A GEORGIAN BELT GRIP

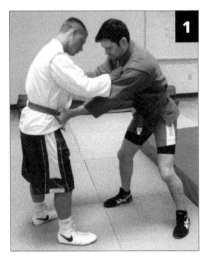

The attacker (on the right) uses his left hand to grip his opponent's belt as an anchor grip to control his opponent.

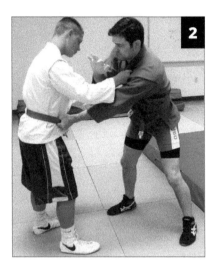

The attacker uses his right hand to start to reach forward.

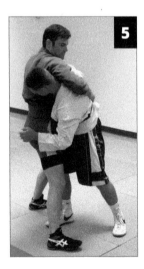

The view has changed to give you a better look at this throw. Look at how the attacker uses his right arm and elbow to drive (or steer) his opponent's upper body down and forward. The attacker's right foot and leg are in front of his opponent and ready to attack.

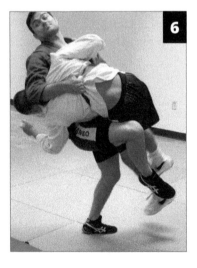

As the attacker continues to force his opponent to bend forward, the attacker uses a powerful sweeping motion with his right bent leg. This sweeping action is also a lifting action. The attacker rotates his body to his right with a lot of force at this point. As he does this, the attacker uses both hands to lift upward on his opponent's belt.

FRONT LEG LIFT THROW USING A GEORGIAN BELT GRIP

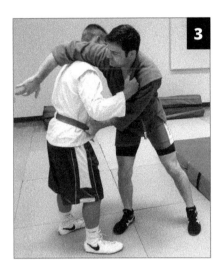

The attacker uses his right hand and arm to reach over his opponent's right shoulder as shown.

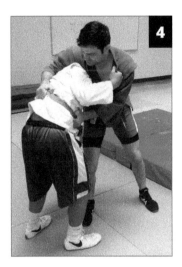

The attacker now has control of his opponent's belt with both hands and is forcing his opponent to bend forward (breaking the opponent's posture and balance).

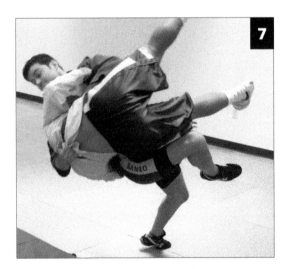

The attacker continues to sweep and lift with his right leg and continues to rotate to his right. All the while, the attacker continues to lift with his hands on his opponent's belt. Doing this throws his opponent as shown.

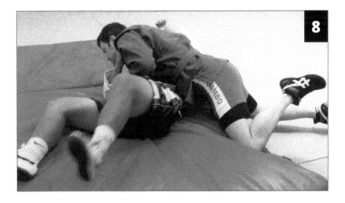

The attacker completes the throw. This throw is a great reason to use crash pads in your gym!

FOOT PROP THROW (USING GEORGIAN BELT GRIP)

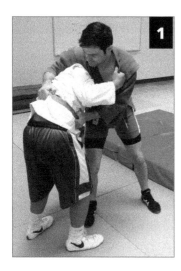

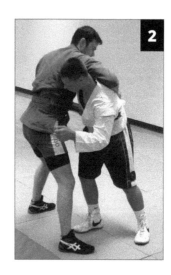

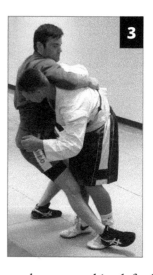

The initial grip and stance for this throw is the same as the previous throw. The attacker uses both hands to grab his opponent's belt as shown.

The view is changed to show the attacker using his right elbow to push (or steer) the back of his opponent's head and upper back. Look at how the attacker's right foot and leg are positioned directly in front of his opponent.

The attacker uses his left hand (gripping the defender's belt) to pull upward as the attacker uses his right elbow, arm, and hand to drive the defender's body forward as shown. At this point, the attacker forcefully moves his right foot in front of the defender's left foot, blocking or propping it. The attacker could also use his right foot to sweep his opponent's left foot.

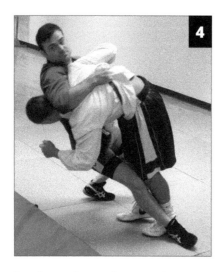

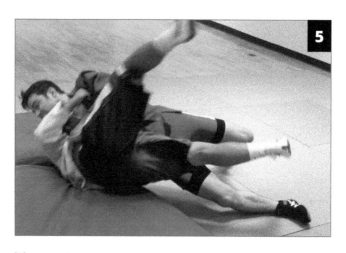

Look at how the attacker uses his right foot to prop or block his opponent's left foot as the attacker turns to his right and starts to throw his opponent.

The attacker throws his opponent.

LEG ENTWINING AND LIFTING THROW

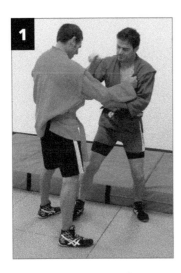

The attacker (on the right) uses a standard grip and uses his left hand to grip his opponent's right sleeve.

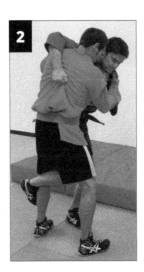

The attacker uses his right hand and arm to reach over his opponent's left shoulder and grip firmly on the defender's jacket. The attacker uses his right foot and leg to entwine his opponent's left leg as shown.

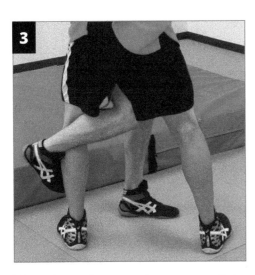

This photo shows a closer view of the leg entwining action that is used by the attacker. Look at how the attacker uses his right foot to hook his opponent's left lower leg for control

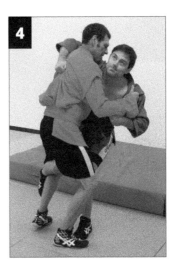

The attacker uses his left foot and leg to step forward and between his opponent's feet and legs. As he does this, the attacker starts to arch his body and rotate strongly to his right.

LEG ENTWINING AND LIFTING THROW

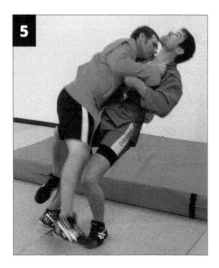

The attacker rotates strongly to his right as he lifts his opponent up and off the mat.

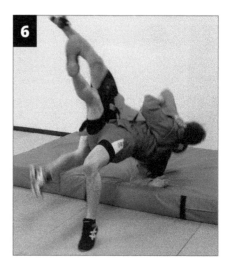

The attacker forcefully rotates into the action of the throw as he drives off of his left foot that is on the mat.

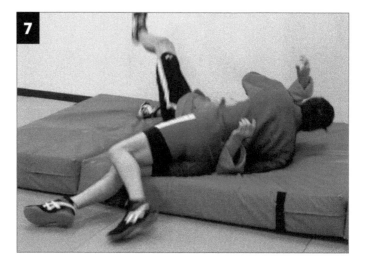

The attacker completes the throw by rotating to his right and onto his opponent.

LEG ENTWINING AND LIFTING THROW USING THE GEORGIAN GRIP

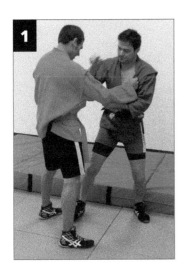
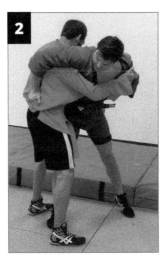

1. The attacker (on the right) uses his left hand to grip his opponent's right sleeve

2. The attacker uses his right arm and hand to reach over his opponent's right shoulder or upper arm and grip the opponent's belt.

3. As the attacker establishes his grip with his hands on his opponent's jacket, the attacker uses his right foot and leg to entwine his opponent's left leg.

4. The attacker uses his right arm and elbow to push his opponent so that the opponent bends forward. The attacker makes sure to plant his left foot firmly on the mat for stability.

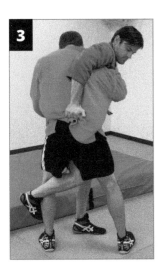
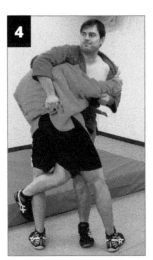
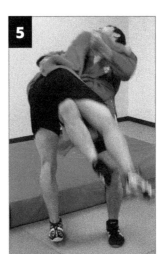

5. The attacker arches backward and rotates to his right forcefully as he uses his right foot and leg to lift his opponent up.

6. The momentum of the forceful rotation of the attacker's body to his right forces the opponent to be thrown as shown. Look at how the attacker continues to rotate to his right as he throws his opponent. Also, notice how the attacker drives off of his left foot that is planted on the mat.

7. As the attacker completes his rotation with his body, he throws his opponent onto the opponent's back.

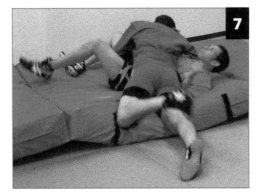

ROLLING LEG ENTWINING THROW

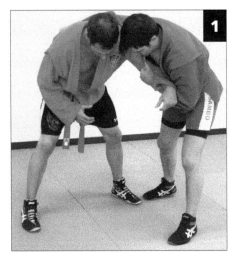

The attacker (on the right) uses a two-on-one grip with both of his hands and arms, controlling his opponent's left arm. This throw often takes place with both sambo wrestlers in a fairly low, crouched, or bent-over position.

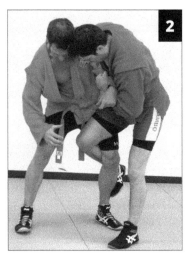

The attacker uses his right foot and leg to entwine his opponent's left leg as shown.

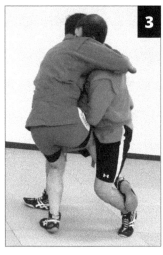

The view is changed so you have a better look at the leg entwining and close body contact. Look at how the attacker (now on the left) positions his left foot so that it is in the middle of his opponent's stance.

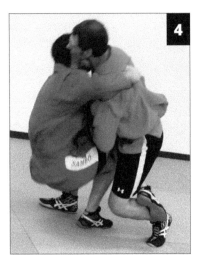

The attacker moves his body forcefully under his opponent's body and starts to roll backward as shown. As he does this, the attacker makes sure to keep control of his opponent with his right foot and leg that entwines the defender's left leg. The attacker uses his right hand and arm to pull his opponent into the throw.

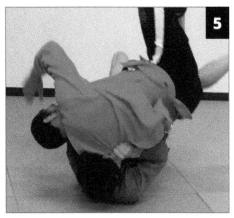

The attacker rolls backward and over his right shoulder, all the while pulling and rolling his opponent over with him.

The attacker completes his backward roll and throws his opponent.

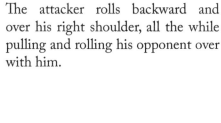

ROLLING ARM-THROUGH-LEGS THROW

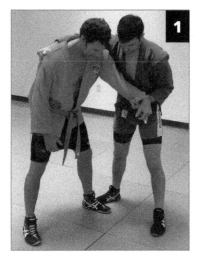

The attacker (on the right) uses his left hand to grab very low on his opponent's left sleeve. The attacker uses his right hand and arm to reach around and grip his opponent's far shoulder at the epaulette.

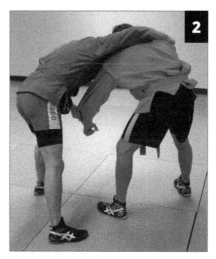

This view from the back shows how the attacker grips his opponent. Often, this throw is used when both sambo grapplers are in a low, bent-over, or crouched position.

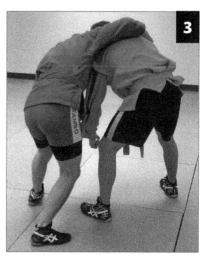

This back view shows how the attacker uses his left hand to start to shove his opponent's left arm through the opponent's legs.

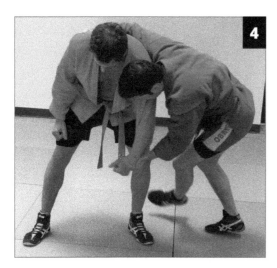

This front view shows how the attacker uses his left hand to shove his opponent's left arm through the defender's legs.

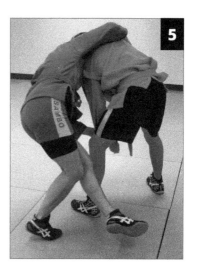

As the attacker uses his left hand and arm to shove the defender's left arm through his legs, the attacker swings or slides his left foot and leg behind the defender. Look at how the attacker's left foot (which is sliding) is on the outside of the defender's left foot and leg.

ROLLING ARM THROUGH LEGS THROW

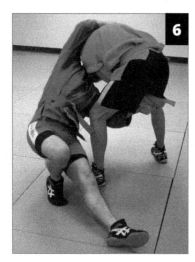

The attacker continues to use his left hand to forcefully drive the defender's left arm through the defender's legs. As he does this, the attacker continues to swing forward with his left foot and leg as shown. The attacker uses his right hand to pull the defender's head and shoulders down and forward.

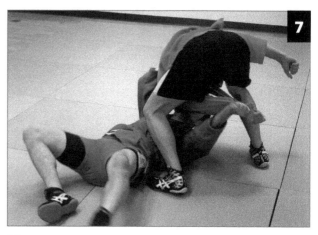

The attacker swings his body through forcefully and uses his left hand to drive the defender's left hand and arm completely through the defender's legs as shown. All the while the attacker continues to use his right hand to pull on his opponent's jacket, forcing the defender's upper body to start to roll forward.

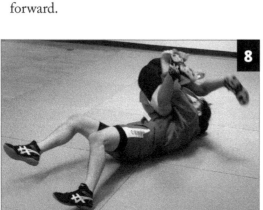

The attacker rolls his opponent over as shown.

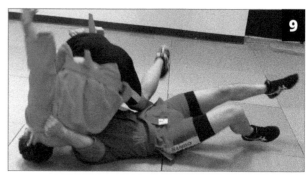

The attacker rolls his opponent and uses his right hand to steer his opponent over (above) and onto his back to complete the throw (below).

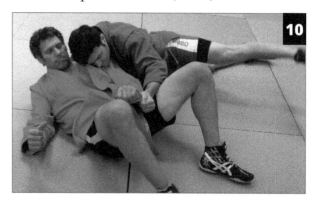

INSIDE LEG GRAB ROLLING THROW

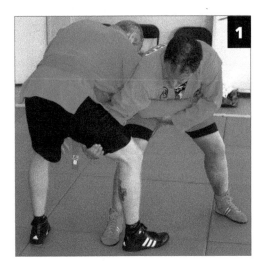

The attacker (on the right) uses his left hand to grip his opponent's right sleeve. After he does this, the attacker uses his right hand and arm to reach over his opponent's right upper arm and grab the inner thigh of the opponent's right leg. Look at how the attacker's right hand is palm up as he grabs his opponent's right leg. Notice that the attacker's right foot is placed forward and very close and inside the defender's foot.

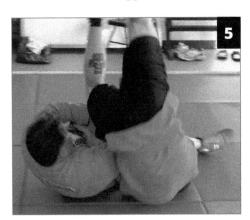

The attacker rolls to his left and rolls over his left side as shown. The momentum caused by this rolling action starts to throw the opponent.

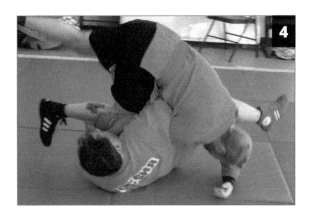

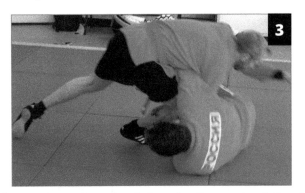

The attacker swings his left leg back and drops to the mat on his left knee. As he does this, the attacker uses both of his hands to pull his opponent forward as shown.

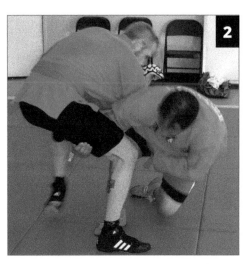

The attacker continues to roll, forcing his opponent to roll over with him.

This photo shows the throw at its peak with the attacker in complete control and the defender being thrown.

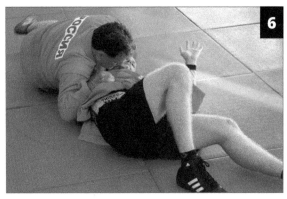

The attacker completes his roll and finishes the throw.

BODY LOCK LIFTING THROW (AS A COUNTER TO A TWO-ON-ONE GRIP)

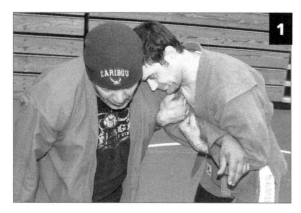

The sambo wrestler on the right controls his opponent's left arm with a two-on-one grip.

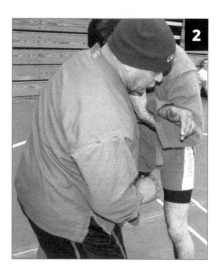

To counter this grip, the sambo wrestler on the left turns his body to his right and toward his opponent. As he does this, the grappler on the left bends his left arm and jams it firmly against his opponent's chest. Doing this nullifies the initial two-on-one grip used by his opponent.

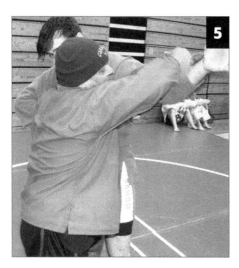

The attacker drives his right hand upward and forces his opponent to release his initial two-on-one grip.

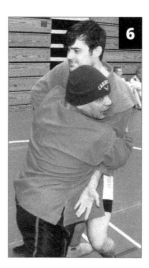

The attacker immediately uses his left hand and arm to reach around his opponent as shown.

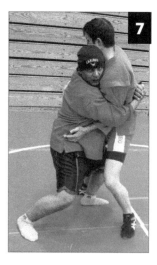

The attacker immediately grasps his hands together in a square grip and hugs his opponent. Look at the close body contact with no space between the grapplers.

BODY LOCK LIFTING THROW (AS A COUNTER TO A 2 ON 1 GRIP)

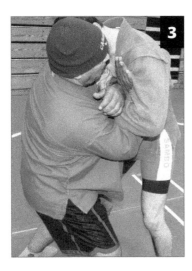

As the grappler on the left (now the attacker) continues to turn to his right and toward his opponent, he uses his right hand to slide up and between his opponent's bent left arm and body.

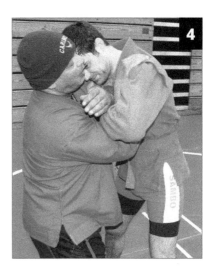

The attacker continues to slide his right hand upward as shown. Often, it is useful for the attacker to place the palm of his right hand on his opponent's left shoulder as shown.

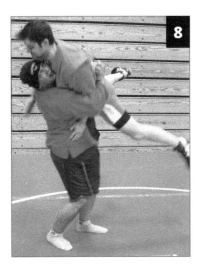

The attacker steps into his opponent and lifts him into the air as shown. The attacker drives to his right and swings his opponent so that the opponent is thrown to the attacker's right front side.

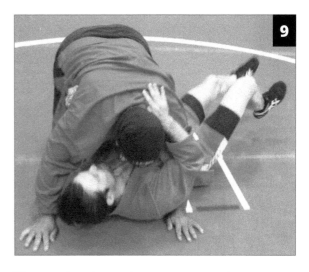

The attacker throws his opponent to the mat.

INSIDE LEG HOOK

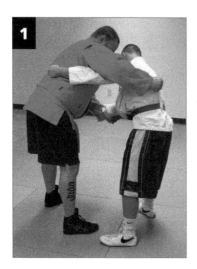

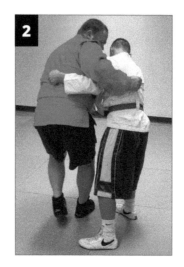

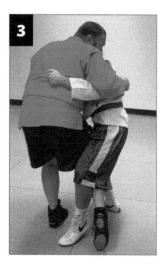

The attacker (on the left) uses his right hand and arm to reach around and grip his opponent's jacket at about the area of the shoulder blade. The attacker uses his left hand to grip his opponent's right sleeve. Look at how the attacker leads with his right foot, which is placed on the inside of his opponent's left foot.

The attacker uses his left foot to step to his left laterally as the attacker uses his right foot to step into the middle of his opponent's stance.

The attacker uses his right foot and leg to reach in and hook the inside of his opponent's left leg.

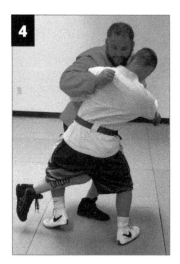

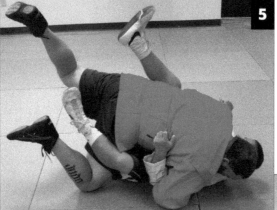

The attacker hooks his opponent's leg and throws him flat on his back.

This view shows how the attacker uses his right foot and leg to hook his opponent's left leg. Look at how the attacker drives forward with his body and into his opponent.

The attacker is now in a strong position to immediately hold his opponent with a front vertical chest hold between the legs.

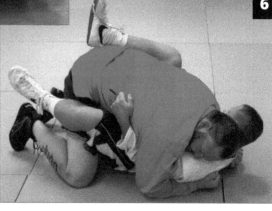

LEG PICK UP AND INSIDE LEG HOOK

This is an effective throw as well as a great transition from standing to the mat or ground to apply a leg or ankle lock.

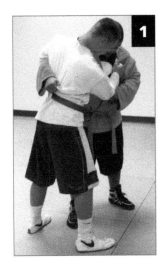

The attacker (on the right) uses his right hand to reach around his opponent's waist and grip his jacket. The attacker uses his left hand to grip his opponent's sleeve at the elbow. Look at how the attacker leads with his right foot, placed between the defender's feet and stance.

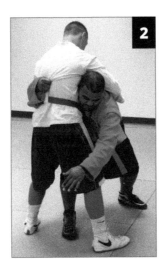

The attacker lowers the level of his body by bending his knees and ducks his head under the defender's right arm as shown. As he does this, the attacker uses his left hand to start to reach for and grab his opponent's right leg.

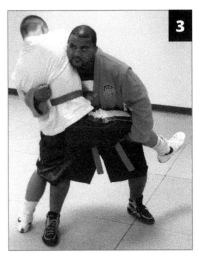

The attacker has ducked his head under the defender's right arm and uses his left hand to grab the defender's right leg at about the knee area. As he does this, the attacker uses his left hand to pull the defender's right leg up to the attacker's left hip area. Look at how close the attacker now is to his opponent.

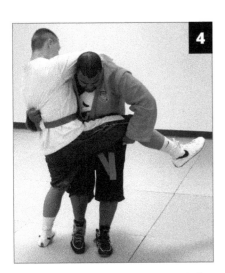

The attacker steps forward with his left foot and leg to provide stability as he continues to use his left hand to pull his opponent's right leg to the attacker's hip.

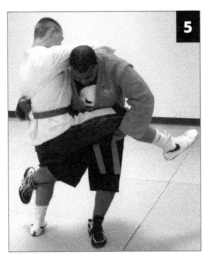

The attacker uses his right leg to hook his opponent's left leg as shown.

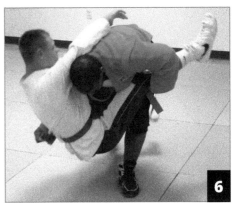

The attacker throws his opponent to the mat.

LEG PICK UP AND INSIDE LEG HOOK

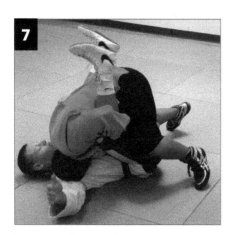

The attacker finishes the throw and can quickly transition to a hold-down if he chooses.

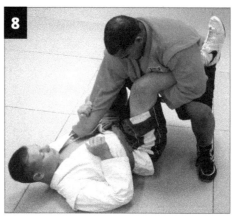

Instead of a hold-down at this time, the attacker chooses to use an ankle lock. The attacker squats low and uses his left hand to hook under his opponent's right lower leg as shown.

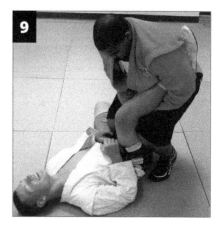

The attacker pinches his knees together and traps the defender's right leg as shown.

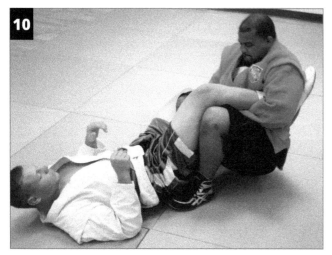

The attacker rolls backward as shown. Look at how he uses his left hand and arm to trap and control his opponent's right leg and ankle and continues to use his knees to trap his opponent's right leg. Look at how the attacker positions his feet so that they are under his opponent's buttocks. Doing this prevents the opponent from grabbing the attacker's leg or ankle as a counter move.

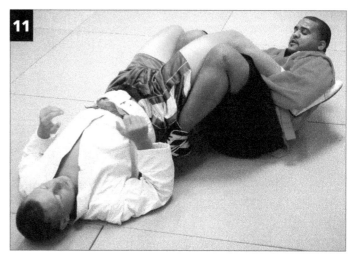

The attacker rolls back and applies the ankle lock.

REAR LEG-LIFT THROW

This throw is sometimes called the hip-shift throw. The idea is for the attacker to shift his (in this case) left hip behind his opponent's right hip and use his left leg to lift or sweep the defender's right upper leg to throw him.

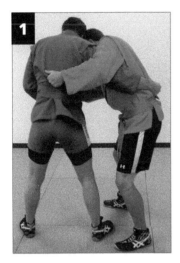

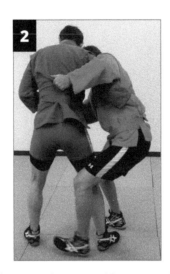

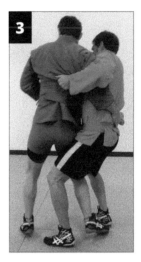

The attacker (on the right) uses his left hand to secure a strong back grip on the middle of his opponent's back. The attacker moves or shifts his left hip, foot, and leg so that they are slightly behind his opponent's right hip, leg, and foot as shown.

The attacker quickly uses the momentum of his shifting movement to start to use his left leg to sweep or lift his opponent's upper right leg (behind the leg as shown).

The attacker makes sure to use his left upper leg to lift or sweep so that it almost appears as though the attacker is using his left knee and upper leg to kick his opponent's right buttocks.

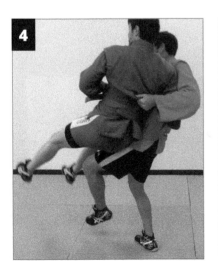

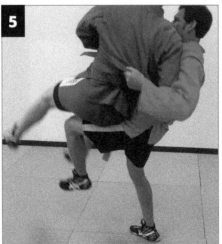

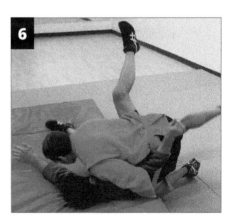

The attacker forcefully uses his left bent knee to lift or sweep his opponent as shown.

This lifting action with the left knee by the attacker produces a strong lifting and sweeping action as shown.

The attacker finishes the throw by throwing his opponent flat on his back.

SLIDING THIGH SWEEP

This is a similar throw to the rear leg-lift throw previously presented. In this throw, the attacker takes a step to build up momentum as he uses his (in this case) left thigh to sweep against his opponent's right upper leg to throw him. This throw is also very similar to the sliding foot sweep that will follow.

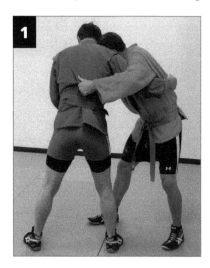

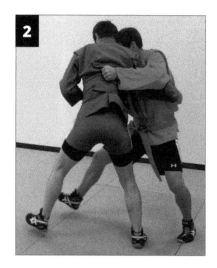

The attacker (on the right) uses his left hand to grip his opponent's jacket in the middle of his back as shown. It is important for the attacker's left hip to be in close proximity to his opponent's right hip. Notice also that the attacker's left foot is about a half step to the left of the defender's right foot and leg. This is necessary for the attacker to have the room to move and sweep his left leg against his opponent's right leg.

The attacker steps laterally to his right in a direct line. Often the defender will take a step (but usually no more than one step) to follow. The faster the attacker steps sideways, the more momentum he will build. I like to use a corny poem to help my athletes learn this throw: "The faster you go, the better you throw."

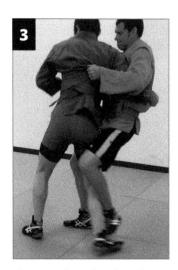

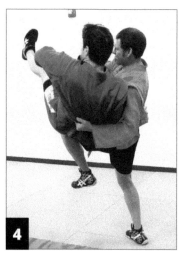

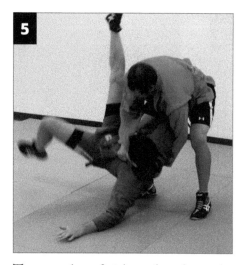

As the attacker finishes his right lateral step, he immediately bends his left leg and starts to use the inside of his left thigh to sweep against the right upper leg and buttocks of the defender as shown.

The attacker uses a strong sweeping motion with his left upper leg to sweep his opponent off of his feet.

The attacker finishes the throw by slamming his opponent to the mat as shown.

SLIDING FOOT SWEEP

This throw is almost identical to the sliding thigh sweep except that the attacker uses his (in this case) left foot to sweep his opponent's right foot so that it is knocked into the defender's left foot and sweeps him off of his feet.

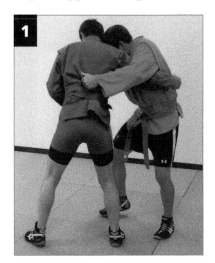

The attacker (on the right) uses his left hand to grip his opponent's jacket in the middle of his back as shown. It is important for the attacker to have close proximity between his left hip and his opponent's right hip. Notice also that the attacker's left foot is about a half step to the left of the defender's right foot and leg. This is necessary for the attacker to have the room to move and sweep his left foot against his opponent's right foot and ankle.

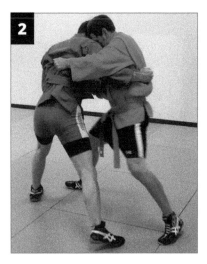

The attacker steps laterally to his right in a direct line. Often the defender will take a step (but usually no more than one step) to follow. The faster the attacker steps sideways, the more momentum he will build. I like to use the corny poem mentioned above to help my athletes learn this throw: "The faster you go, the better you throw."

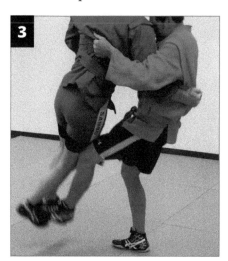

The attacker uses his left foot (actually the inside of his left foot) to sweep against the outside of the defender's right foot and ankle. This action, coming off the fast side moving action created by the attacker sweeps the defender off of his feet as shown.

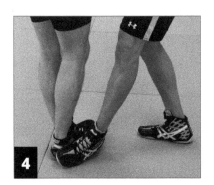

This is a close view of how the attacker uses the inside of his left foot to sweep the outside of his opponent's right foot and ankle.

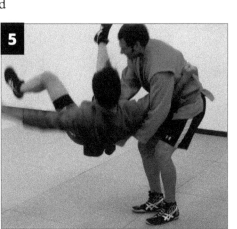

The momentum of the lateral moving bodies and the sweeping action of the attacker's left foot and leg create a strong throw as shown.

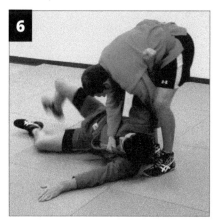

The attacker throws his opponent.

FOOT KICK THROW

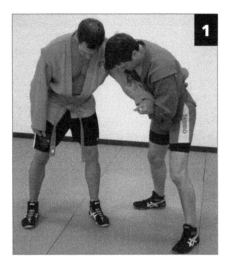

The attacker (on the right) uses a two-on-one grip on his opponent's left arm as shown. The attacker leads with his right foot so that it is positioned a bit behind and to the outside of his opponent's left foot.

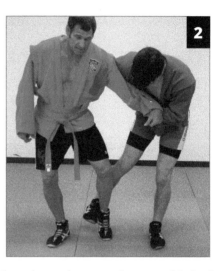

The attacker closes the space between his body and his opponent's by using his left foot to back step so that it is in line with his opponent's left foot and pointing in the same direction. As he does this, the attacker uses his right instep (or the laces of his sambo shoes) and places it behind his opponent's foot at the heel or ankle area.

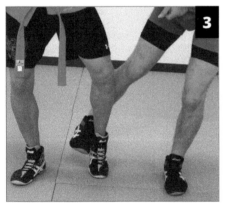

This close view shows how the attacker uses his right instep to hook behind his opponent's left ankle or foot.

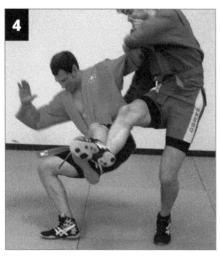

The attacker uses his right foot and leg to kick or sweep his opponent's left foot and leg forward, throwing him.

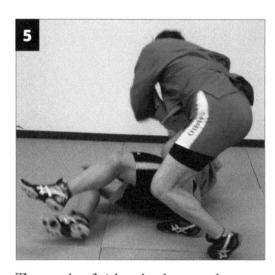

The attacker finishes the throw as shown.

INSIDE FOOT SWEEP

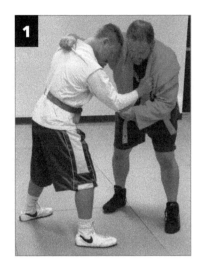

The attacker (on the right) uses his right hand to grip his opponent's collar or lapel as shown and uses his left hand to grip his opponent's sleeve at the elbow.

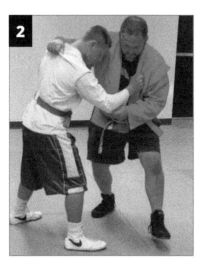

The attacker steps to his left as shown.

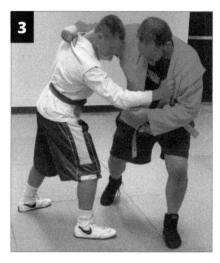

The attacker is now positioned so that his right hip is aimed directly at his opponent's middle.

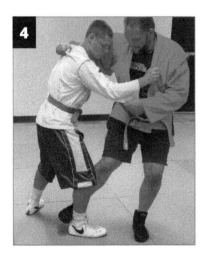

As the attacker moves to his left, he uses his left foot to sweep at the inside and rear of his opponent's right foot as shown.

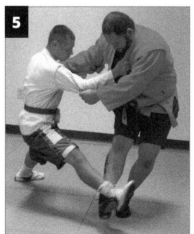

Doing this enables the attacker to both sweep and hook with his right foot and leg. As he does this, the attacker uses his hands and arms to push his opponent down, throwing his opponent as shown.

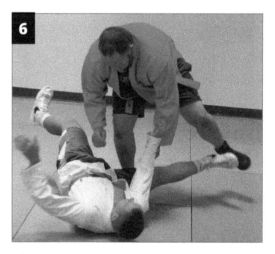

The attacker completes the throw, resulting in a total victory.

LEG SCISSORS THROW

This is a good throw by itself but it is also a good way to transition from a standing position to a straight leg or ankle lock on the mat or ground.

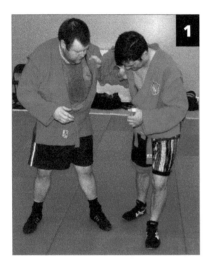

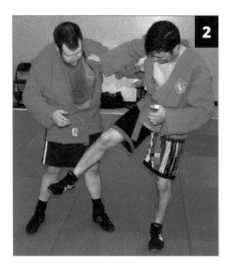

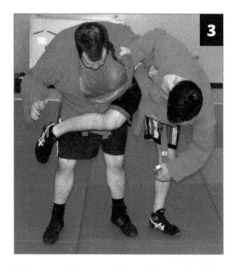

The attacker uses his right hand to grip onto his opponent's left lapel. The attacker is positioned so that he is standing at his opponent's left side as shown.

The attacker uses his right foot and leg to reach across his opponent as shown.

The attacker positions his right leg so that his knee is bent downward and his right foot is hooked and anchored on his opponent's right hip.

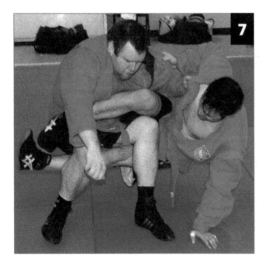

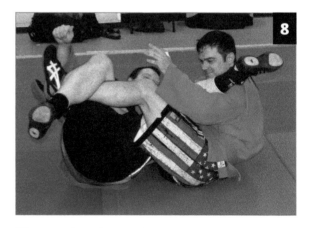

The attacker scissors his legs so that they throw his opponent back as shown.

The attacker throws his opponent on his back and the attacker lands on his buttocks so he can transition more effectively into a leglock. Look at how the attacker immediately uses his left hand to start to hook his opponent's left lower leg. Look at how the attacker uses his feet and legs to control his opponent's feet and legs after the throw is completed.

LEG SCISSORS THROW

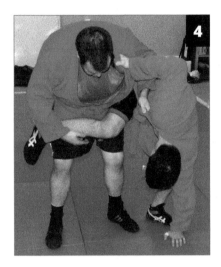

The attacker places his left hand on the mat for stability as he bends over. The attacker's left foot is still placed on the mat directly to the side of the defender's left foot.

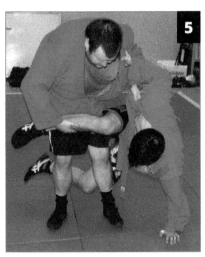

The attacker swings his left leg behind his opponent's legs as shown.

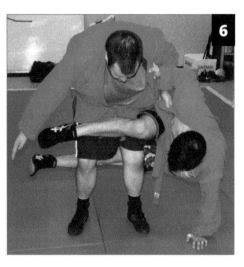

The attacker's left leg is positioned directly behind his opponent's knees, and the attacker's right leg is positioned in front of his opponent's upper legs and hips.

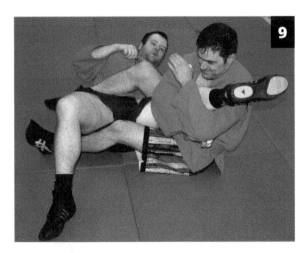

The attacker uses both hands to trap and hug the defender's left leg to the attacker's chest and body as shown.

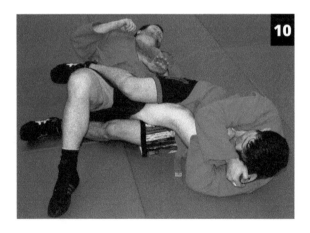

The attacker rolls to his left side as he drives his hips forward to create a knee bar and secures the straight knee lock or knee bar.

INNER THIGH THROW (HIP STYLE)

The attacker uses a strong hip placement combined with a strong leg sweep (between his opponent's legs) to create a powerful throwing attack. The inner-thigh throw, in its many variations, is a popular and effective throw in sambo as well as judo.

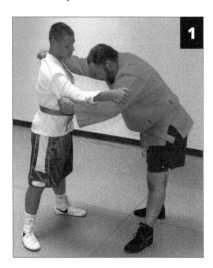

The attacker (on the right) uses his right hand to grip onto his opponent's collar and uses his left hand to grip his opponent's right sleeve at the elbow as shown.

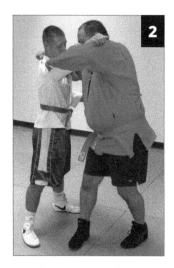

The attacker uses his right foot to step across his opponent's body and uses his left foot to back step as shown. As he does this, the attacker uses his left hand to pull up and forward on his opponent's sleeve.

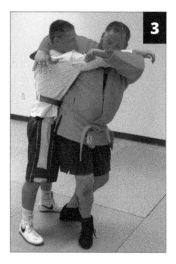

The attacker fits into the throw as shown, continuing to use his left hand to pull strongly on his opponent's sleeve. Look at how the attacker's hips are securely positioned in front of his opponent.

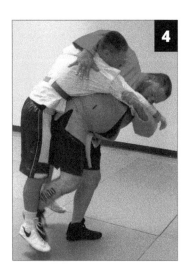

The attacker continues to pull with his left hand on his opponent's left sleeve as he starts to use his right leg to sweep up between his opponent's legs. Look at how the defender is being thrown over the attacker's right hip.

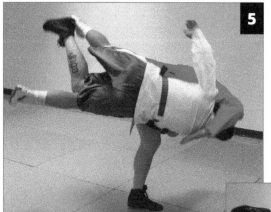

The attacker continues to use his right foot and leg to sweep between his opponent's legs as shown. Doing this throws the defender.

The attacker continues his throwing action and finishes the throw.

INNER THIGH THROW (LEG STYLE)

In this application of the inner thigh throw, the attacker emphasizes a spinning back step and a strong leg sweep and does not place as much emphasis on throwing his opponent over his hip as in the previous application of the inner-thigh throw. This application that places emphasis on the attacker's leg is often used when the defender is bent over or in a low crouched position as shown

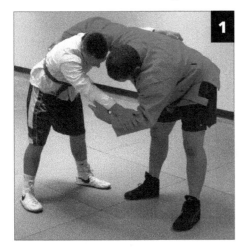

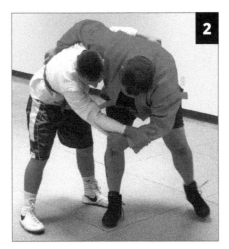

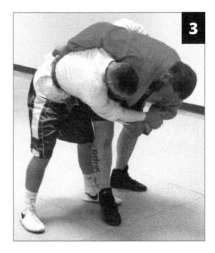

The attacker and defender are bent over with their hips far apart from each other. The attacker uses his right hand and arm to reach over his opponent's left shoulder and grip the defender's jacket or belt. The attacker uses his left hand to grip low on the defender's right sleeve. The attacker leads with his right foot.

The attacker positions his right foot so that it is on the inside of the defender's left foot as shown. As he does this, the attacker starts to spin and back step with his left foot.

The attacker uses his left foot to back step and places his left foot on the outside of his opponent's left foot. As he does this, the attacker prepares to use his right foot to sweep the inside of the defender's left leg.

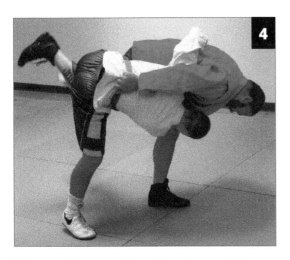

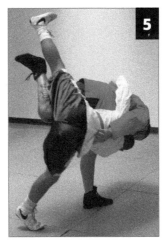

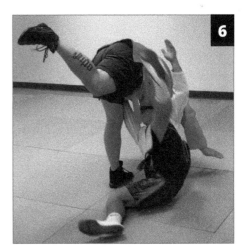

The attacker uses his right foot and leg to sweep on the inside of the defender's left leg.

The attacker continues to use his right foot and leg to sweep on the inside of his opponent's left leg and throws him.

The attacker finishes the throw.

ROLLING INNER THIGH THROW (WITH ARM OVERHOOK)

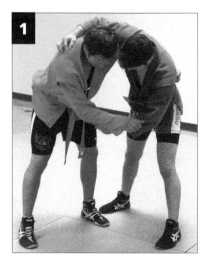

The attacker (right) uses his left hand to grip low on his opponent's right sleeve. Note how he is leading with his right foot.

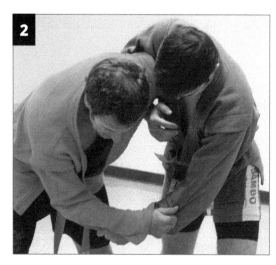

The attacker quickly uses his right hand and arm to hook over his opponent's left shoulder and upper arm as shown.

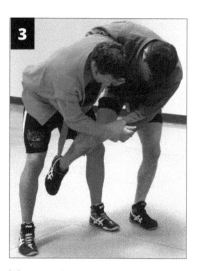

The attacker uses his right foot and leg to start to sweep on the inside of his opponent's left upper leg.

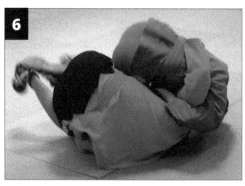

The opponent rolls over his right shoulder. Doing this forces his opponent to roll over as well.

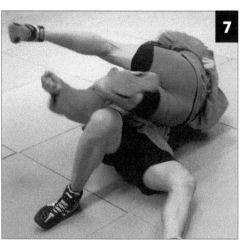

The attacker completes his roll, throwing his opponent.

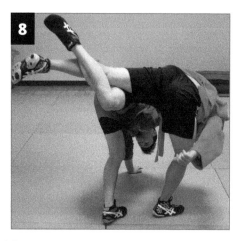

This view from the back side of the throw shows how the attacker uses his right leg to sweep the inside of his opponent's left leg. Look at how the attacker uses his left hand to post on the mat for stability as he starts his rolling action into the throw.

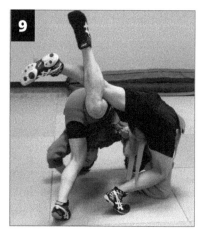

This photo shows the back view of how the attacker continues his rolling action and controls his opponent's leg through the entire throwing action.

ROLLING INNER THIGH THROW (WITH ARM OVERHOOK)

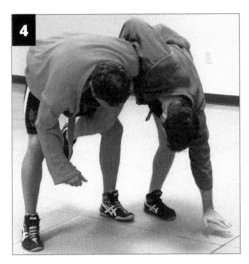

The attacker places his left hand on the mat as he continues with the attack. Look at how the attacker's head is driving forward.

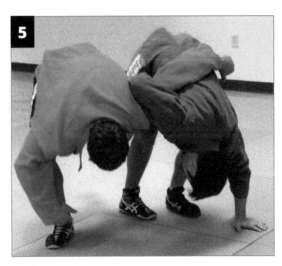

The attacker has his left hand posted on the mat as he starts to roll forward and continues to sweep with his right foot and leg on his opponent's left leg.

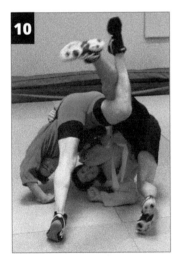

Here is the throw at its peak.

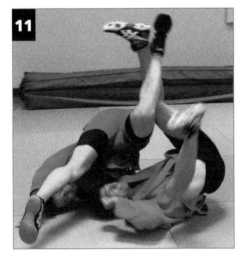

The attacker continues his rolling action over his right shoulder and throws his opponent as shown.

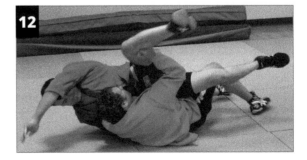

The attacker completes the throw.

INNER THIGH THROW TO ANKLE PICK

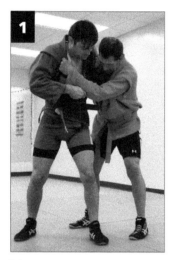

The attacker (on the left) initiates an inner-thigh throw by using his right hand to grip fairly low on his opponent's left sleeve.

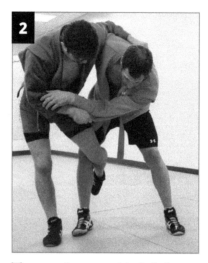

The attacker uses his left leg to attack the inside of his opponent's right leg as shown. Look at how the attacker uses his left hand to grip at his opponent's collar or upper back on the jacket.

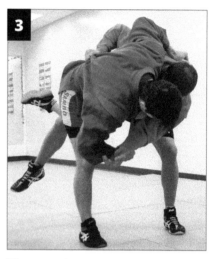

The attacker attempts to throw his opponent with the inner-thigh throw but the defender starts to hop to his left to avoid the attack.

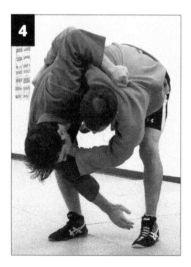

As the defender hops to his left to avoid the throw, the attacker uses his right hand to reach out to grab his opponent's left ankle as shown.

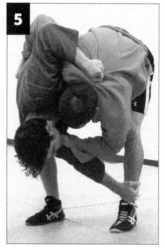

The attacker uses his right hand to grab his opponent's left ankle.

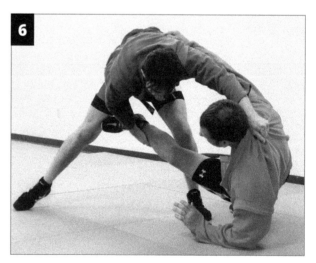

The attacker uses his right hand to grab and pull his opponent's left ankle. Doing this throws the opponent as shown.

ROLLING LEG-LIFT THROW

There are many variations of this excellent throw. This application is a popular one and has a high rate of success.

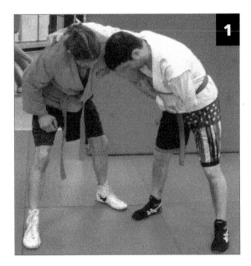

The attacker (on the right) uses his left hand to grip his opponent's left arm as shown and uses his right hand and arm to reach over his opponent's left upper arm and shoulder to grip the jacket at the opponent's upper-back area. The attacker is crouched forward with his head wedged in his opponent's left-shoulder area.

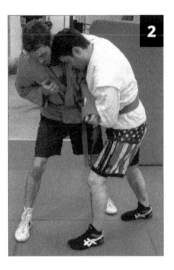

The attacker uses his right foot and leg to jam on the inside of the defender's right upper thigh. Look at how the attacker uses his right foot to hook and control his opponent's right knee.

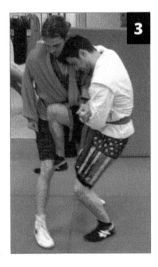

The attacker closes the space between the bodies by using his left foot to step directly across and in front of the defender as shown.

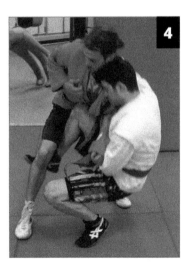

The attacker starts to squat and roll backward as shown.

ROLLING LEG LIFT THROW

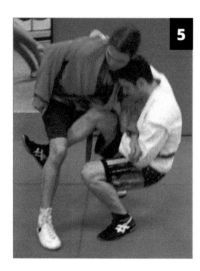

This photo shows how the attacker controls his opponent as the attacker continues to roll backward.

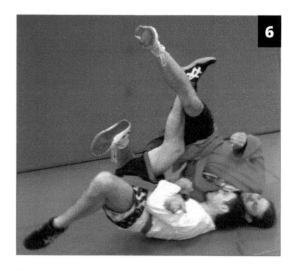

The attacker rolls onto his back and uses his right foot and leg to lift and throw his opponent.

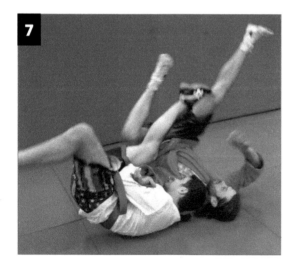

The momentum of the attacker's rolling action continues and the attacker rolls over his right shoulder as he throws his opponent.

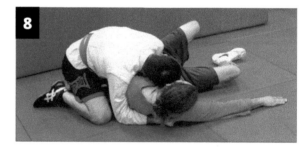

The attacker rolls over his right shoulder and onto his opponent to transition immediately into a hold-down.

ROLLING ANKLE PICK TO STRAIGHT KNEE LOCK

This is an effective and often-used throwing attack that is also a transition to a straight leglock.

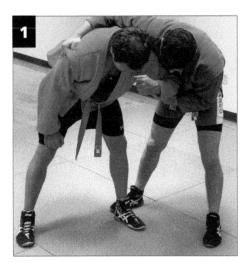

The attacker (on the right) uses his left hand to grip and control his opponent's left arm as the attacker uses his right hand to grip on his opponent's jacket at the upper-back area as shown. The attacker leads with his right foot and his left foot is placed out and in front of his opponent's left foot.

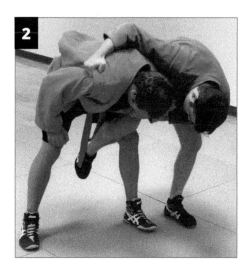

The attacker uses his right foot and leg to sweep the inside of his opponent's left leg.

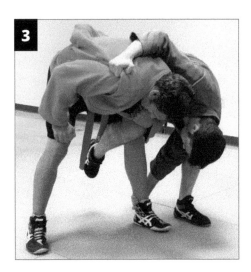

The attacker actually props his right foot and leg on the inside of his opponent's left inner thigh to control the defender's movement through the entire rolling action and after the throw is completed. As he does this, the attacker uses his left hand to reach down and grab the outside of his opponent's left ankle as shown. Look at how the attacker is starting his forward roll at this point.

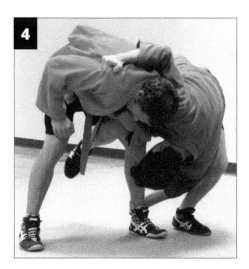

The attacker rolls over his left shoulder as shown. Look at how the attacker uses his right hand to continue to grip and pull his opponent forward and into the action of the rolling throw.

ROLLING ANKLE PICK TO STRAIGHT KNEE LOCK

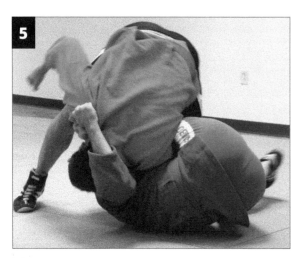

The attacker continues to roll over his left shoulder and rolls his opponent over with him.

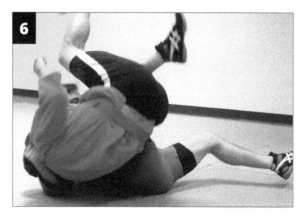

The attacker continues to roll and throws his opponent.

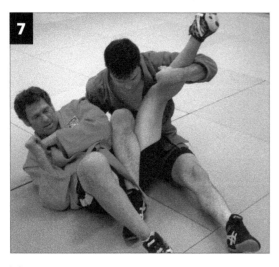

The attacker completes his roll and throws his opponent. As he does this, the attacker rolls up and onto his buttocks and continues to use his left hand to grip and control his opponent's left lower leg as shown. Look at how the attacker's right leg is positioned over his opponent's left upper leg for control.

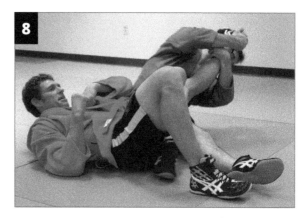

The attacker uses both hands to grab and hook his opponent's extended (and vulnerable) left leg close to the defender's left foot and ankle as shown. At this point, the attacker starts to roll to his left side.

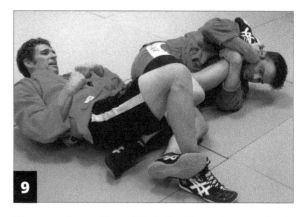

The attacker rolls to his left side as he uses both hands and arms to trap and hug his opponent's extended left leg to his torso. The attacker arches his hips and bars his opponent's straight knee.

INSIDE LEG GRAB ROLLING THROW

This is both a throw and a transition to get an opponent onto the mat to apply a straight leglock. The leglock is a good one, but if the attacker is unable to secure the leglock at the end of the move, the throw will score points.

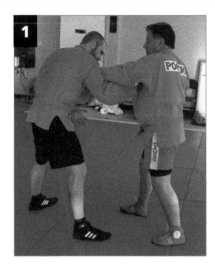

The attacker (on the right) uses his left hand to grip and control his opponent's right lapel as shown.

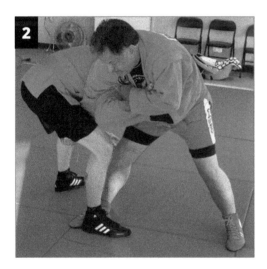

The attacker steps forward with his right foot so that it is placed on the inside of his opponent's right foot as shown. The attacker uses his right arm and hand to reach over his opponent's right upper arm (at about the side of the deltoid). As he does this, the attacker uses his right hand to hook and grab (palm up) on the inside of his opponent's right upper leg.

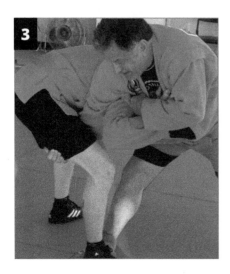

This close view shows how the attacker uses his right hand and arm to reach over his opponent's right upper arm and grab on the inside of his opponent's right upper leg. The attacker continues to uses his left hand to grip his opponent's jacket at the right lapel.

INSIDE LEG GRAB ROLLING THROW

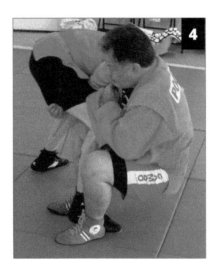

The attacker immediately steps forward with his left foot so that it is placed on the outside of his opponent's right foot as shown. The attacker squats low and drives his hips forward so that he starts to roll backward. Look at how the attacker continues to use his right hand to grab and control his opponent's right upper leg. Look at how the attacker has now changed his grip with his left hand and uses his left hand to grip his opponent's right sleeve.

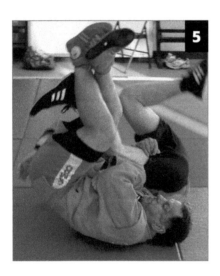

The attacker rolls backward as shown. As he does this, the attacker crosses his ankles together. Doing this traps and controls his opponent's right leg.

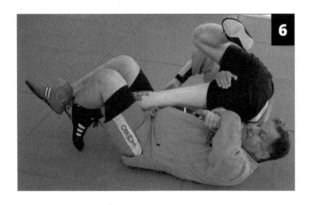

The attacker rolls backward and onto his back. As he rolls onto his back, the attacker arches his body, trapping his opponent's right leg and straightening it as shown. The attacker uses both of his hands to control his opponent as shown. Doing this stretches the opponent's right leg and bars it at the knee joint, creating pain. If the opponent escapes the straight knee bar, the attacker can continue to roll backward and onto the defender, scoring points for the throw.

ANKLE LIFT THROW

This is a good example of how a throw in sambo can be started from any position.

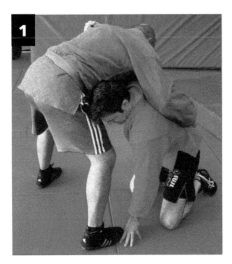

The attacker (on the right) is kneeling and is being dominated by his standing opponent. Look at how the attacker uses his right hand to grip high on his opponent's left lapel.

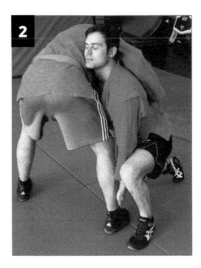

The attacker uses his left hand to grab (palm up) his opponent's right ankle. As he does this, the attacker positions his head up and under his opponent's right shoulder as shown. The attacker places his left foot on the mat as shown for stability and support.

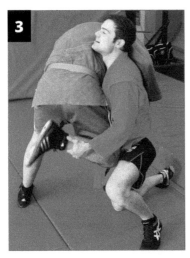

The attacker uses his left hand and arm to lift his opponent's right ankle, causing the defender's right knee to bend as shown. The attacker starts to stand up.

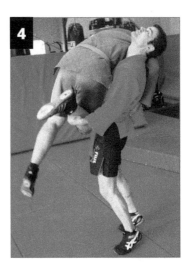

The attacker stands and lifts his opponent up as shown. Look at how the attacker arches his back and drives his hips forward to help lift his opponent up and off the mat.

ANKLE LIFT THROW

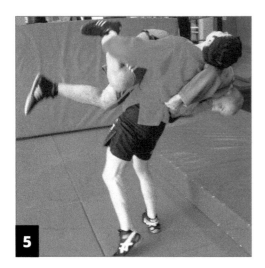

The attacker rotates to his right as he lifts and throws his opponent. The attacker continues to use his right hand that is gripping his opponent's left lapel to pull, and the attacker uses his left hand that is grabbing the defender's right ankle to continue to lift. Look at how the attacker "steers" with his head as he rotates and throws his opponent.

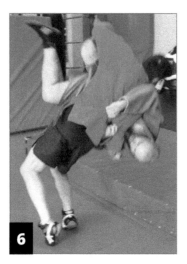

The attacker continues to rotate and turn to his right and throws his opponent as shown.

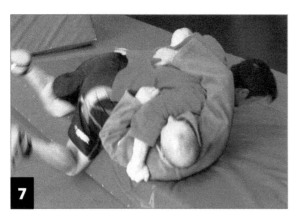

The attacker finishes the throw with a hard landing for the defender, who ends up flat on his back.

LEG PICK UP TIGHTWAIST AND THIGH SWEEP THROW

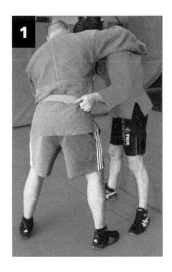

The attacker (on the right) is being dominated by his opponent's strong right-hand back grip as shown.

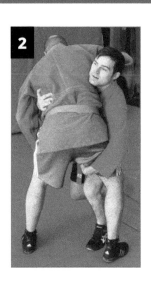

The attacker ducks his head under his opponent's right armpit and shoulder. As he does this, he uses his right hand to grab firmly around his opponent's waist and his left hand and arm to reach around his opponent's right upper leg and grab the inner thigh. Look at how the attacker uses his left foot to step forward for stability.

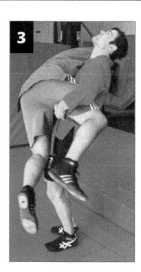

The attacker uses his left hand and arm to lift his opponent up and into the air. Look at how the attacker arches back and drives his hips forward. The attacker starts to rotate his body and arch and lean to his right.

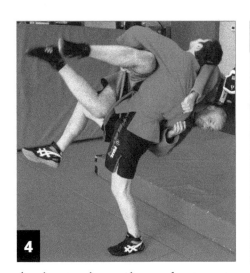

As the attacker arches and rotates to his right, he uses his right bent leg to sweep his opponent's left upper leg and thigh. As he does this, the attacker rotates and drives hard to his right. Doing this, the attacker lifts, sweeps, and rotates his opponent over the attacker's body as shown.

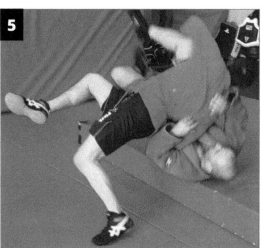

The attacker continues to rotate to his right, throwing his opponent.

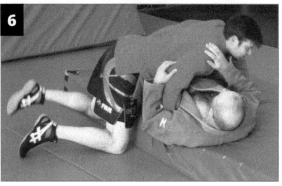

The attacker throws his opponent flat on his back and can transition immediately into a hold-down.

TIGHTWAIST REAR SPLIT THROW

This is an effective technique where the attacker shifts or slides his body behind his opponent and throws him. There are many variations of this throw, but this sequence of throws is a common application.

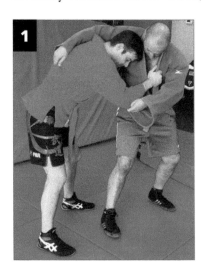

The attacker (on the left) is leading with his left hip and his opponent is leading with his right hip. The opponent uses his right hand and arm to use a back grip on the attacker.

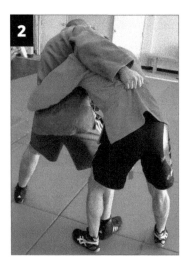

This photo from the back side shows how the attacker uses his left hand and arm to reach around his opponent's waist and grab his opponent's left hip or belt at the left hip area. Doing this creates a "tightwaist" and gives the attacker strong control of his opponent's hips.

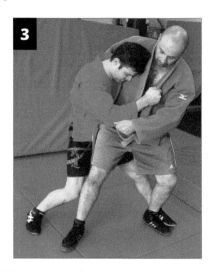

The attacker (now on the left) slides or shifts his body to his left and behind his opponent. As he does this, the attacker slides his left foot behind his opponent's left foot and leg as shown. Look at how the attacker uses his head to drive into his opponent's right shoulder area.

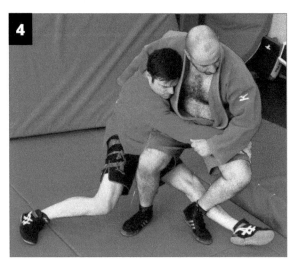

The attacker continues to shift to his left and behind his opponent, and as he does this, he uses his left foot and leg to sweep his opponent's left leg. Look at how the attacker uses his right hand and arm to grab and control his opponent's left hip or upper leg. The attacker's momentum drives his opponent down, throwing him.

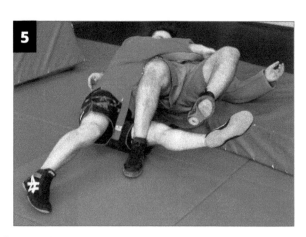

The attacker continues to sweep with his left foot and leg as he drives his opponent to the mat onto his back. The attacker makes sure to turn his body to his left as he throws his opponent so that the attacker's chest is turned down. Doing this ensures that the attacker lands chest to chest with his opponent and that the score will be awarded to the attacker.

ANKLE-PICK THROW

Ankle picks serve two effective purposes. First, ankle picks are good throws that score points. Second, ankle picks are excellent transition moves to ankle locks. I like to coach my athletes to do what we call "ankle to ankle" throws. In other words, follow up an ankle-pick throw with a fast ankle lock. This series of photos shows this.

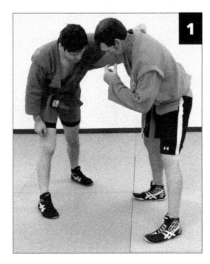

The attacker (on the left) uses his left hand to grab high on his opponent's right lapel.

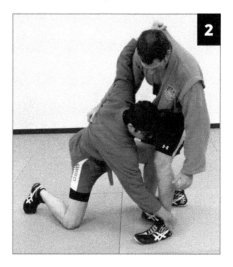

The attacker lowers his level by stepping in deeply with his left foot as shown. As he does this, he uses his right hand to reach down and grab (pick) his opponent's left ankle. Look at how the attacker uses his left arm to continue to grip his opponent's right lapel high near the defender's right shoulder. Doing this creates a "high and low" controlling effect. Look at how the attacker's left hand is "high" and his right hand is "low," controlling his opponent's upper body and lower body as the attacker drives forward into the throw.

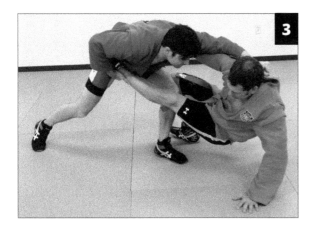

The attacker uses his right hand to pick his opponent's left ankle and uses his left hand to drive his opponent down as shown.

ANKLE PICK THROW

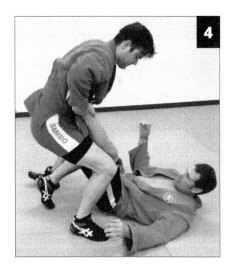

The attacker throws his opponent to the mat and continues to drive forward. As he does this, the attacker uses his right hand to move his opponent's left ankle under the attacker's right armpit area. Look at how the attacker uses his right foot to step forward so that his right foot is near his opponent's left hip. The attacker steps forward with his left foot so that it will be placed between his opponent's legs.

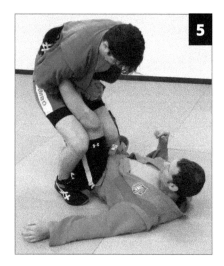

The attacker steps forward so that his feet and legs trap his opponent's left extended leg as shown. As he does this, the attacker squeezes his legs and knees together, trapping his opponent's left leg. The attacker uses his right hand and arm to trap his opponent's ankle in the attacker's armpit and forms a square grip with his hands to start a straight ankle lock.

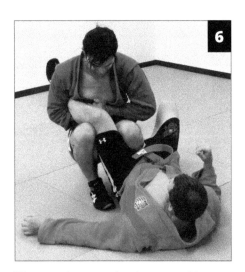

The attacker uses his knees and legs to trap and control his opponent's left leg as the attacker rolls back to apply the ankle lock.

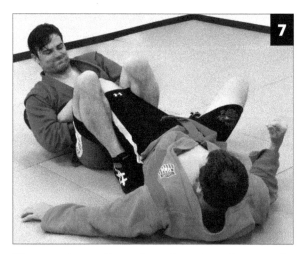

The attacker rolls back and applies the straight ankle lock to get the tap out.

There a just a few things about throwing techniques to discuss before we go on to the next chapter.

A major feature of the throwing techniques used in sambo is that, in as many cases as possible, the attacker terminates his throw so that he can immediately transition to a submission technique to finish off his opponent. A sambo wrestler doesn't view a throw as a single item or entity. The match may end with a total victory from a throw, but in most cases, it doesn't. The concept of sambo is to integrate the throwing techniques directly with the submission and holding techniques. In this sense, a sambo wrestler looks at a throw as part of the "total package." The rules of the sport require (and emphasize) that the sambo wrestler throwing his opponent exhibit control. Controlling the opponent's movement from the throw's inception to its finish is fundamentally important. This is a subtle but major difference between sambo's philosophy (and ultimately, its practical application) in regard to throwing techniques and that of judo.

Learning and developing throwing techniques is not an easy task. It takes a lot of time, patience, and intelligent practice. There are no shortcuts in the development and mastery of throwing techniques. If you want to be successful at sambo, get used to the idea that every sambo match starts with both wrestlers standing up facing each other, and it takes two people to make a throw. In a very real sense, throws are submission techniques, just like armlocks and leglocks. If you throw an opponent with control and force, you will take a lot of the fight out of him and may even score a total victory. Even if your preference is for groundfighting (as mine is), it is still vital that you develop your ability at throwing techniques to a high level of functional skill.

The possibilities for throwing techniques are limited only by what the human mind can conceive and the ways the human body can move. We've touched on a few of those possibilities as we've considered a wide variety of technical skills that are used by sambo wrestlers at all levels of experience and weight class, whether they are male or female, and in a variety of situations. Take what's been presented here, make it work for you, and continue to learn, explore, and become skilled in as many throwing techniques as possible. But, above all, take Maurice Allan's wise advice and put it into practice: "Make the technique work for you." Now, let's turn our attention to lower-body submissions: the ankle, leg, and hip locks of sambo.

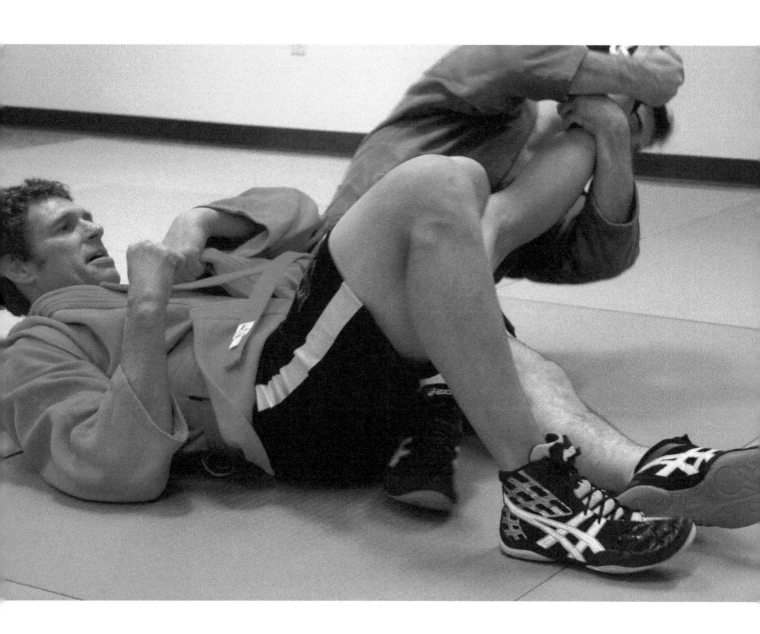

Chapter Three: The Leglocks, Ankle Locks and Hip Locks of Sambo

"Nobody's leg should be safe."

LOWER BODY SUBMISSIONS (ANKLE, LEG, AND HIP LOCKS)

A defining feature of sambo is its aggressive, innovative, and effective use of lower body submissions. There are few, if any, other grappling or fighting sports that have such a sophisticated approach to leg, ankle, and hip locks. This section of the book will focus on as many lower body submissions as possible, all with a common theme of functional efficiency.

There are three joints that are targeted in sambo's lower body submissions. They are (1) the ankle, (2) the knee, and (3) the hip. Let's analyze the basic concepts of attacking these three target joints.

TECHNICAL TIP: Ankle locks are the most popular of all lower body submissions. An opponent's foot or ankle is easy prey as a follow-up or transition from a throw or takedown.

ANKLE LOCKS

Ankle joint locks are common and effective in sambo. While all the leg and hip locks used in sambo competition are good, ankle locks often prove to be the workhorse of all lower body submission techniques and have a high rate of success in all levels of competition. It seems as though the foot (the ankle) is an inviting target, just dangling on the end of an opponent's leg waiting to be attacked. And, from a defensive point of view, it seems as though it's more difficult for most people to defend their legs and, most especially, defend their ankles from being attacked.

It's important to point out that the rules of sambo do not permit the ankle joint to be twisted; all locks must be applied in a straight line with the leg. In other words, heel hooks and toeholds are not permitted in sambo. This is done for the safety of the athletes. It's a good rule but just about every sambo wrestler and coach I know also practice heel hooks and toeholds, including me. For this reason, some of these ankle joint locks will be included but for the most part, ankle locks applied in a straight line with the leg will be emphasized.

Often, the ankle joint that is being attacked is stretched beyond its normal range of motion, and this causes pain. Also, many ankle locks work because the attacker uses the sharp part of his forearm (the "blade" of his forearm) to trap his opponent's ankle and roll it so that the Achilles' tendon is strained.

Ankle Lock Using Square Grip

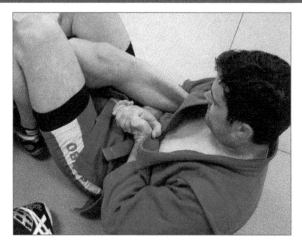

This photo shows the basic application of the ankle lock using a square grip. The attacker grasps his hands together forming a "square." There are other ways the attacker can grip or grasp his hands together to trap and apply pressure to the defender's ankle, but the square grip can be applied quickly and effectively, and as a result is often used.

Ankle Lock Using Figure-Four Grip

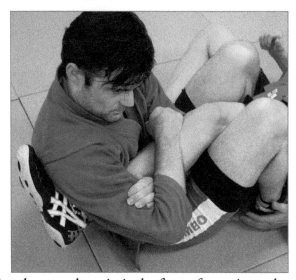

Another popular grip is the figure-four grip as shown in this photo. There are several variations, and for more information on the many grips that can be used, you can refer to my book *Tap Out Textbook* published by Turtle Press.

IMPORTANT POINTS ABOUT ANKLE LOCKS

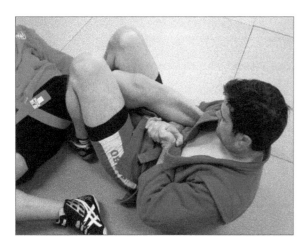

1. Trap Opponent's Leg with Your Knees

The attacker (right) pinches his knees together and uses his legs to trap and control his opponent's left leg. Doing this allows the attacker to isolate and control his opponent's leg, giving the attacker more time to apply the ankle lock.

2. Attacker Jams or Tucks His Feet under His Opponent's Hip or Buttocks

The attacker jams or tucks his feet under his opponent's hips or buttocks to prevent the opponent from grabbing the attacker's foot, ankle, or leg as a counter attack. The most common way to counter an ankle lock is with an ankle lock. If the attacker tucks his feet under his opponent's hips or buttocks, he lessens the chance that his opponent will grab his ankle and apply an ankle lock or leglock of his own.

Attacker Uses Foot to Control Opponent

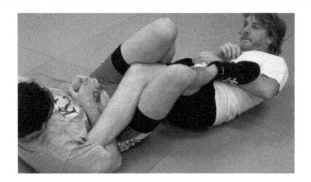

Sometimes, the attacker (shown on left) will use one or both feet to push, kick, or manipulate his opponent's hands, arms, legs, hips, or any other part of the body. However, when doing this, make sure not to allow your opponent to grab your foot or ankle and attack it.

Foot Placement for Ankle Locks

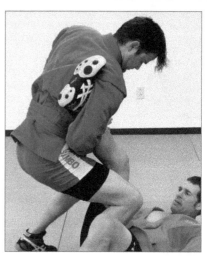

For maximum control and effect, the attacker (on the left) positions his opponent's foot so that the laces of the defender's shoes (the defender's instep) are placed on the back of the attacker's shoulder as shown. Doing this gives the attacker a lot of control and also isolates the defender's foot, putting the defender's ankle in direct line to be attacked.

While the straight ankle lock is the only form of ankle or foot lock allowed in the sport of sambo, there are other ankle and foot locks that are effective and commonly used in other fighting sports by sambo grapplers. Presented here are two of them.

Basic Heel Hook

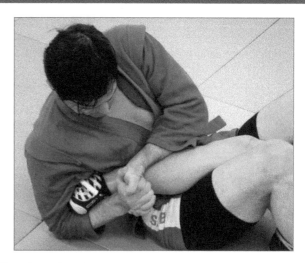

The heel hook is currently not allowed in sambo competition, but this move is nonetheless practiced by most every sambo grappler on the planet.

Basic Toehold

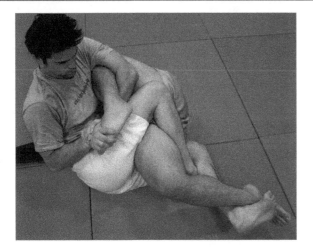

Like the heel hook, the rules of sport sambo do not allow toeholds as this move causes the ankle joint to be twisted, inflicting pain. However, the toehold is a useful ankle lock and should be studied and practiced.

DEFENSE AGAINST ANKLE AND LEGLOCKS

The best defense against ankle and leglocks is for the defender to always be aware of where his feet are and continually use his feet and legs in the same way he uses his hands and arms. The following photo shows a popular and effective defense against an ankle lock.

BASIC DEFENSE AGAINST THE STRAIGHT ANKLE LOCK

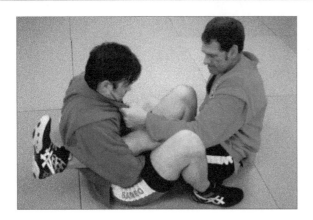

The defender (right in photo) uses one or both hands to grab and pull on his opponent's jacket at the lapels. As he does this, the defender jams his left foot and leg

(the leg the attacker is attacking) forward (leading with his heel as shown) so that the attacker no longer has the defender's foot placed in his armpit area. This is a common (and effective) defense against ankle locks.

KNEE LOCKS

Like ankle locks, knee locks are also used commonly in sambo. And, just like ankle locks, the rules of sambo do not permit the knee joint to be twisted or cranked. When applying a knee lock, the lower leg and upper leg must be aligned (even when applying bent knee locks). Again, this is a good rule for the safety of the athletes, and this rule has saved many sambo wrestlers from ACL tears and other ligament and cartilage injuries.

Fundamentally, there are two types of knee locks. They are (1) straight knee locks or "knee bars" where the knee is stretched or straightened and levered or "barred" over part of the attacker's body (or appendage) or over part of the defender's body or appendage and (2) bent knee locks where the attacker bends the defender's knee and applies pressure. A subset of the bent knee lock is a compression lock. A compression lock occurs when the attacker bends the knee and jams or places an appendage on the inside of the bent joint and applies pressure.

Straight Leg Lock (Knee Bar)

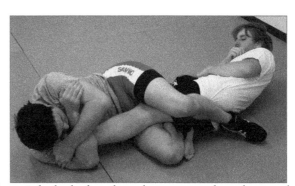

A straight leglock or knee bar occurs when the attacker traps and stretches his opponent's leg and levers it over his pubic bone (that serves as the fulcrum). Often called a "knee bar" because the defender's knee is "barred" across the attacker's pubic bone and pressure is applied.

Bent Knee Lock

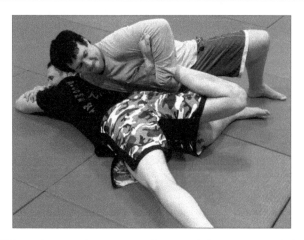

When the attacker traps and controls his opponent's leg and forces it to bend at the knee, a bent knee lock takes place.

Compression Bent Knee Lock

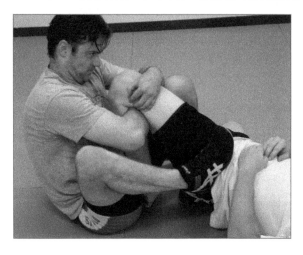

Often, what are called "compression" leg or knee locks take place when the attacker uses his hand, arm, foot, or leg to jam or wedge behind his opponent's bent knee. Often, the best bent knee locks are compression locks. This photo shows how the attacker's right arm is wedged behind his opponent's left knee as pressure is applied.

HIP LOCKS

From my personal experience through the years, hip locks have been allowed and then not allowed in the rules of sambo, but as of this writing, hiplocks are allowed in the rules of competitive sambo. Basically, a hip lock occurs when the hip or upper leg is abducted, externally or internally rotated, or stretched outside of its normal range of motion. Hip locks often also compromise the lower back in many situations so these submission techniques can be painful and, when applied, painful in a hurry!

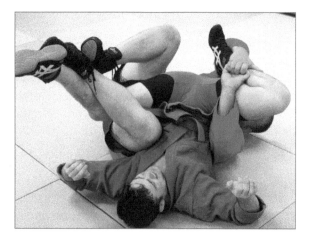

TECHNICAL TIP: Often, a lower body submission hurts everything, not only the joint being attacked. Also, most ankle, leg, and hip locks combine more than one element of application. A good example is that most bent knee locks are used in conjunction with compression locks.

CONTROL THE POSITION AND GET THE SUBMISSION

Submission techniques don't just happen by luck. You have to make the submission technique happen and put your opponent into a position so that it will happen with a high rate of success. A common approach to ankle, leg, or hip locks (as well as armlocks, for that matter) is that the attacker must control his opponent before he can apply the submission technique. To control an opponent, it is vital that the attacker control the movement of his opponent's body and then focus in on controlling the specific appendage or body part that will be attacked.

This is true in both lower body submissions as well as upper body submissions.

First, Control the Opponent's Position and Movement

Limit your opponent's movement. Using a "ride," hold-down, or any method to limit and control how your opponent moves is necessary.

This photo shows one way to control an opponent's movement. The attacker is using a hip hold-down to immobilize his opponent and control him.

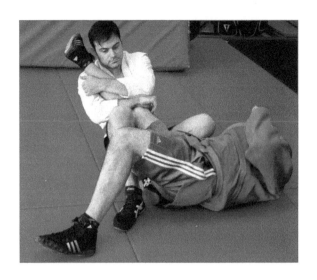

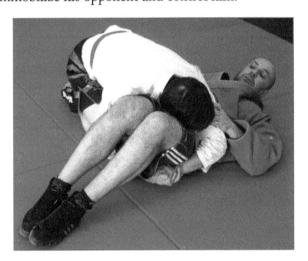

Second, Trap and Isolate the Opponent's Ankle, Leg, or Hip

To apply any lower body submission, the attacker must trap his opponent's leg or ankle (in the case of lower body submissions) in order to isolate and control it. After the leg or ankle is trapped, it is much easier to lever it (straighten or bend the leg or ankle) against a fulcrum to cause pain in the joint.

The following photo shows the attacker using his hands and arms to trap or hug his opponent's right leg. Trapping the leg being attacked isolates it and controls not only the appendage being attacked, but controls the movement of the defender so that the attacker can more effectively apply the leglock.

Third, Apply the Submission Technique

The natural progression from controlling and trapping your opponent's body is to lever, crank, wrench, bend, or apply the submission technique.

This photo shows the attacker applying a straight leg lock (knee bar) and levering the defender's right leg against the pubic bone (the fulcrum) of the attacker.

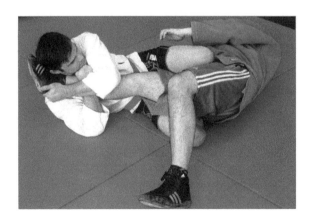

TECHNICAL TIP: All submission techniques involving a joint of the human body are simply an application of the theory of a lever and fulcrum. The lever is placed over the fulcrum and pressure is applied. When done with accuracy and skill, it works.

LEG LACING AND GRAPEVINES

Leg lacing is also called leg wrapping, leg entwining, leg wrestling, leg rides, or other names. There are numerous varieties and applications of leg lacing, but two are commonly used. Generally, the term "leg lacing" refers to the attacker wrapping his legs around his opponent's leg from the bottom up (from the foot area up the length of the leg). However, this isn't always the case.

1. Leg Lace from Bottom Up

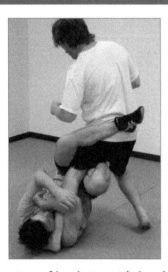

In this application of leg lacing, it's handy to visualize someone lacing his boot strings all the way up the boot so that it fits tightly on the foot and leg. The grappler standing is "wearing" a boot (the grappler on the mat) and the grappler on the mat is using his feet and legs (as well as his hands and arms) to "lace" himself tightly on his opponent's leg. Doing this traps and controls an opponent's leg so that the attacker can better apply a lower body submission or take his opponent to the mat to transition to a finishing hold.

TECHNICAL TIP: When controlling an opponent, make it as uncomfortable as possible. If your opponent is more concerned with the pressure, pain, or discomfort you are applying on him, he's less likely to mount a decent defense or escape.

2. Leg Lace from Hip Down

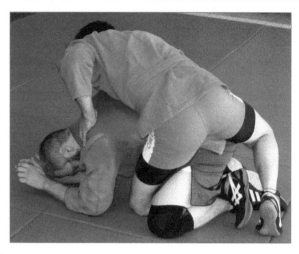

The grappler on top is using his left leg to lace or entwine his opponent's left leg as a method of control to apply a bent leglock. Some people call this a near leg ride, grapevine, or a leg lace (or other name), so it really doesn't matter what terminology you use; the important thing is to use it so that it works for you.

3. Grapevines

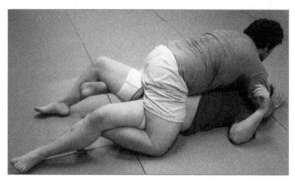

When a sambo wrestler uses both of his legs to wrap (entwine) both of his opponent's legs, that is often called a grapevine. When applied right, a grapevine can be painful and force an opponent to submit from the pressure and pain. Even if the grapevine doesn't get the tap out, it sure can be uncomfortable. Actually, "grapevine" is a pretty generic term, but it's used often when specifying this particular situation. This photo shows the top grappler using his legs to grapevine his opponent's legs. Often, what is called a grapevine is applied from this position, with the defender either on his back or on his front. In either position, it's a bad place for him to be.

STRAIGHT ANKLE LOCK

The straight ankle lock is a basic skill that works at all levels of competition. The best advice is to learn this technique and then drill on it every practice. What is presented here is the basic application of the straight ankle lock using a square grip.

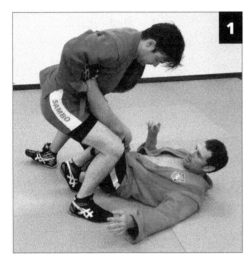

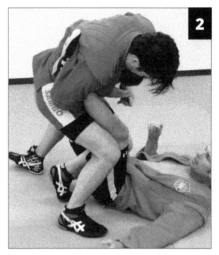

1. The attacker uses his right hand to grab his opponent's left foot (at the heel). As he does this, he pulls the defender's left foot to the attacker's left hip area. This helps extend and stretch the defender's left leg, making it more vulnerable. The attacker uses his right foot to step close to the defender's left hip so he will be closer to his opponent in anticipation of continuing the attack.

2. The attacker uses his right hand and arm to hook under his opponent's extended left lower leg as shown. The attacker makes sure that the defender's left foot is placed so that the defender's left instep is tucked in and behind the attacker's right armpit. Doing this places the defender's left foot and ankle in the correct positon to be attacked.

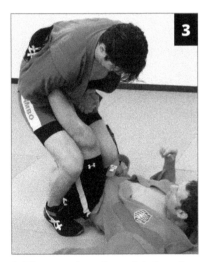

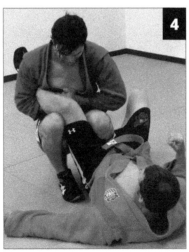

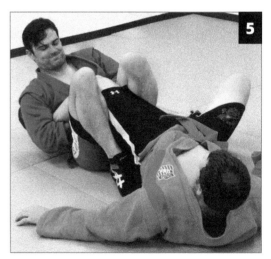

3. The attacker clasps his hands together, forming a square grip with his hands. As he does so, he steps in with both feet and legs and uses his knees and legs to pinch the defender's extended left leg. This traps, isolates, and controls the defender's left leg. Note how the defender's left foot is firmly controlled in the attacker's right armpit area. The attacker starts to bend so that he will be better able to roll back to apply the ankle lock.

4. The attacker rolls back and applies the ankle lock. It is important that the attacker make sure not to let go with one hand to place on the mat as he rolls back.

5. As the attacker rolls back, he arches his hips and applies the ankle lock.

ANKLE TO ANKLE: ANKLE PICK TO ANKLE LOCK

Another variation of the ankle pick was presented in the chapter on throwing techniques (validating the fact that many throws in sambo are excellent transitions to a submission technique). This variation is a near ankle pick, meaning that the attacker focuses on the opponent's foot nearer to the attacker.

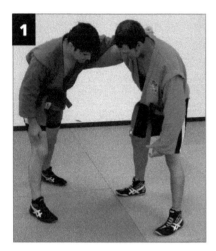

The attacker (left) uses his left hand as an anchor grip and keeps his right hand in reserve as his probing hand.

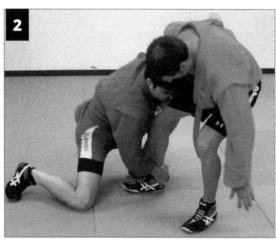

The attacker uses his left foot and leg to do a deep lunge step as he uses his right hand to grab (pick) on the inside of his opponent's right heel as shown.

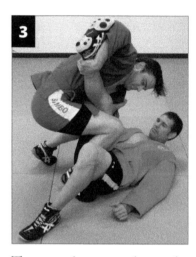

The attacker completes the ankle pick throw and makes sure to use his right hand to pull his opponent's right leg out straight as shown. Look at how the attacker uses his right foot and leg to step in between the defender's legs.

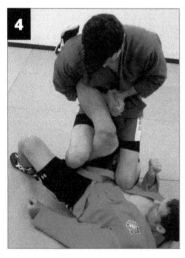

The attacker uses his hands to form a square grip. As he does this, the attacker pinches his knees and legs together, trapping his opponent's right leg as shown.

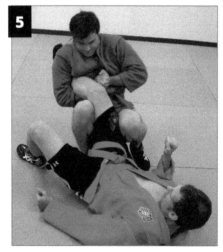

The attacker rolls back and applies the ankle lock.

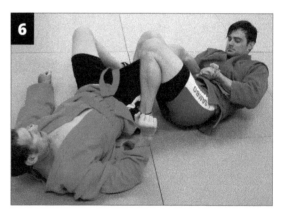

The angle of the photo has been changed so that you can see how the attacker rolls back to apply the ankle lock. Look at how the attacker's feet are tucked under the defender's buttocks and hips. Doing this prevents the defender from attempting to grab the attacker's foot or ankle as a counter ankle lock.

ROLL TO TIGHTEN ANKLE LOCK

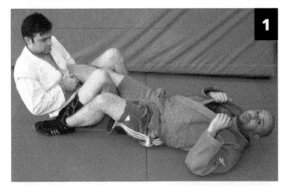

This move is used often to increase the effect of an ankle lock, using the momentum of the rolling action to tighten the effect of the ankle lock. It is called various names including the "gator roll," "death roll," or "trap and roll."

1. The attacker (left) has already started to apply a straight ankle lock using his left hand and arm to attack his opponent's right ankle as shown.

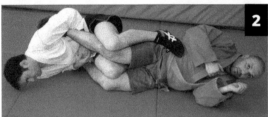

2. If the opponent resists too much or if the attacker feels that he doesn't have enough control to make the ankle lock work, the attacker will roll to his right side. Rolling in the direction away from the arm that controls his opponent's ankle works to tighten the effect of the ankle lock. (If the attacker rolls the other way and gains more control, that's okay as well. Experiment to see which way works best for you.)

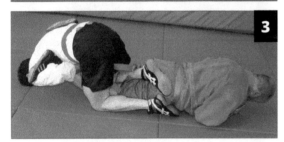

3. The attacker continues to roll to his right, and as he does, he continually gains more control of his opponent's right ankle. Doing this tightens the ankle lock.

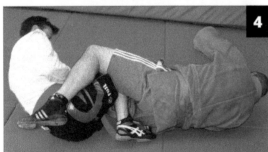

4. The attacker continues to roll. Make sure not to try to roll too fast or too slow. The attacker will roll only as far as necessary to force his opponent to tap out or submit.

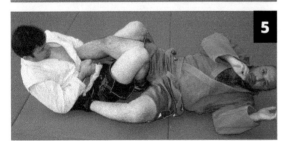

5. An important point is that as the attacker rolls, he makes sure to pinch his knees and legs together tightly to trap and control his opponent's right leg as shown.

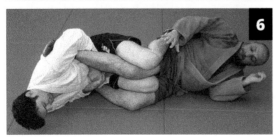

6. Often, the defender will tap out in mid-roll as shown in photo 6.

REVERSE ROLLING ANKLE LOCK

For some reason that makes no sense to this author, some sambo wrestlers will take such a defensive position where they lie flat on their front in the hope that the referee will call a halt to the action. If your opponent lays on his front in this belly-down hiding position, say a silent "thank you" and then take advantage of the situation.

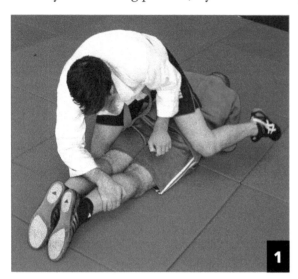

The attacker (on top) immediately changes his position so that he faces the defensive grappler's feet as shown. Doing this is "facing the business end" of the ankle lock.

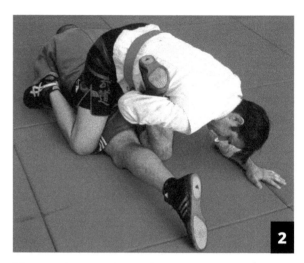

The attacker uses his right hand and arm to hook and control his opponent's right ankle as shown. If possible (as shown in this photo), it's a good idea for the attacker to hook his opponent's ankle and force his knee to bend. Doing this gives the attacker more control of the right ankle.

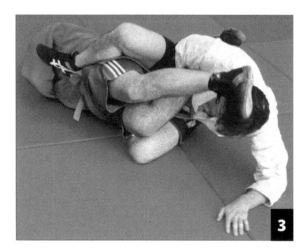

The attacker rolls to his left hip as shown. Look at how the attacker starts to use his feet and legs to trap his opponent's legs and hips and his right hand and arm to cinch the ankle lock in tighter as he rolls.

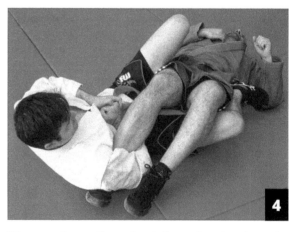

The attacker rolls to his left, and as he does, he arches his hips and finishes the ankle lock as shown.

REVERSE BUNDLE ANKLE LOCK

When the attacker grabs both of his opponent's legs or ankles and traps them, it is called "bundling." Much as someone picks up a bundle of sticks, the attacker bundles his opponent's legs together and attacks them.

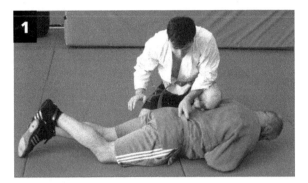

The attacker controls his defensive opponent from the top as shown. He immediately places his left knee on his opponent to start his attack.

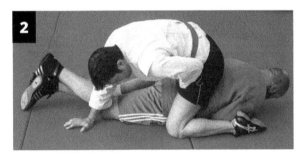

The attacker moves so that he faces the feet of his opponent as shown.

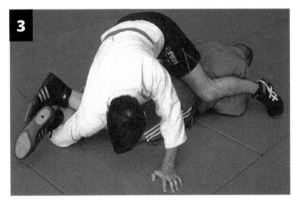

The attacker uses his right hand and arm to hook under both of his opponent's feet and lower legs.

TECHNICAL TIP: Again, it should be pointed out that when the defender assumes the extreme defensive position of lying on his front (and in many cases, crossing his ankles), this shows the attacker that his opponent is simply hiding and hoping the referee will call a halt to the action to save him. This extreme defensive position is more common than one might expect, so it's a good idea to train on these ankle locks when encountering an opponent in this position. Conversely, when defending from the bottom, it's not a good idea to lie on the front and hide in this way. Hoping that the referee will blow his whistle and call a halt to the action and get you out of trouble is not a good tactic.

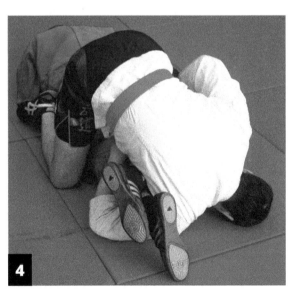

This view shows how the attacker uses his right hand and arm to bundle his opponent's feet and lower legs.

REVERSE BUNDLE ANKLE LOCK

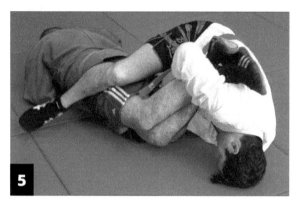

5

The attacker rolls to his left side, all the while using his right hand and arm to tighten the hold of his opponent's trapped lower legs and ankles.

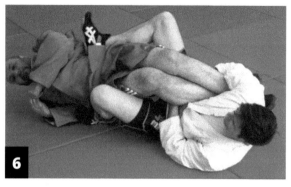

6

The attacker continues to roll and starts to use his legs and knees to squeeze and pinch his opponent's legs so that they stay trapped together as shown.

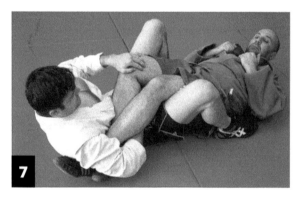

7

The attacker completes his roll and immediately uses his left hand to grab and pull his opponent's right knee so the attacker can separate the lower legs of his opponent and allow room for the attacker to slide his right hand up between the defender's trapped lower legs.

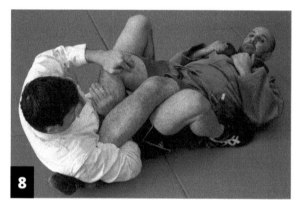

8

The attacker slides his right hand up to trap his opponent's left lower leg as shown.

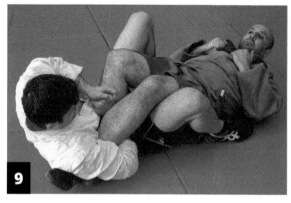

9

The attacker immediately grasps his hands together to form a square lock and apply the straight ankle lock.

REVERSE BUNDLE ROLL TO DOUBLE ANKLE LOCK

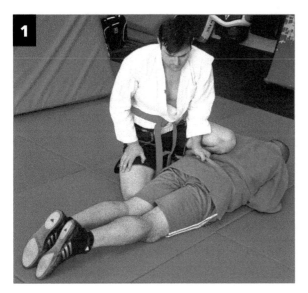

The attacker controls his defensive opponent from the top as shown.

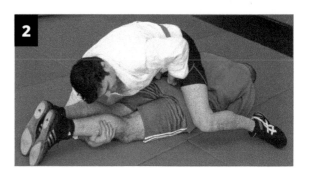

The attacker uses both hands and arms to trap and hug the defender's legs to the attacker's torso.

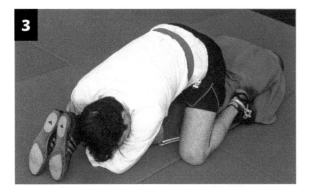

The attacker moves so that he faces the same direction as his opponent's feet. As he does this, the attacker uses his right hand and arm to hook and trap his opponent's lower legs.

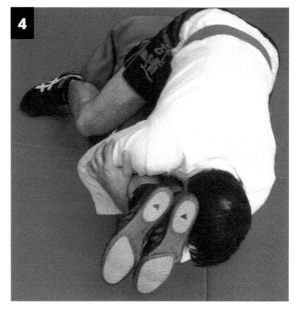

This view shows how the attacker hugs his opponent's lower legs. Doing this traps the defender's legs together.

REVERSE BUNDLE ROLL TO DOUBLE ANKLE LOCK

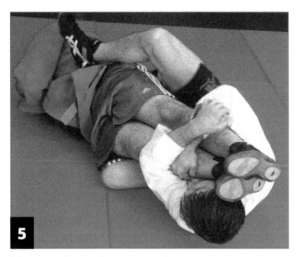

5

The attacker rolls to his left maintaining control of his opponent's trapped legs.

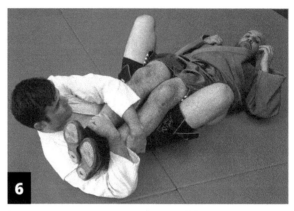

6

The attacker rolls over as shown. The attacker slides his right hand so that it is closer to the defender's ankles as shown. The attacker maintains control of the defender's lower legs with his left hand and arm. Doing this, the attacker continues to have control over his opponent's lower legs.

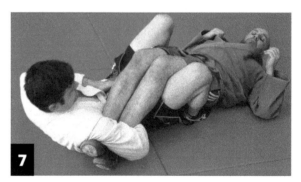

7

The attacker quickly uses his right hand and arm to hook over the defender's ankles, setting them up for the double ankle lock. The attacker forms a square grip with his hands and applies pressure on both ankles.

DOUBLE LEG ATTACK TRANSITION TO LEG LACE ANKLE LOCK

This technique is a good example of a transition from standing to the ground or mat.

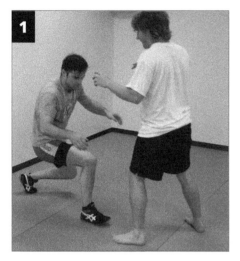

The attacker (left) starts to shoot in with a double leg throw or takedown.

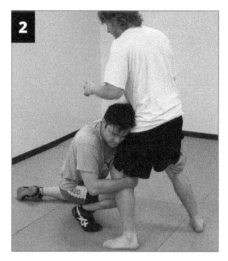

The attacker uses this double leg attack to get in close enough so that he can swing under his opponent to lace his legs. Look at how the attacker drives in deep using his hands and arms to grab his opponent's legs above the knees.

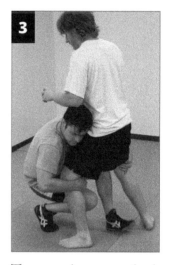

The attacker uses both of his hands and arms to grab his opponent's legs to anchor himself so that he can immediately bend (and "get round") and roll or swing under his opponent and between his opponent's legs.

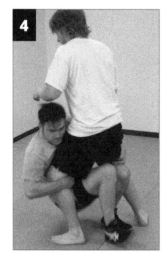

The attacker swings or rolls his body between his opponent's legs as shown.

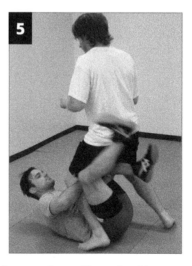

As the attacker rolls under his opponent, he makes sure to swing both of his feet and legs completely through his opponent's legs. Look at how the attacker uses his right hand and arm to hook and trap his opponent's left lower leg.

DOUBLE LEG ATTACK TRANSITION TO LEG LACE ANKLE LOCK

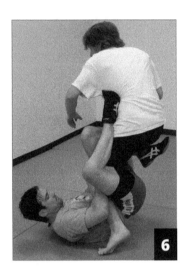

The attacker uses his right hand and arm to trap and control his opponent's left lower leg. The attacker uses his left bent knee to jam between his opponent's legs and places his right foot and leg on his opponent's left upper leg and hip area as shown. This is the start of the leg-lace movement.

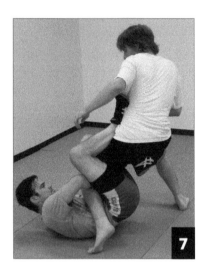

The attacker uses his feet and legs to push his opponent.

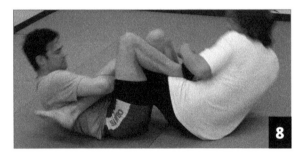

The attacker pushes his opponent onto the opponent's back or buttocks as shown. As he does this, the attacker slides his right hand and arm down closer to the defender's left ankle.

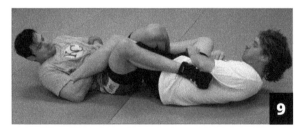

The attacker applies the straight ankle lock from this position.

BASIC HEEL HOOK

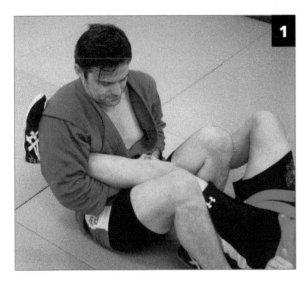

The attacker (left) uses his right hand and arm to trap and isolate his opponent's left lower leg.

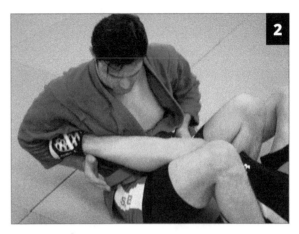

The attacker uses his hands to trap his opponent's left heel and ankle in the attacker's right elbow. The attacker hugs his opponent's left foot in tightly to the right side of his body so that the entire lower leg is trapped by the attacker's hands, arms, and body as shown. Look at how the attacker forms a square grip with his hands, with the attacker's left forearm over the top of the defender's left ankle and the attacker's right forearm positioned under the defender's left heel. Doing this allows the attacker to securely trap, isolate, and control his opponent's left lower leg. Also, look at how the attacker inches his knees and legs together, further trapping and controlling his opponent's left leg.

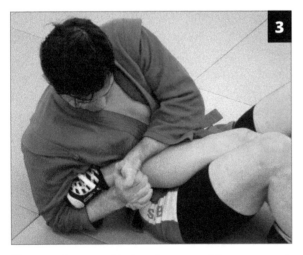

The attacker slides his right arm back so that his opponent's left heel is hooked and trapped on the inside of the attacker's right elbow as shown. Look at how the attacker moves his right hand up and under his opponent's left heel and ankle.

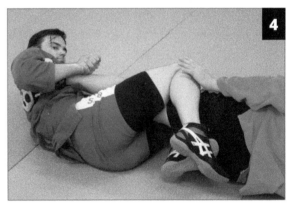

The attacker rolls to his left to apply pressure to the heel hook. When practicing this move, make sure to apply this lock slowly and allow your partner time to tap out.

TECHNICAL TIP: A painful and effective variation of the ankle lock is the heel hook. This move was permitted in sambo competition up until the late 1970s (as I recall) but was eventually banned from the rules of sport sambo for safety reasons. A heel hook can not only do a lot of damage to an opponent's ankle, it can also tear the ligaments of the opponent's knee. However, since so many sambo grapplers compete in other combat sports (such as MMA, catch wrestling, and submission grappling), every sambo wrestler should study and practice heel hooks (as well as toeholds). There are many variations of the heel hook and the basic application is presented here.

SINGLE LEG RIDE TO CRADLE HOLD-DOWN AND THEN TO A TOEHOLD

This series has been included to illustrate how good groundfighting can (and often does) blend one move into another; if the initial attack doesn't work, there is another move that the attacker can use. This is "chain wrestling" or "chain grappling" in action. A basic (but effective) single leg ride has been selected to start this series of moves.

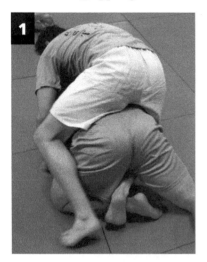

The attacker (on top) uses a single leg ride with his right foot and leg hooking under his opponent's right hip and upper leg.

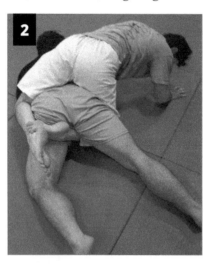

The attacker lifts up so that his opponent comes off the mat. As he does this, the attacker uses his right foot to hook and control his opponent's left ankle.

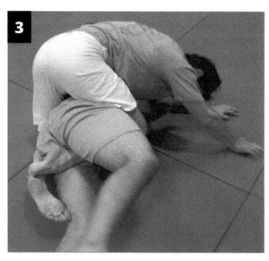

The attacker moves his body to his right as he slides his right foot up his opponent's leg. Doing this starts the action to turn his opponent over.

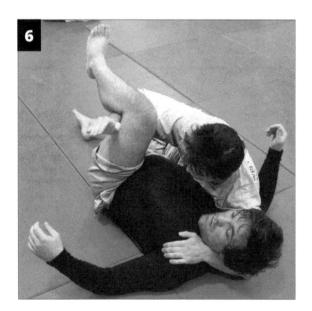

The attacker uses his right hand and arm to hook under his opponent's left knee as shown.

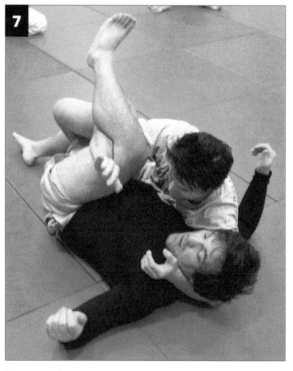

The attacker starts to grasp his hands together.

SINGLE LEG RIDE TO CRADLE HOLD-DOWN AND THEN TO A TOEHOLD

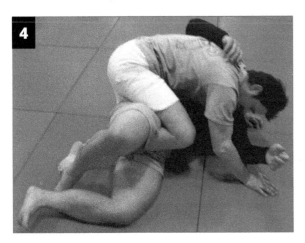

The attacker turns his opponent over onto the defender's left side as shown. This is a good example of how the attacker can use his feet and legs to control his opponent and is often called "leg wrestling."

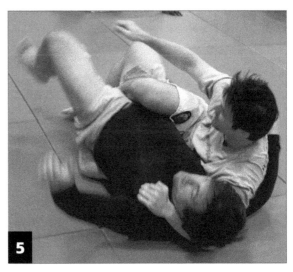

The attacker turns his opponent onto his back as shown. Look at how the attacker positions his left arm under his opponent's head. The attacker uses his right hand and arm to start to reach out for his opponent's left leg.

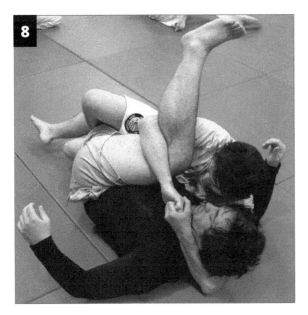

The attacker grasps his hands together. Doing this, the attacker can hold his opponent to the mat to score points and control him until the referee signals to the attacker that he must continue on to apply a submission technique.

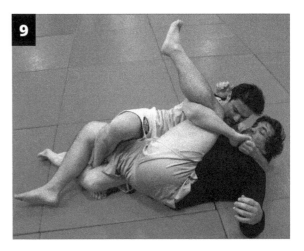

This photo shows the cradle hold-down. Look at how the attacker uses his legs to lace his opponent's legs and how the attacker uses his hands (using a "C" or "hook" grip) to form the cradle hold. The attacker's torso is firmly placed on his opponent's right torso, making this a hold-down that can score points in the rules of sambo. When the referee signals that four points have been scored by the attacker, the referee will tell the attacker to "go for the submission."

SINGLE LEG RIDE TO CRADLE HOLD-DOWN AND THEN TO A TOEHOLD

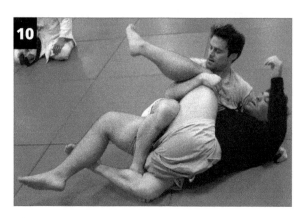

The attacker now goes for the submission technique and releases his grip with his hands. As he does this, the attacker turns to face his opponent's left lower leg and foot. Look at how the attacker continues to lace and control his opponent's right leg.

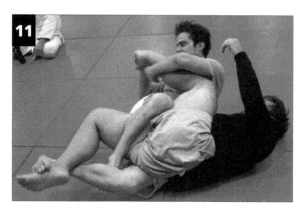

The attacker uses his right hand to grab the top of his opponent's left foot at the area of the toes. The attacker uses his left hand and arm to hook under his opponent's left lower leg to grab the opponent's left ankle. This is the start of a toehold.

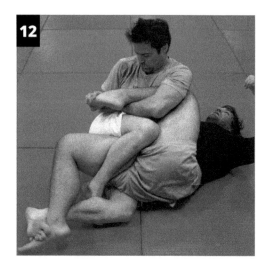

Look at how the attacker uses his right hand to grab the defender's left lower foot (at the toes). The attacker places his left hand on his right forearm to trap his opponent's left ankle. Doing this forms the toehold as shown.

IMPORTANT: The attacker could have used a straight ankle lock instead of a toehold. The toehold is considered a "twisting" ankle lock and is not allowed in the rules of sambo but is shown in this series of moves to illustrate the point that it is a good idea for sambo wrestlers to study and practice a variety of submission techniques and finishing holds, even if they are not currently allowed in the rules of the sport of sambo.

SINGLE LEG RIDE TO HIP LOCK

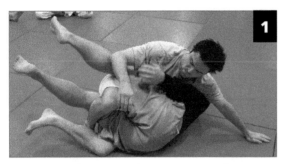

Continuing from the previous series: if, for some reason, the attacker chooses not to use a toehold or ankle lock, he can go for a hip lock from this position. This photo picks up from where the attacker releases the cradle hold-down.

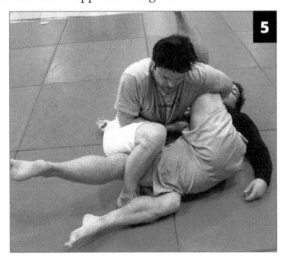

The attacker uses his right hand and arm to push his opponent's left leg up so that the attacker can move his right hand and arm through and between his opponent's legs as shown.

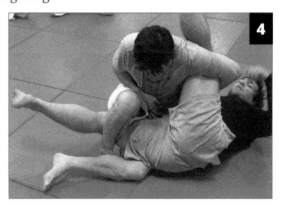

The attacker grasps his hands together, trapping his opponent's left upper leg. As he does this, the attacker starts to lean back so that pressure will be applied to his opponent's left hip.

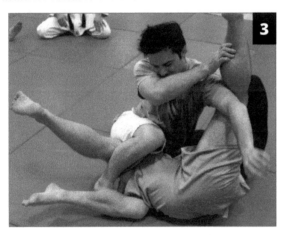

The attacker uses his right hand to grab the lower left leg of his opponent. Look at how the attacker uses his legs to lace and control his opponent's right leg.

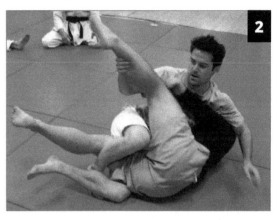

The attacker uses his left hand and arm to hook and control his opponent's left upper leg as shown.

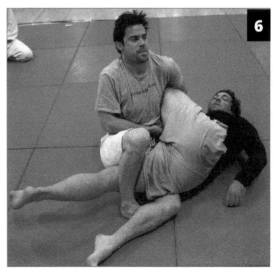

The attacker leans back and applies pressure to his opponent's left hip, stretching it out of its normal range of motion and causing pain in the joint.

BACK ROLL HIP LOCK

Called the "banana split" or "spladle" in wrestling, this move is actually a painful hip lock. This application is an effective and commonly used one and there are several other effective variations. For more information on this hip lock and other variations, refer to *Tap Out Textbook* published by Turtle Press.

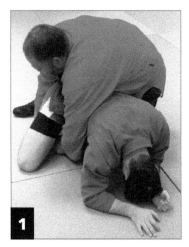

The attacker (on top) uses both of his hands and arms to reach over his opponent's lower back and grab the defender's right leg. As he does this, the attacker uses his left leg to hook and lace his opponent's left leg using a near leg ride.

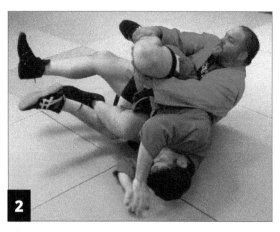

The attacker uses both hands and arms to reach around his opponent's right leg and grab his opponent's right ankle.

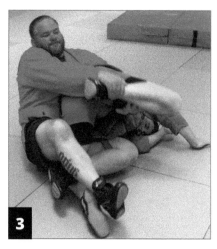

This view shows how the attacker rolls to his back and onto his buttocks as he uses both his legs and feet to entwine and lace his opponent's left leg as shown. Look at how the attacker pulls on his opponent's right ankle and leg. Doing this tilts the defender over his left side and onto his back.

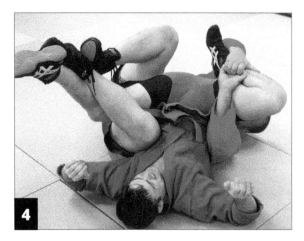

The attacker rolls onto his back and grasps his hands together as shown. The attacker's left foot and leg are wrapped around the defender's extended left leg and the attacker uses his right foot to push onto his left foot as shown. Doing all of this splits the defender's legs wide apart.

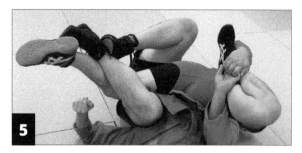

This close view shows how the attacker grasps his hands together, trapping his opponent's right leg and ankle. The attacker uses his right foot to push on the back of his left foot to create more pain in the defender's hip and leg and split the defender's legs wider apart.

ROLLING STRAIGHT LEG LOCK FROM A FRONT CHEST HOLD-DOWN

A common (and effective) transition from a hold-down to a leglock takes place after the attacker (on top) scores four points for his hold-down and the official instructs him to go for the submission. This straight knee bar is an example of an effective transition from a hold-down to a submission. This is also an effective attack when fighting an opponent who is on his back in the guard position.

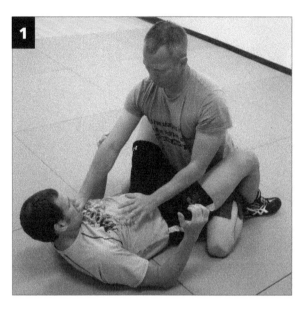

The attacker (on top) has just scored four points for his hold-down and is going to attempt a leglock from this position.

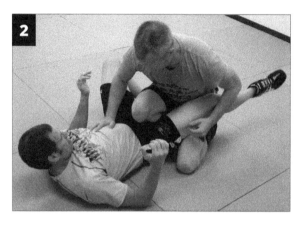

The attacker brings his right knee and shin up off the mat and places it on his opponent's crotch as shown. As he does this, the attacker uses his left hand to start to reach down his opponent's right leg.

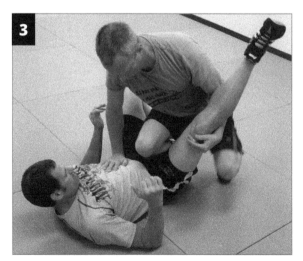

The attacker uses his left hand to reach over his opponent's right leg as the attacker drives his right shin down hard between his opponent's legs. As he does this, the attacker starts to come up off the mat with his left knee.

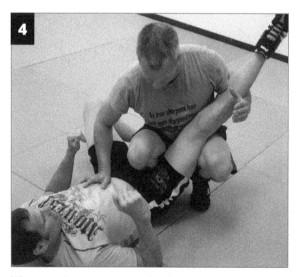

The attacker squats on both feet as shown and uses his knees and legs to pinch and trap his opponent's right upper leg as shown.

ROLLING STRAIGHT LEGLOCK FROM A FRONT CHEST HOLD-DOWN

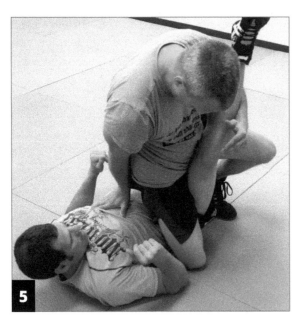

The attacker slides his right knee and leg over his opponent's right hip as shown. As he does this, the attacker uses his left hand and arm to trap his opponent's right leg to the attacker's chest.

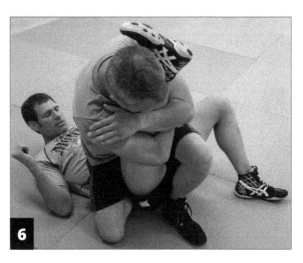

The attacker uses both hands and arms to hug his opponent's right leg to the attacker's chest as the attacker rotates and rolls to his right and over his opponent's right hip

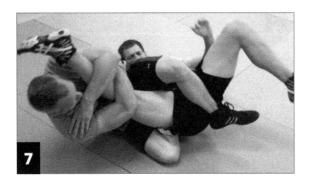

The attacker continues to roll to his right side as he uses both hands to hug and trap his opponent's extended right leg to the attacker's chest.

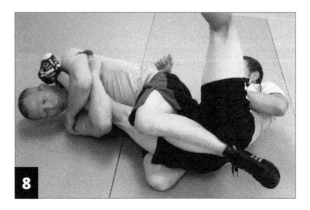

The attacker rolls onto his right hip and arches his hips. Doing this "bars" the defender's extended right knee over the attacker's pubic bone. (Important: The attacker must not roll onto his back.) Look at how the attacker tucks his feet so that they are hooked onto the defender's buttocks and continue to trap the defender's right leg.

BRIDGE-AND-ROLL ESCAPE FROM VERTICAL HOLD-DOWN INTO ROLLING STRAIGHT KNEE BAR

Here is a technique that serves as an example of how a sambo wrestler can escape from a hold-down and counter with a leglock.

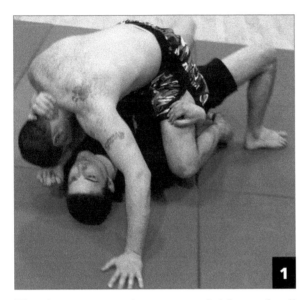

The bottom grappler uses a bridge-and-roll escape from his opponent's vertical hold-down. The bottom grappler uses his left hand to hook around his opponent's head and uses his right hand and arm to hook under his opponent's left upper leg as shown. As he does this, the bottom grappler bridges up off the mat, pushing on the mat with his fee and shoulders.

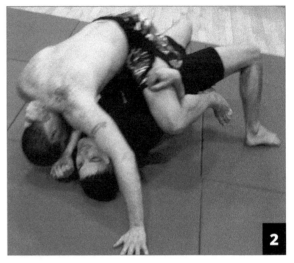

The bottom grappler drives off of his feet and shoulders as he rolls to his left, all the while using his right hand on his opponent's head to hook and control it. The bottom grappler continues to use his right hand and arm to hook under his opponent's left leg.

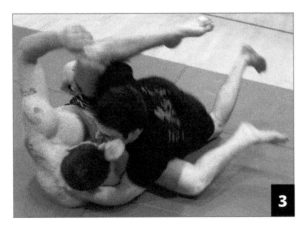

The bottom grappler rolls to his left and rolls his opponent over as well.

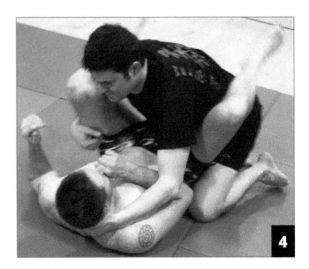

The bottom grappler is now on top and is the attacker.

BRIDGE AND ROLL ESCAPE FROM VERTICAL HOLD-DOWN INTO ROLLING STRAIGHT KNEE BAR

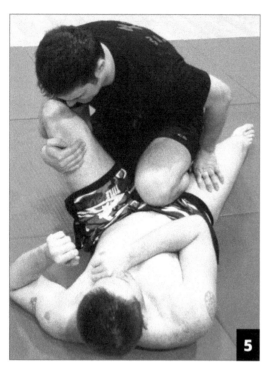

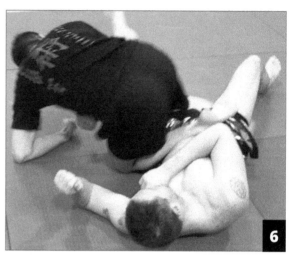

The attacker rotates his body so that it rolls to his right and over his opponent's left leg. Look at how the attacker's left bent knee is jammed across the bottom grappler's left hip area.

The attacker drives his left knee and shin up and between his opponent's legs as shown. The attacker continues to use his right hand to hold and control his opponent's right upper leg.

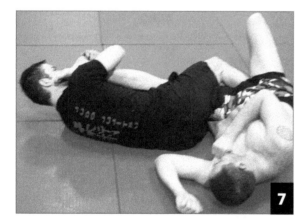

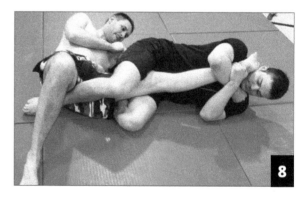

The attacker rolls and as he does, he uses both hands and arms to catch and trap his opponent's left leg as shown. The attacker finishes on his left side (and not on his back). As he does this, the attacker arches with his hips, creating a knee bar on his opponent's extended left leg.

This view shows how the attacker finishes the straight leg lock and gets the tap out.

HEAD ROLL STRAIGHT LEG LOCK

This roll is similar to the popular and effective head roll cross-body armlock, but instead of an armlock, a straight leglock is used.

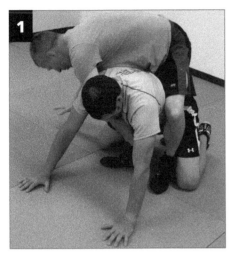

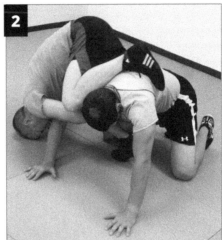

1. The attacker (on top) rides his opponent and uses his left hand to hook over his opponent's left shoulder to control his arm.

2. The attacker posts his head on the mat as shown for stability (this is important—the top of the head must be on the mat). As he does this, the attacker moves his left foot and leg up and behind his opponent's head as shown. Look at how the attacker uses his left arm to hook and trap his opponent's right upper arm.

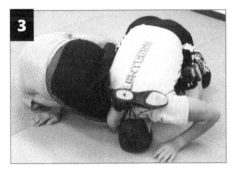

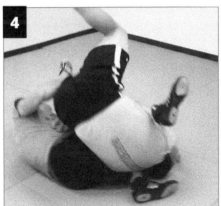

3. The attacker rolls onto his left hip. Look at how the attacker uses his right foot that is placed at the bottom grappler's left hip as an anchor.

4. The attacker uses his right hand to grab his opponent's leg or ankle to help pull it over as the attacker rolls his opponent over his head.

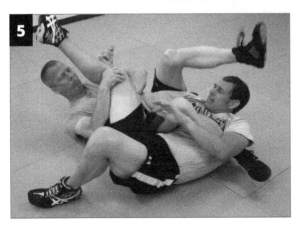

5. The attacker rolls his opponent over and immediately uses both hands and arms to catch and trap the defender's right leg.

6. The attacker uses his hands and arms to hook and trap the defender's right leg. As he does this, he stretches the defender's right leg and arches his hips to create a straight leg lock.

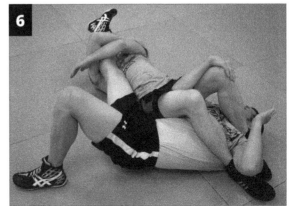

FAR HIP ROLL TO STRAIGHT KNEE LOCK

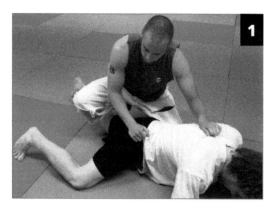

The attacker (top) controls his opponent as shown.

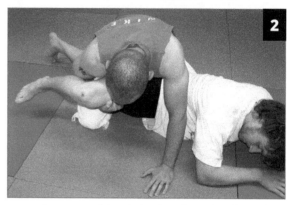

The attacker uses his right hand to hook under his opponent's right upper leg. It may be necessary for the attacker to place his left hand on the mat for stability.

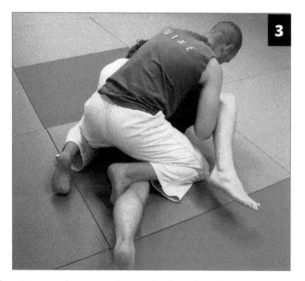

As the attacker uses his right hand to hook under and trap his opponent's right leg, the attacker places his right shin and knee over his opponent's left leg as shown.

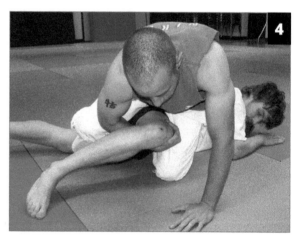

The attacker uses his right hand and arm to scoop his opponent's right leg as the attacker starts to roll over his left side.

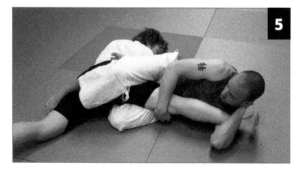

The attacker rolls over his left side and ends up lying on his left side as shown. As he does this, the attacker uses both hands and arms to trap and catch his opponent's extended right leg. The attacker makes sure to have the defender's straight leg positioned so that the defender's knee is resting in the attacker's pubic area. Doing this ensures that the knee bar will take place.

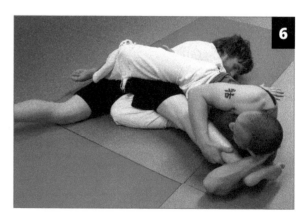

The attacker arches with his hips to apply pressure to the straight knee, creating a barring action on the knee to cause pain.

BOTH KNEES BREAKDOWN TO STRAIGHT LEG LOCK

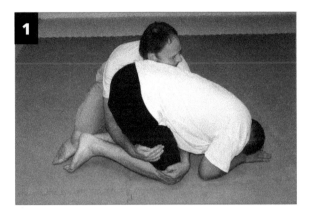

The attacker uses both of his hands and arms to reach around and grab his opponent's right leg.

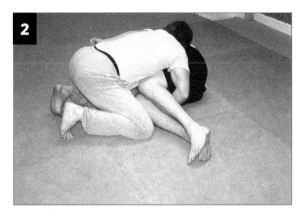

The attacker pulls with both hands and arms on his opponent's legs as the attacker drives his body into his opponent. Doing this breaks the defender down and puts him on his right side or on his back.

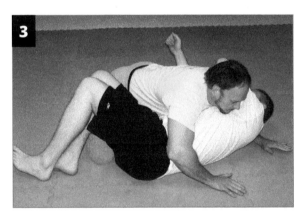

The attacker moves his body so that his torso is above his opponent's hips and the attacker's torso is positioned directly on top of his opponent's torso as shown. The attacker could immediately initiate a hold-down at this point if he chooses.

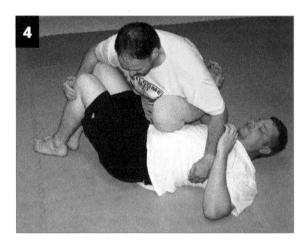

The attacker moves his left knee up and on the right side of his opponent's torso.

BOTH KNEES BREAKDOWN TO STRAIGHT LEGLOCK

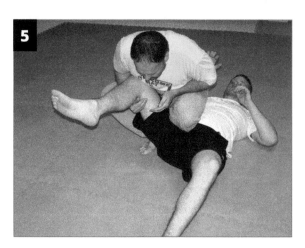

The attacker jams his left knee and shin on his opponent's right hip area as the attacker uses both hands and arms to scoop and trap the defender's right upper leg.

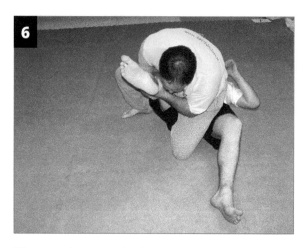

The attacker uses both hands and arms to hug and trap the defender's extended right leg to the attacker's chest. As he does this, the attacker starts to roll to his left side as shown.

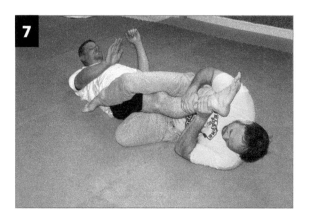

The attacker rolls onto his left side as shown and immediately arches his hips, creating a straight knee bar. Look at how the attacker places his feet and legs on his opponent's hip and buttocks to prevent the defender from grabbing the attacker's foot or ankle as a counter attack.

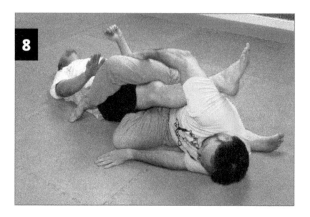

If the defender doesn't submit from the initial straight knee lock, the attacker can use his right hand and arm to hook over the defender's right lower leg. The attacker uses his right hand to grab his own upper leg and arches his hips forward. Doing this creates a nasty straight knee lock.

HIP HOLD-DOWN TO STRAIGHT KNEE LOCK

This is another example of how a sambo wrestler can transition from a hold-down to a leglock.

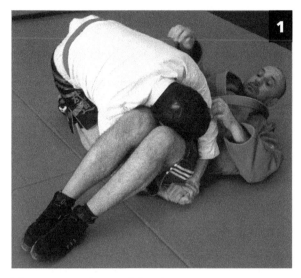

The attacker (on top) holds his opponent with a hip hold-down.

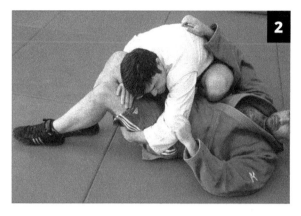

When the official scores the points for the hold-down and instructs the top grappler to go for the submission, the attacker immediately places his left bent knee and shin on the right side of his opponent's torso. The attacker continues to use his hands and arms to control his opponent's legs and hips.

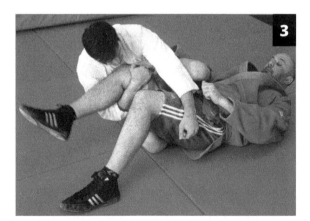

The attacker slides his right bent knee under his opponent's right buttocks. As he does this, the attacker starts to roll back onto his right back side as shown. Look at how the attacker uses his right hand and arm to hook and trap his opponent's right leg at about the knee.

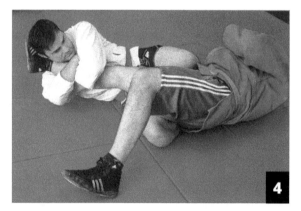

The attacker rolls back on his right side as he uses both hands and arms to hook and trap his opponent's right leg as shown. As he does this, the attacker arches his hips to create the pressure on the stretched and straight knee joint.

LEG SCISSORS TRANSITION TO STRAIGHT LEG LOCK

Some transitions take place with the attacker positioned on the mat and his opponent standing. This is an example of this type of transition and it illustrates how a sambo wrestler can score from just about any position.

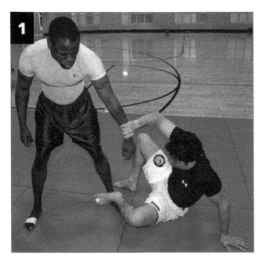

The attacker (on bottom) is positioned on his left hip and he has used his right hand to grab his opponent's left wrist. Look at how the attacker places his left foot on the front of his standing opponent's left ankle. The attacker's right leg is positioned slightly behind his opponent's left heel.

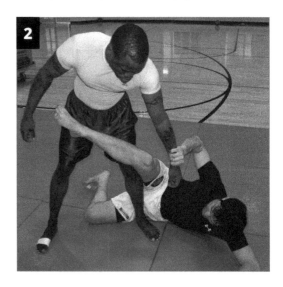

The attacker slides his body so that his hip area is positioned behind his opponent's left leg as shown. The attacker swings his right leg up and in front of his opponent's upper legs. Doing this traps the standing opponent's left leg.

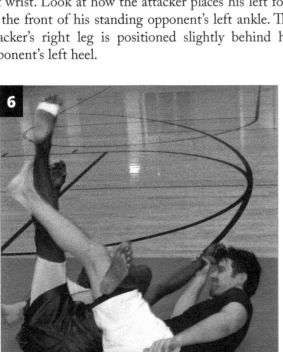

The attacker scissors his opponent and takes him onto his back.

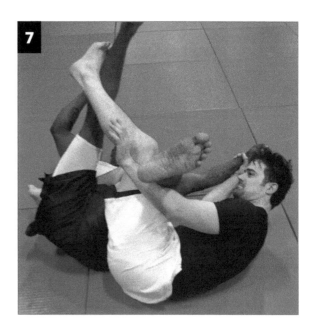

The attacker immediately uses his left hand and arm to reach out and grab his opponent's left leg.

LEG SCISSORS TRANSITION TO STRAIGHT LEGLOCK

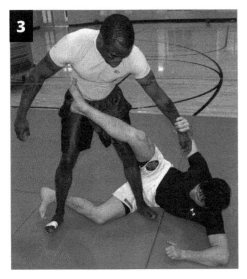

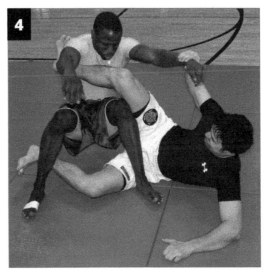

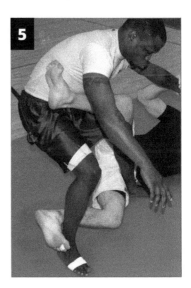

The attacker swings his left foot and leg and hooks the standing grappler's right lower leg at the ankle as shown. Look at how the attacker continues to use his right hand to hold his opponent's left wrist. You can see how the attacker has positioned his body so that he will be able to create a sweeping or scissors motion to take his opponent to the mat.

The attacker uses his legs to sweep or scissor his opponent, forcing the defender to fall to the mat on his back.

This photo shows how the attacker places his feet and legs so that he will be able to sweep and scissor his standing opponent. Look at how the attacker's right foot is placed as the defender's right hip area and how the attacker's right foot is cocked and catches the standing grappler behind his right ankle.

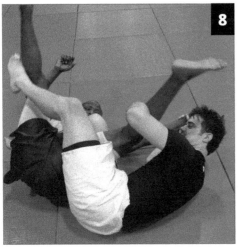

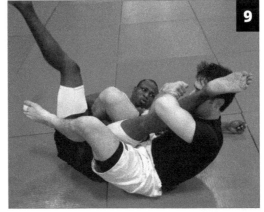

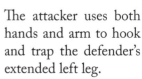

The attacker uses both hands and arm to hook and trap the defender's extended left leg.

The attacker uses his left hand and arm to hook and start to trap the defender's left leg as shown.

The attacker rolls back slightly and arches his hips, creating a knee bar.

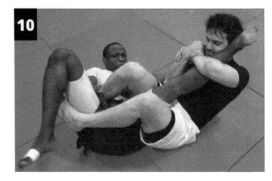

ANKLE FAKE TO ROLLING LEG LACE AND LEGLOCK

This is an effective transition from standing to the mat or ground and illustrates how transitions are not throws and are not takedowns, but are definitely effective in getting an opponent off of his feet and onto the mat, and then forcing him to submit.

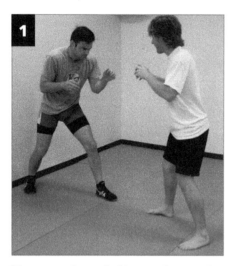

The attacker (left) is facing his opponent in a standing position.

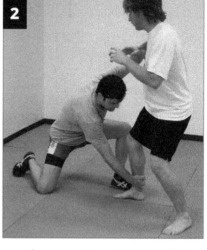

The attacker steps in with his left foot and leg with a deep lunge step and uses his right hand to grab at the inside of his opponent's right ankle. This ankle pick is a diversion to force the opponent to react.

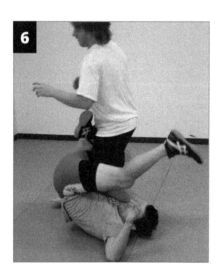

This view shows how the attacker uses his right knee and shin to jam between his opponent's legs. Look at how the attacker swings his left leg upward on the outside of the defender's left hip area and spins on his upper shoulders.

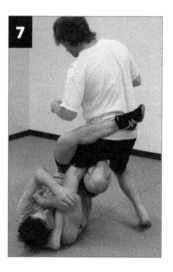

The attacker laces his opponent's left leg. Look at how his right bent knee and shin are jammed between the defender's legs and trapping the inside of the defender's left upper leg. The attacker uses his left leg and foot to trap the defender's left upper leg with the left foot placed solidly on his opponent's left rear hip area. Note how the attacker uses both hands and arms to hook and trap the defender's lower left leg. This is a classic example of a "leg lace" in action.

ANKLE FAKE TO ROLLING LEG LACE AND LEGLOCK

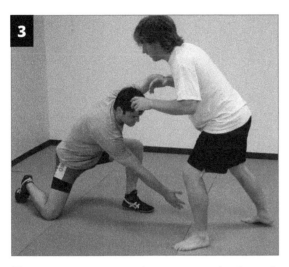

The opponent reacts by stepping back with his right foot and leg to avoid the ankle pick attack. Doing this leaves the opponent's left leg vulnerable.

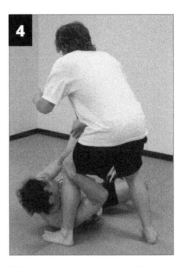

The attacker immediately uses his right hand and arm to hook around his opponent's left leg at about the knee as shown. As he does this, the attacker rolls in sideways so that his right shoulder is very close to or touching the defender's left lower leg.

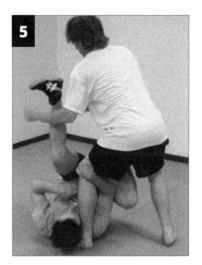

The attacker rolls on his right shoulder so that he is now able to use his right bent knee to swing up and between his opponent's legs. The attacker starts to swing his left foot and leg upward. Look at how the attacker uses his right hand and arm to hook and trap his opponent's left leg.

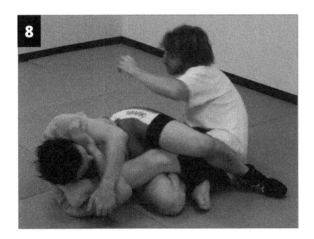

The attacker uses his feet and legs to force his opponent backward and onto his buttocks as shown. The attacker continues to control his opponent with the leg lace. At this point, the defender's left leg is vulnerable to the attacker's straight knee lock. Look at how the attacker is lying on his right side and using both of his knees and legs to pinch together and trap his opponent's left leg.

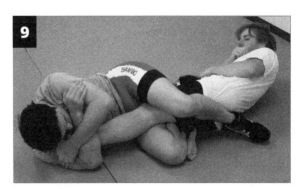

The attacker arches his hips to apply pressure to the knee joint, causing pain and getting the submission.

ROLLING KNEE BAR

This move is a good leglock but it is also a good way to get off of the bottom if an opponent is riding you. There is more than one variation of this rolling knee bar but this one has a high rate of success.

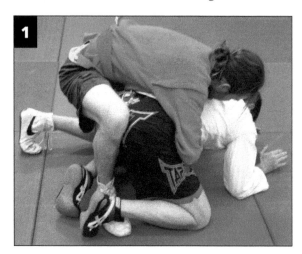

The attacker (on bottom) is being controlled by his opponent in a ride.

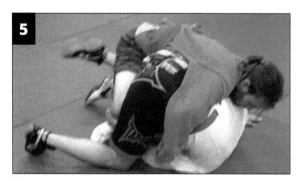

The bottom grappler uses left foot to hook and trap his opponent's right ankle as shown. As he does this, the bottom grappler uses his right hand to grab the top grappler's right ankle.

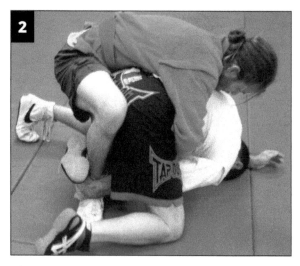

The attacker rolls over his right shoulder, forcing his opponent to roll over also. As he does this, he continues to control his opponent's right ankle.

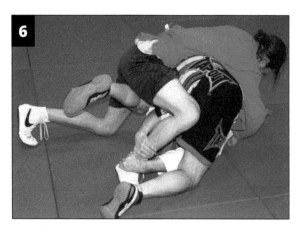

As the attacker rolls over his right shoulder, he grabs his opponent's ankle with his left hand so that both hands of the attacker are grabbing and controlling the defender's right ankle.

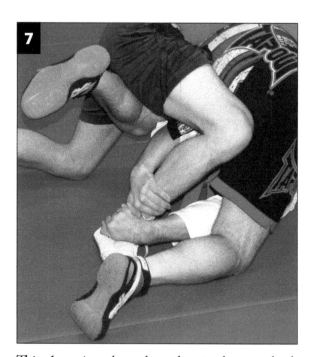

This close view shows how the attacker uses both hands to grab his opponent's right ankle. Also, look at how the attacker now uses his right foot and leg to help lift his opponent at the opponent's right thigh area. Doing this allows the attacker to control his opponent better during the roll.

ROLLING KNEE BAR

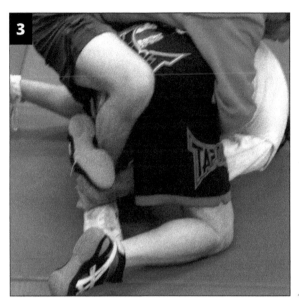

This photo shows a close view of how the attacker (on bottom) uses his left foot to hook and trap his opponent's right lower leg and ankle. You can see how the attacker uses his right hand to grab and control the top grappler's right ankle as well.

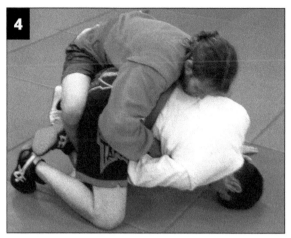

The bottom grappler posts on the top of his head so he can better roll his opponent over the right shoulder of the bottom grappler. As he does this, the bottom grappler continues to control his opponent's right ankle.

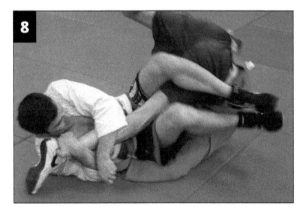

The attacker has rolled over his right shoulder and rolls his opponent over with him. Look at how the attacker finishes the rolling action by placing both of his feet and legs on his opponent's buttocks. Doing this gives the attacker more power from his legs in order to roll his opponent over, but more importantly, this leg placement helps prevent the defender from grabbing the attacker's ankle as a counter attack.

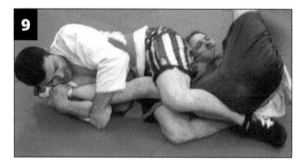

The attacker completes the roll and finishes on his right side as shown. As he completes the roll, the attacker arches his hips and applies the knee bar on the defender's right leg.

STRAIGHT KNEE BAR TO FAR SIDE OF OPPONENT FROM SIDE CONTROL

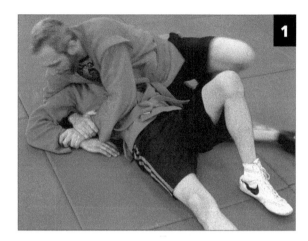

The top sambo wrestler controls his opponent from the side. In this case, he is attempting a bent armlock on the bottom grappler's right arm. The attacker (on top) uses this bent armlock attack as a diversion in order to attack his opponent's leg. The attacker turns his body so that he faces his opponent's legs.

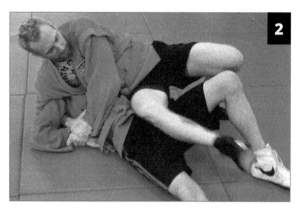

The attacker uses his left foot to post onto the mat for stability and then moves his right leg up and over his opponent's left hip and leg.

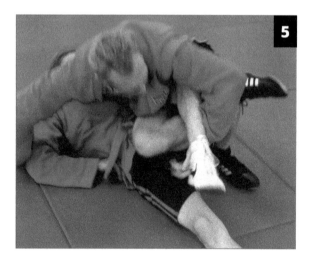

The attacker leans forward and uses his left hand and arm to hook and control his opponent's left leg as shown.

STRAIGHT KNEE BAR TO FAR SIDE OF OPPONENT FROM SIDE CONTROL

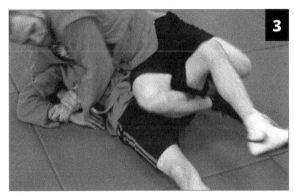

The attacker uses his right foot and leg to hook the inside of his opponent's left upper leg as shown.

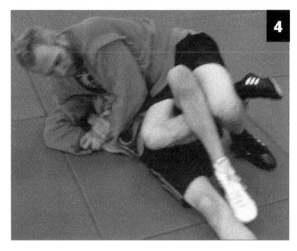

The attacker reinforces his leg control by entwining or lacing his legs, forming a triangle with his feet and legs to trap his opponent's left leg.

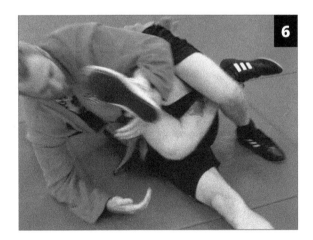

The attacker rolls to his right side as he continues to use his left hand and arm to hook and control his opponent's left leg.

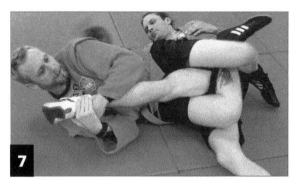

As the attacker rolls onto his right side, he uses both hands and arms to grab and trap his opponent's left leg, stretching and extending it. The attacker arches with his hips and applies the knee bar.

STRAIGHT KNEE BAR TO NEAR SIDE FROM SIDE CONTROL

This leglock is similar to the previous one except that the attacker rolls back and applies the knee bar from the near side of his opponent.

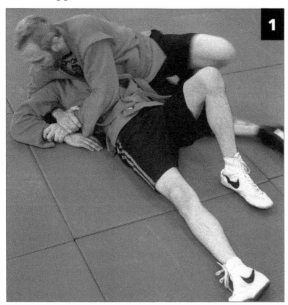

The attacker (on top) controls his opponent from the side with a bent armlock attack directed at the defender's right arm.

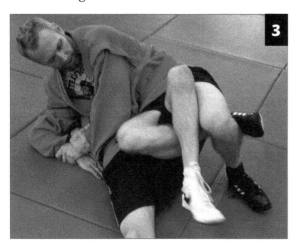

The attacker turns and faces his opponent's feet and uses his left foot to post on the mat for stability. As he does this, he swings his right foot and leg over his opponent's left hip and leg.

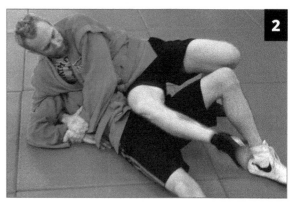

The attacker reinforces his leg control by lacing his opponent's left leg. As he does this, the attacker sits on his opponent's left hip area.

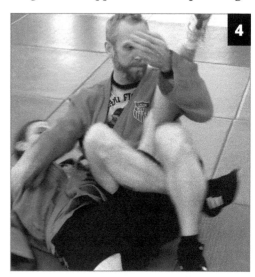

The attacker uses his left hand and arm to hook and control his opponent's left leg. As he does this, the attacker starts to roll backward.

The attacker rolls backward and uses both hands and arms to hook and trap his opponent's left leg. As he rolls back, the attacker immediately arches his hips and applies pressure on the extended left knee and leg of his opponent.

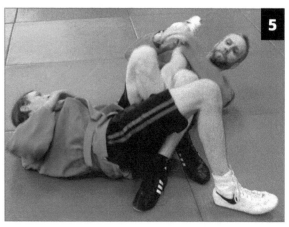

KICK BACK STRAIGHT KNEE BAR

This is effective if the attacker (top) is being prevented from getting close enough to apply a front chest hold by the defender on bottom.

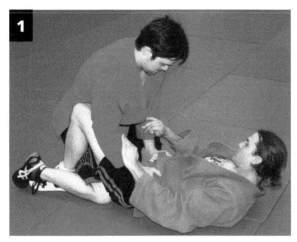

The attacker (top) is being prevented by his opponent from getting close enough to apply a hold-down. The attacker uses his right foot and leg to grapevine his opponent's left leg.

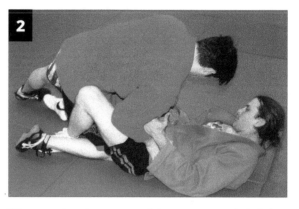

The attacker has trapped his opponent's left leg and uses both of his hands to push down on his opponent's hips. As he does this, the attacker starts to move his left foot and leg back to clear his foot from his opponent's right leg.

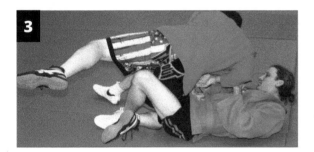

The attacker does a kick back with his left foot and leg, swinging it backward as shown. The attacker continues to use his right foot and leg to grapevine and control his opponent's left leg.

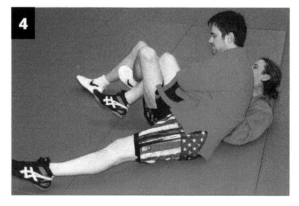

The attacker kicks back and sits on his buttocks. As he does this, the attacker uses his right foot and leg to lift his opponent's left leg up and off the mat.

KICK BACK STRAIGHT KNEE BAR

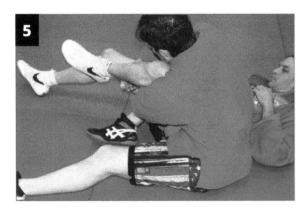

The attacker uses both hands and arms to hook and trap his opponent's left leg to the attacker's chest as shown.

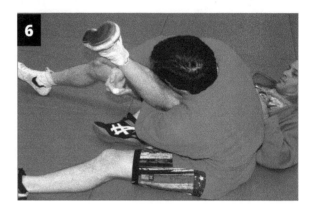

The attacker rolls to his left side.

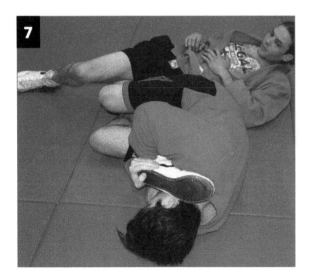

The attacker rolls to his left side as he continues to use his hands and arms to hug and trap his opponent's left extended leg to his chest. As the attacker's left side touches the mat, he arches his hips and bars his opponent's left knee.

TECHNICAL TIP: When applying straight leglocks, make sure that you are lying on your side and not on your back. By lying on your side, you have much better leverage in both trapping and then levering your opponent's leg and arching your hips (using the strength of your body) to stretch and apply the straight knee bar.

KICK BACK STRAIGHT LEGLOCK AGAINST OPPONENT'S LEG SCISSORS

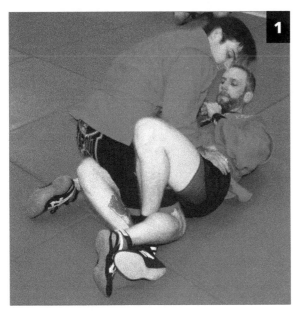

The defender (bottom) crosses his legs together in a leg scissors or half guard. The attacker (top) positions his right foot over his opponent's ankle (in this photo, the right ankle) in order to trap it.

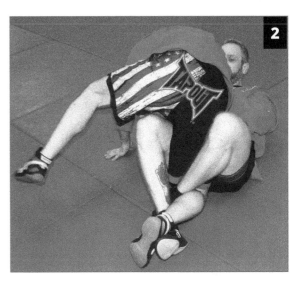

The attacker starts to swing his left foot and leg over to his back as shown.

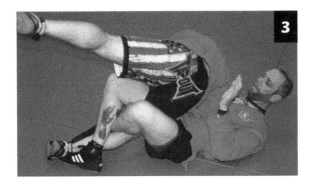

The attacker continues this kick back action with his left foot and leg. As he does this, the attacker continues to use his right foot to trap his opponent's ankle and lower leg area.

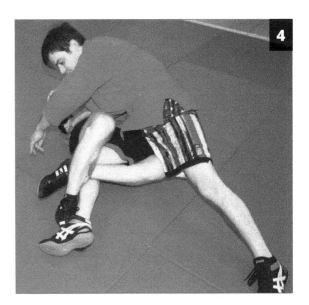

The attacker completes his kick back and starts to reach forward with his left hand.

KICK BACK STRAIGHT LEGLOCK AGAINST OPPONENT 'S LEG SCISSORS

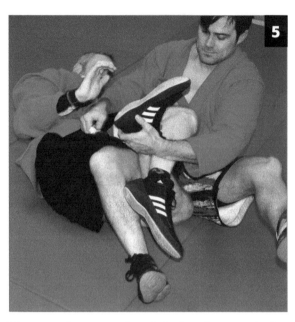

The attacker uses his left hand to grab his opponent's left heel. As he does this, the attacker sits back onto his buttocks, giving him stability. As he sits back onto his buttocks, the attacker pulls his opponent with him so that the defender on bottom will lay on his left side as shown.

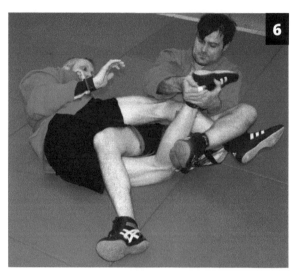

As the attacker pulls his opponent over, the defender on bottom will often move his legs over as well. When this happens, the attacker moves his left foot and leg over and hooks the defender's extended right lower leg as shown. Look at how the attacker continues to use both of his hands to pull back on his opponent's left foot.

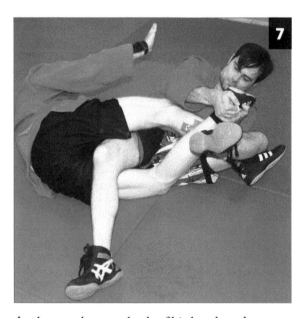

As the attacker uses both of his hands and arms to pull on his opponent's left foot, the attacker uses his left foot and leg to continue to hook over his opponent's right lower leg and drive it downward toward the mat. Doing this enables the attacker to better straighten out the defender's left leg.

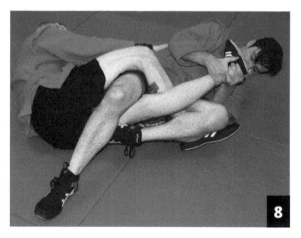

The attacker rolls back onto his left rear side and uses both hands to pull on his opponent's extended left foot and leg. This creates a straight knee bar.

TRANSITION FROM A STRAIGHT LEGLOCK TO A BENT LEGLOCK

Sometimes, the attacker may not be in the best position to secure a straight leglock or knee bar, or the defender may have managed to pull his leg back and out of position as a defensive maneuver. In this case, the sambo wrestler may switch to a bent leglock.

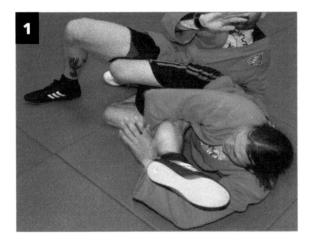

The attacker (on the right) realizes that his opponent has pulled his left leg back enough that the attacker is now unable to secure a straight leglock. The attacker starts to move his left hand and arm so that he will swing his left hand over his opponent's extended left lower leg. The attacker continues to use his right hand and arm to hook and trap his opponent's extended left leg as shown.

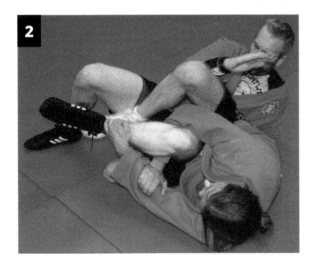

The attacker uses his left hand to grab his opponent's lower left shin area or ankle. The attacker places his right forearm in the back of his opponent's left knee and immediately uses his left hand to push downward on his opponent's left lower leg. Doing this forces the left leg to bend at the knee as shown. As he does this, the attacker starts to move his right leg up so that he will swing it over his opponent's left lower leg.

TRANSITION FROM A STRAIGHT LEGLOCK TO A BENT LEGLOCK

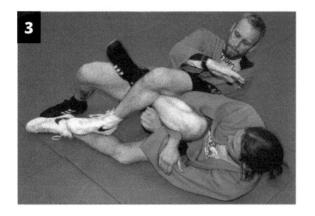

The attacker swings his right leg over his opponent's leg near the ankle as shown. Doing this helps bend the defender's left leg even more. Look at how the attacker continues to use his hands and arms to hug and trap his opponent's left bent leg.

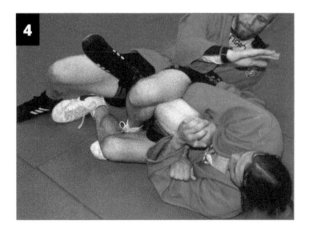

The attacker secures the bent leglock by moving his left leg over his right lower leg area forming a triangle with his feet and legs.

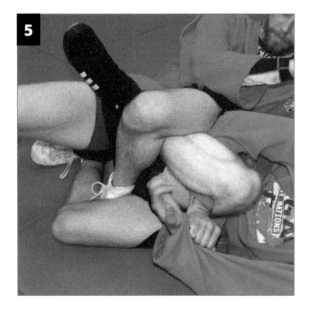

This view shows how the attacker forms a triangle with his feet and legs and uses his hands and arms to trap the defender's bent left leg. Doing this creates a strong bent leglock.

KICK BACK TO BENT LEGLOCK

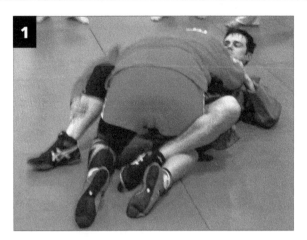

The attacker (on top) may have scored his points for his hold-down and has been instructed by the referee to go for his submission. The attacker raises up from his hold-down but makes sure to use his right foot and leg to hook and control his opponent's left leg.

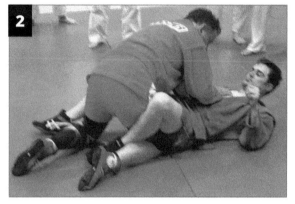

The attacker raises up enough so he will be able to swing his left leg back in a kick-back motion. Look at how the attacker continues to use his right foot and leg to trap his opponent's left leg.

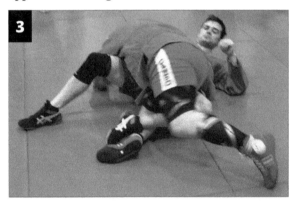

The attacker swings his left leg back in a kick back motion. Look at how he continues to use his right foot and leg to trap his opponent's left leg.

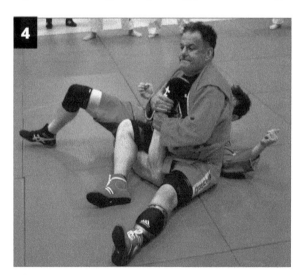

The attacker completes his kick back and sits on his buttock for stability. As he does this, the attacker immediately uses both of his hands and arms to grab his opponent's left foot or lower leg as shown. Doing this forces the opponent's left knee to bend.

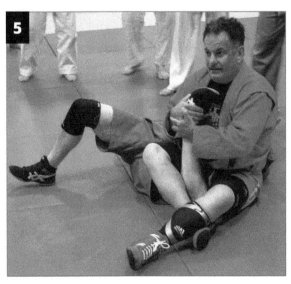

The attacker continues to use his hands and arms to grab his opponent's left ankle and pulls the ankle toward the attacker's body. The attacker can add further pain to the hold by leaning back. The attacker uses his feet and legs to from a triangle to further control his opponent's bent left leg.

KICK BACK TO A COMPRESSION BENT LEG LOCK

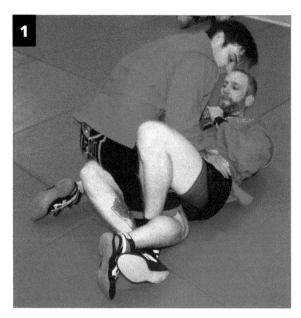

The defender (on bottom) crosses his feet or legs together forming a leg scissors or half guard. The attacker uses his right foot to hook over the top of his opponent's crossed feet. Doing this traps the defender's lower legs and ankles.

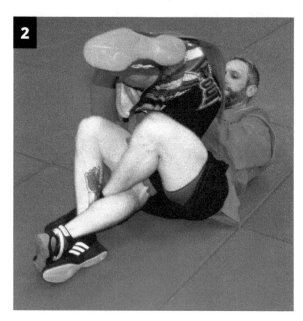

The attacker swings his left foot and leg back in a kick-back motion as shown.

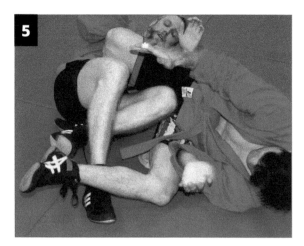

The attacker uses his left foot and bent leg to drive into his opponent's lower leg at the lower shin as shown. As he does this the attacker uses his right foot and shin to hook under his opponent's bent right knee and push forward with it. This movement of the attacker's legs can create pain in the defender's right leg, but not always.

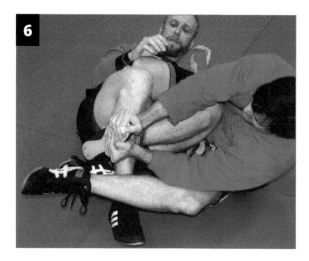

The attacker uses both hands to grab his right foot (as shown, near his toe area) and pull upward. As he does this, the attacker uses his left foot and lower leg to drive into his opponent's lower leg. This creates a compression lock.

KICK BACK TO A COMPRESSION BENT LEGLOCK

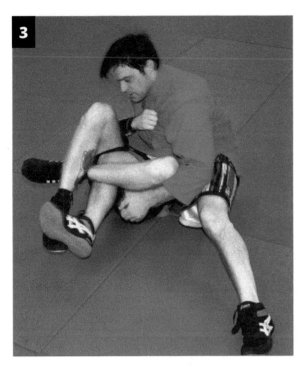

The attacker completes his kick back and sits on his buttocks for stability. Look at how the attacker continues to use his right foot to hook and trap his opponent's right foot. This trapping action prevents the defender from further movement, especially with his legs.

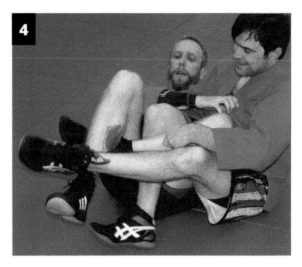

The attacker moves his left foot and leg over his opponent's right lower leg; as he does this, the attacker withdraws his right foot from his opponent's right ankle.

TECHNICAL TIP: Whether it's a leglock, armlock, hold-down, throwing technique, or transition, it is vital to aggressively pursue your goal. But, equally important, don't be so focused on one thing that you miss other opportunities. This is why it is important to train hard and train smart. Training smart means that you look for opportunities as well as learn how to create opportunities for yourself in practice; and then take that attitude and those skills into every fight or match.

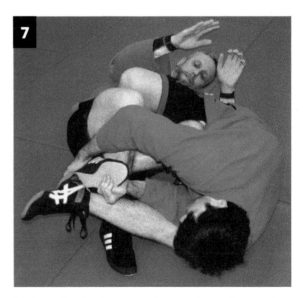

If the defender has not submitted yet, the attacker uses his right hand to grab his right heel and pull even harder. The attacker continues to use his left foot and leg to drive into his opponent's lower leg. This movement creates pain in the defender's bent right leg from the compression lock.

BREAKDOWN TO BENT KNEE LOCK AND TOEHOLD

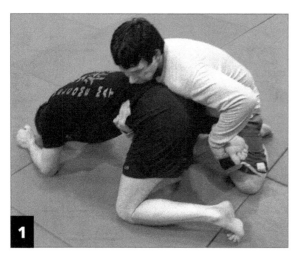

The attacker (on top) uses his right hand and arm to grab and hook under his opponent's waist and hip as shown. As he does this, the attacker uses his left hand to grab his opponent's right ankle and pull up and back on it.

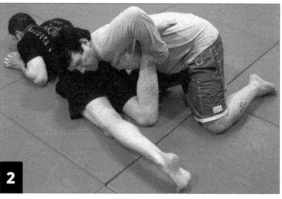

The attacker breaks his opponent down to the mat, continuing to use his left hand to hold and control his opponent's right ankle or lower leg.

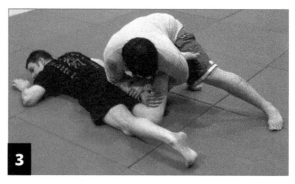

The attacker uses his hands and arms to form a figure-four hold on his opponent's lower right leg as shown. Look at how the defender's right foot is trapped under the attacker's left armpit area.

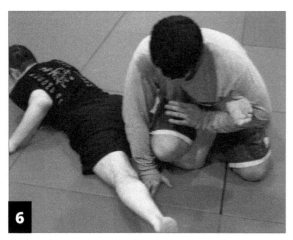

The attacker slides his right knee behind his opponent's bent right knee and upper leg as shown. Look at how the attacker has now moved his hands so that his left hand and forearm hook under his opponent's lower right leg and ankle. Doing this traps and secures the bottom grappler's right ankle.

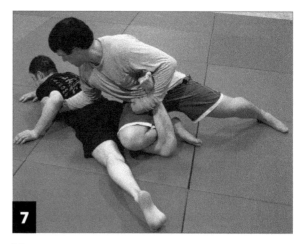

The attacker uses his right knee and shin to wedge behind his opponent's right knee as he uses his left hand and forearm to hook and trap his opponent' right ankle. As he does this, he uses his right hand and arm to hook under his opponent's left upper arm.

BREAKDOWN TO BENT KNEE LOCK AND TOEHOLD

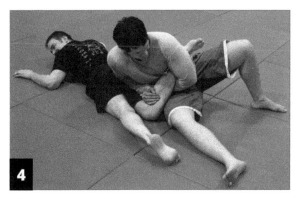

4

The attacker sits through with his right foot and leg and is now stabilized on his right hip and side as shown. The attacker can crank his opponent's bent right knee sideways as shown and get the tap out. This is a painful knee crank and is useful in submission grappling and MMA. It may not always be permitted in sambo, depending on the mat official.

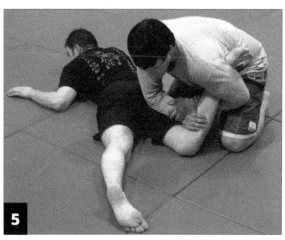

5

The attacker can continue on to a compression bent knee lock by moving up and onto his knees as shown. Look at how the attacker continues to control his opponent's lower bent right leg with his figure-four hold.

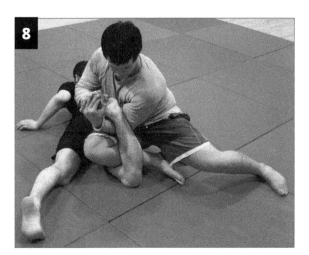

8

The attacker leans to his right and toward his opponent's upper body. Doing this creates a nasty bent leglock.

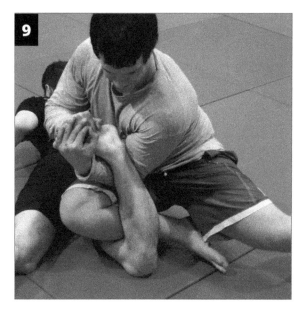

9

In submission grappling or MMA, the attacker can continue on to a toehold from this position. Here is a case of "double trouble" where the attacker applies both a bent leglock. This photo shows how the attacker uses his hands to grab and secure the toehold. There are a variety of toeholds and this is an effective one.

FAR LEG KNEE JAM BENT LEGLOCK

Here is another situation where the defender (on bottom) is lying on his front. Even if he is lying on his front for a split second, the attacker can take advantage of this situation.

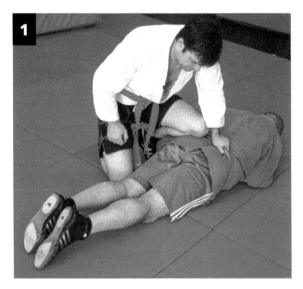

The attacker (top) starts to slide his left bent knee over his opponent's left hip or upper leg area.

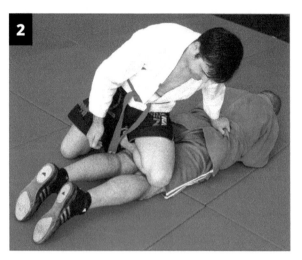

The attacker slides his left knee and shin across his opponent's upper legs so that his left shin is jammed on the defender's knee area (actually, just above the defender's knees).

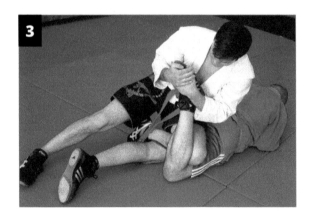

The attacker uses both of his hands and arms to grab and pull the defender's right foot up, bending it as shown. As he does this, the attacker continues to drive his left shin down and into the defender's bent knee, creating pain in the joint.

IMPORTANT: The attacker could have jammed his left knee and shin in the defender's near (left leg) if he so chose. Either way is good, but this application of the bent leglock was presented to illustrate how the attacker can use his left leg to trap and control his opponent's lower body as well as use his left leg to directly apply the leglock.

SIT ON OPPONENT KNEE JAM BENT LEGLOCK

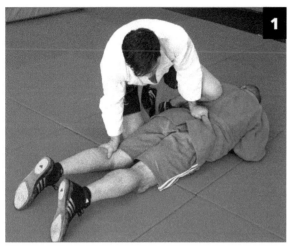

The attacker starts to move his left bent leg over his opponent as shown.

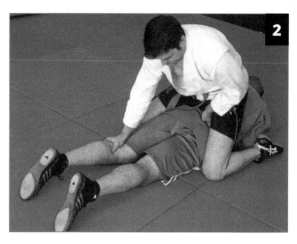

The attacker sits on his opponent's back and faces the same direction of his opponent's feet.

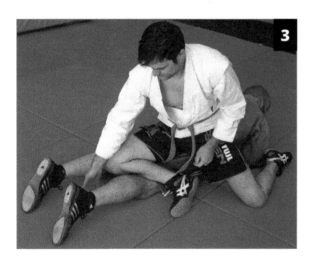

The attacker moves his right knee over his opponent and positions it so that the attacker's bent right knee and shin are jammed behind the defender's right knee as shown. As he does this, the attacker starts to reach with his right hand to grab his opponent's right lower leg or foot.

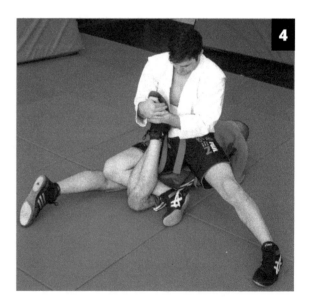

The attacker now uses both hands and arms to grab onto his opponent's right foot (at the shoelaces as shown) and pull. The action of the attacker's right knee and shin jammed behind the defender's bent right knee and the pulling action of the attacker on the defender's right foot create a nasty compression bent leglock.

LEG CRANK BENT LEGLOCK

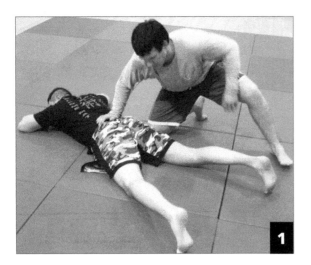

The attacker (on top) positions himself close to his opponent's right leg.

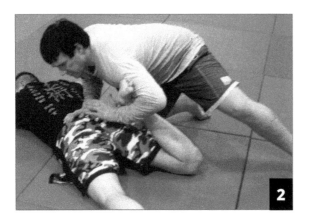

The attacker uses his left hand and arm to hook under his opponent's right lower leg and ankle. Doing this bends the defender's right leg at the knee joint.

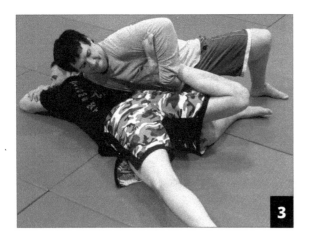

The attacker sits through with his right foot and leg so that the attacker is lying on his right side as shown. The attacker immediately leans to his back, and by doing this, the opponent's right knee is pulled up and off the mat and pulled toward the attacker. This cranking action is painful and causes the defender to submit. This is a useful bent knee lock for submission grappling and MMA but may not be permitted by some sambo mat officials. In this case, the attacker can forego this application and go on to apply the following leg-entwining bent leglock.

LOCK

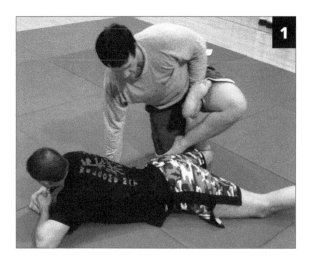

Picking up from #2 from the previous leglock, the attacker slides his left foot and leg around the back of the defender's right lower leg as shown.

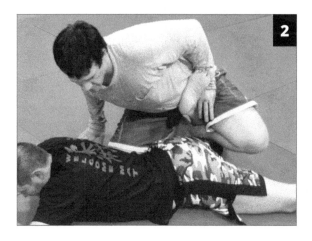

The attacker drives his left foot and leg down, and as he does this, the defender's right shin and ankle are wedged in the left hip area of the attacker as shown. The attacker leans forward and applies pressure to the bent knee and leg.

NEAR LEG LACE TO BENT LEGLOCK

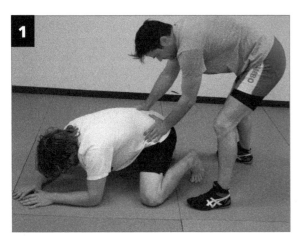

The attacker (standing) controls his opponent, who is on all fours.

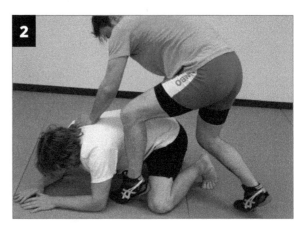

The attacker moves forward and starts to drive his left foot and leg over his opponent's left hip and upper leg as shown.

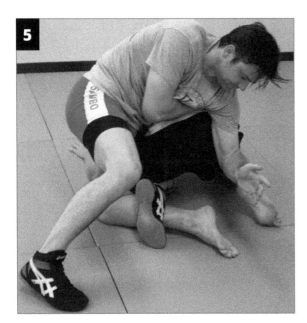

The attacker turns to his right so that he is facing the back end of his opponent. As he does this, the attacker uses his left elbow to push against his opponent's buttocks and uses his left hand and arm to reach down to start to grab his opponent's left lower leg and ankle.

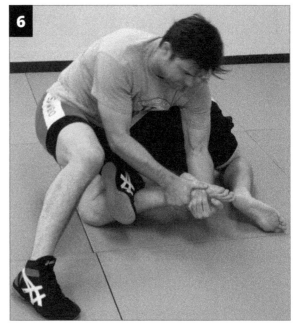

The attacker uses both hands to grab his opponent's left ankle and instep. As he does this, the attacker uses both hands to pull his opponent's left foot up and off the mat.

NEAR LEG LACE TO BENT LEGLOCK

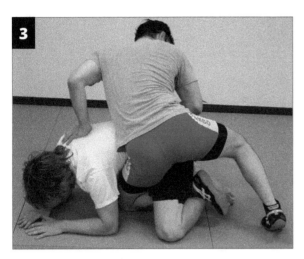

The attacker drives his left foot and leg down and over his opponent's left hip and upper leg. As he does this, he moves his left foot so that it laces or entwines his opponent's left lower leg and foot.

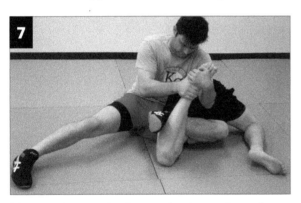

The attacker sits back onto his buttocks and uses both hands to pull back on the defender's left foot. Look at how the attacker uses his right foot and leg to post out wide for stability.

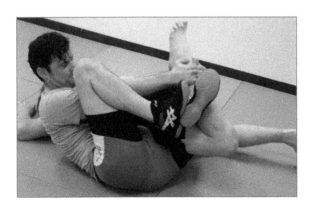

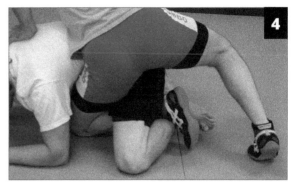

This shows how the attacker laces his left foot and leg around his opponent's left leg and ankle. Look at how the attacker uses his left foot to hook and trap his opponent's left lower leg and ankle.

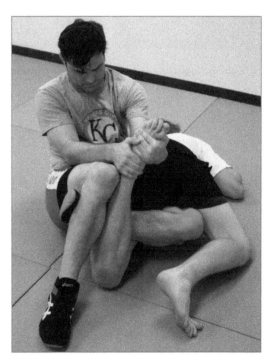

A variation for finishing (above) is for the attacker to form a triangle with his feet and legs and use both hands to pull on the defender's left foot. This triangle control with the legs prevents the defender from escaping and holds the left bent leg in place very well.

Another variation (left) is for the attacker to use his right foot to push on his right heel or foot as he uses both hands to pull on his opponent's left foot. The combined pushing and pulling action creates a painful finish. Look at how the attacker rolls onto his back, increasing the torque applied to the bent leglock.

CROWBAR BENT KNEE LOCK

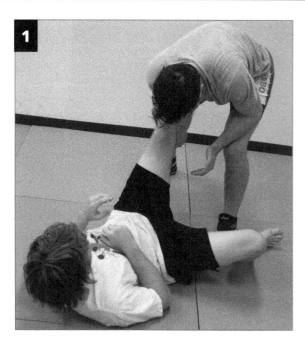

The attacker (standing) bends over his opponent.

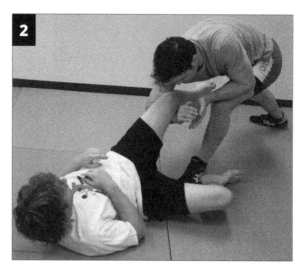

The attacker uses his right hand and arm to hook over his opponent's left lower leg. As the attacker does this, he steps forward with his left foot as shown.

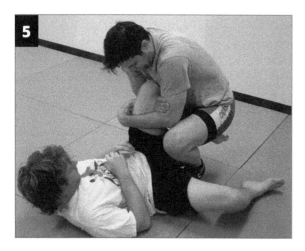

This side view shows how the attacker squats and traps his opponent's left bent leg.

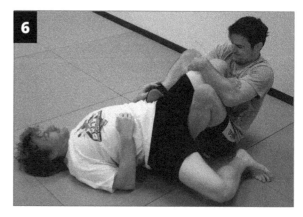

To apply pressure to the bent knee lock, the attacker rolls back onto his buttocks. This raises the defender's left leg and hips up and off the mat, creating a painful bent knee lock.

CROWBAR BENT KNEE LOCK

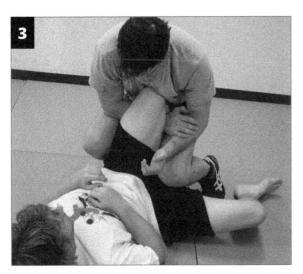

The attacker closes the space between his body and his opponent's by stepping in and squatting. As he does this, the attacker slides his right forearm under the knee of his opponent and starts to grab his left forearm with his right hand as shown. As he does this, the attacker moves his body forward and traps his opponent's left lower leg to the attacker's chest and torso.

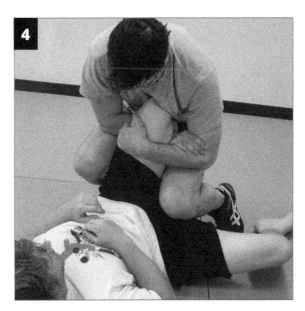

The attacker uses his right hand to grab his left forearm and forms a figure four with his hands and arms, trapping his opponent's left leg. The attacker uses his right hand to grab and hold his opponent's left upper leg. Look at how the attacker is squatting and uses his knees and legs to pinch together and trap his opponent's left leg.

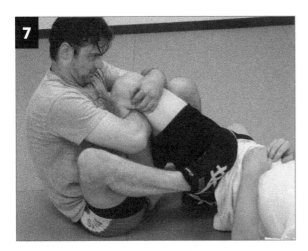

This view from the other side shows how the attacker uses his right forearm to wedge directly under the defender's left knee. Look at how the attacker places his right foot on his opponent's hip. The defender's right shin and lower leg is wedged and trapped in the attacker's chest. The attacker uses his right foot to push on the defender's left hip to add pressure to the compression bent knee lock. This is a painful bent knee lock.

TRANSITION TO CROWBAR COMPRESSION BENT KNEE LOCK

While the crowbar bent knee lock is painful when applied from a groundfighting situation, the momentum created by the transition from standing to groundfighting seems to add to the pain level for the defender.

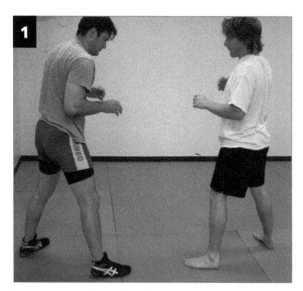

The attacker (left) faces his opponent in a standing position.

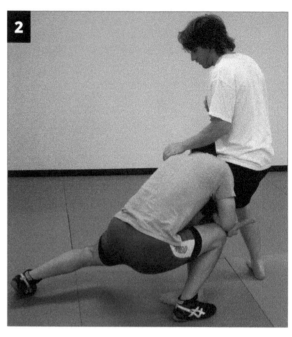

The attacker does a drop step in with his right foot and leg and uses both hands and arms to grab his opponent's left upper leg.

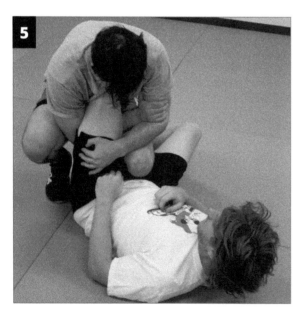

The attacker immediately follows through and applies the crowbar compression bent knee lock.

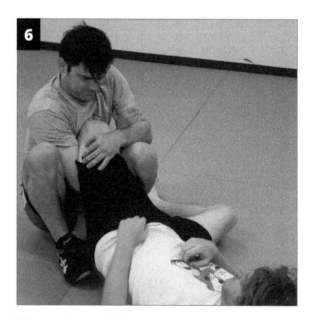

The attacker rolls back to apply pressure to the compression bent knee lock.

TRANSITION TO CROWBAR COMPRESSION BENT KNEE LOCK

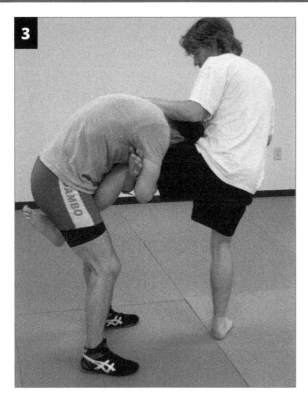

The attacker lifts his opponent's left leg up and off the mat.

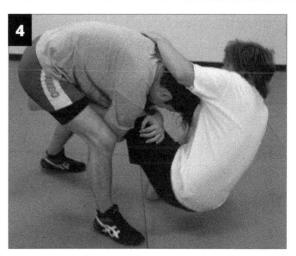

The attacker dumps his opponent down to the mat as shown.

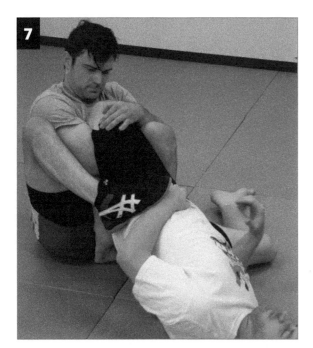

To control his opponent as well as to add pressure to the leglock, the attacker uses his right foot to push on his opponent's hip.

ROLLING STRAIGHT LEGLOCK

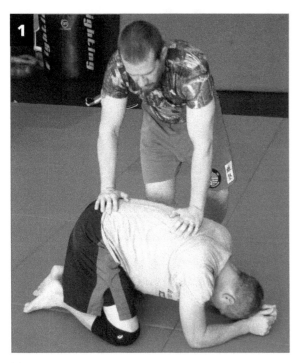

The attacker stands to the side of his opponent as shown.

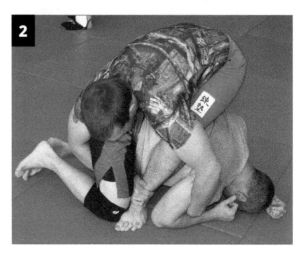

The attacker steps over his opponent with his left foot and leg. As he does this, the attacker uses his right hand to grab his left ankle. The attacker uses his left hand and arm to hook around his opponent's left upper arm as shown. Look at how the attacker starts to lean toward his left shoulder.

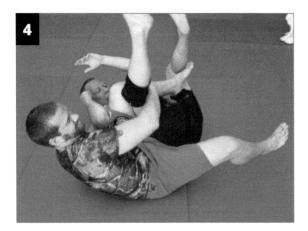

As the attacker finishes his roll, he continues to use his right hand to hold onto his left ankle. Doing this traps his opponent's right leg.

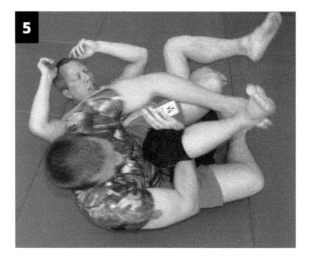

The rolling action has positioned the attacker on his right side as shown. As he completes the roll, the attacker uses his right hand to release his grasp of his left ankle and immediately uses his right hand to hook under his opponent's right knee. As he does this, the attacker starts to use his right hand and arm to hook and trap his opponent's right lower leg.

ROLLING STRAIGHT LEGLOCK

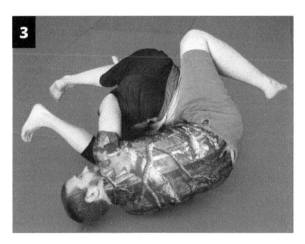

The attacker rolls over his left shoulder, and as he does, he forces his opponent to roll as well. The attacker continues to use his right hand to hold onto his left ankle during the roll. Doing this enables the attacker to roll more compactly and better control his opponent's left upper leg during the roll.

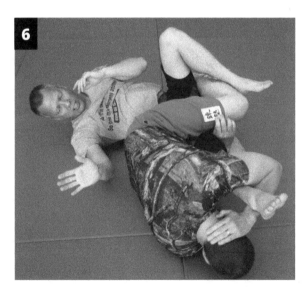

The attacker uses both hands to hook and trap his opponent's right leg, extending it straight. The attacker arches his hips and applies the straight knee lock.

SOME FINAL COMMENTS ON LOWER BODY SUBMISSIONS

Sambo is a fast-paced and aggressive fighting sport. As a result, the people who do sambo are more often than not attracted to submission techniques. Some sambo wrestlers have skill at both leglocks and armlocks, but in many cases athletes tend to favor one over the other. In either case, a fighter or grappler who enjoys making people submit is always a difficult guy to fight. One of my athletes, Jarrod Fobes, once commented that "nobody's leg should be safe." That's pretty good advice for a sambo wrestler who specializes in lower body submissions.

It's also important to remember that combat sports are more up-close and personal than other sports. From my early days as an athlete and then as a coach, I have believed that what we do is a fight, not a game. Because of this, I've always told my athletes that if you make an opponent surrender to you, he will never forget you and will never forgive you. He'll always remember that you're the person who made him give up.

As a final comment on lower body submissions, it's been my experience (as well as the experience of others) that sambo wrestlers or grapplers often do not tap out or signal submission quickly enough when a lower body submission has been put on them. Some athletes have said that they don't feel the pressure or pain until the very last instant, and by then it may be too late to avoid an injury. Significant tendon or ligament injury can take place if a grappler doesn't submit in a timely manner. This is one of the reasons the rules of sambo recognize a yell or verbal submission in addition to tapping out.

Okay, now it's time to turn our attention to upper body submissions: the armlocks of sambo.

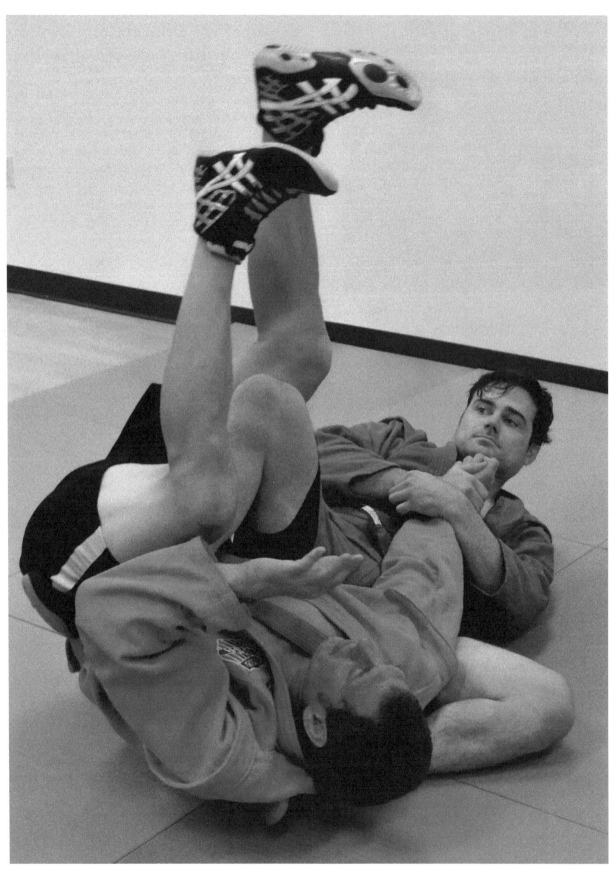

Chapter Four: The Armlocks of Sambo
"It's always a good day when you can armlock your opponent."

THE ARMLOCKS OF SAMBO

When the Soviet sambo grapplers first appeared on the world stage in the 1950s and 1960s, they brought with them a not-so-secret weapon: armlocks. It seemed as though these Soviet sambo grapplers could apply an armlock from almost any position, either in groundfighting or from a standing position. Isolated for many years from outside observers, the sambo exponents had developed the theory and practice of armlocks to a high degree of sophistication. And when the Soviet sambo men used a variety of armlocks with success against top-ranked Japanese judo men in international competition, the importance of stretching or bending an opponent's arm gained a new-found respect. Objectively, from both historical and technical points of view, it's apparent that the judo exponents from Japan gave birth to the initial development and standardization of armlocks, but it was the Soviet sambo exponents who refined armlocks into the precision-like weapons they became (and remain). In the 1960s through to the present, European judo athletes and coaches, as well as later exponents of every combat sport, have continued to develop and refine armlocks. So, it's safe to say that sambo has a great history and tradition of aggressive, realistic, and functional armlocks. As one of my athletes, Derrick Darling, said, "It's always a good day when you can armlock your opponent."

This chapter focuses on the armlocks (upper-body submissions) of sambo. Initial emphasis will be placed on the basic concepts of the three primary armlocks and then we will move into a variety of functional and realistic applications for these primary armlocks.

THE PRIMARY ARMLOCKS

From a sambo perspective, there are three primary armlocks. From these three fundamental and core armlocks, there are countless variations and applications. The three fundamental armlocks of sambo are: (1) the cross-body armlock, (2) the bent armlock, and (3) the straight armlock.

Cross-Body Armlock

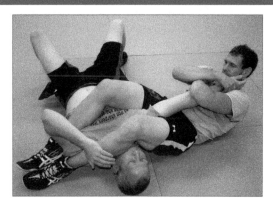

The primary feature of the cross-body armlock is that the attacker traps and stretches his opponent's arm across the attacker's pubic bone. In this photo, the attacker uses both of his hands and arms to trap the defender's right arm. The attacker also pinches or squeezes his knees and legs together so that the defender's right arm (closer to the defender's right shoulder) is trapped as well. The attacker "levers" or straightens the defender's right arm across the attacker's pubic bone. The defender's right elbow is jammed against the attacker's crotch and pubic bone. The attacker arches upward so that he applies more pressure from his hips and pubic area against the extended and stretched right arm of the defender. The cross-body armlock is one of the most versatile weapons in any sambo wrestler's arsenal. There are a variety of applications of the cross-body armlock.

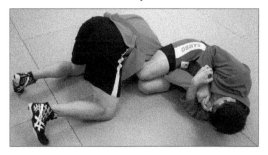

This photo shows the attacker lying on his left side as he applies the cross-body armlock.

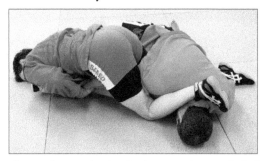

This photo shows the both the attacker and defender lying belly down as he applies the cross-body armlock.

Called udehishigi juji gatame (juji gatame for short) in Kodokan judo, this armlock has made its mark on international judo, sambo, and mixed martial arts as well as many other fighting sports and self-defense systems. The Japanese name, udehishigi juji gatame translates to mean "arm-breaking cross lock." A fitting name for this excellent technique.

For anyone interested in studying this armlock in serious depth, please get a copy of *Juji Gatame Encyclopedia*, written by this author and published by YMAA Publication Center. I'm not trying to peddle my book (although I have no qualms about doing that), but the book has over four hundred pages with over one-thousand photos of nothing but the cross-body armlock, and I honestly believe it's the most comprehensive presentation of this armlock on the market.

Bent Armlock

The bent armlock is one of the sneakiest and most painful armlocks ever invented (and sneaky is a good thing in sambo). The bent armlock can be done in two directions: (1) upward and (2) downward.

Bent Armlock (Upward Direction)

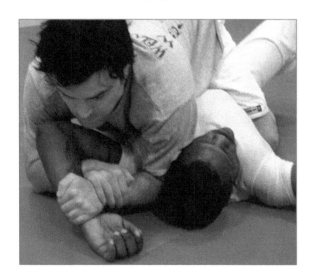

The attacker traps the defender's bent left arm with the defender's left hand pointed in the same direction as the defender's head.

Bent Armlock (Downward Direction)

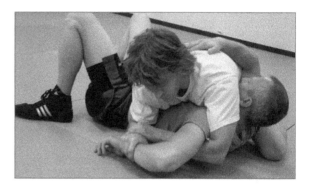

The attacker traps his opponent's bent left arm with the defender's left hand pointed in the same direction as the defender's feet.

Bent Armlock (Compression)

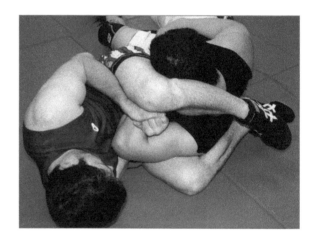

A variation of the bent armlock, most often applied in the downward direction, is the compression armlock. In this armlock, the attacker wedges one of his appendages between the defender's upper left arm and the defender's lower left arm and applies pressure.

TECHNICAL TIP: While the primary armlocks of sambo are directed at the opponent's elbow joint, it's often the case that the opponent's shoulder is compromised as well. This is especially the case in the bent armlock, where there is considerable pressure applied on the opponent's shoulder as well as his elbow.

Straight Armlock

This group of armlocks includes a variety of armlocks, the most recognizable feature of which is that they are all applied with the attacker straightening his opponent's arm and levering it against a fulcrum. These armlocks are also called "armbars" because the arm (specifically the elbow) is straightened and "barred" over a fulcrum. Shown here are some basic examples of straight armlocks.

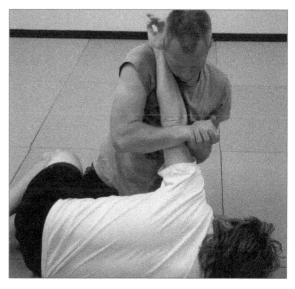

This application of the straight armlock is a good example of "barring" the arm. The attacker uses his head and right shoulder to trap his opponent's left arm at the wrist area as the attacker uses a square grip to trap and bar his opponent's extended and straightened left arm.

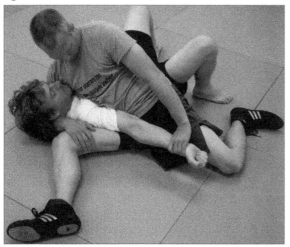

The attacker stretches his opponent's right arm out straight and bars it over his right upper leg. This application is the most fundamental way of doing the straight armlock, but it has stood the test of time and works at all levels of sambo competition.

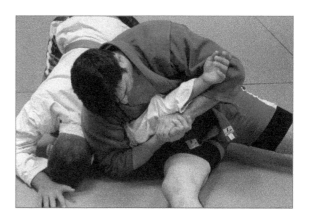

The attacker applies this variation of the straight armlock so that his opponent's left elbow is turned upward and pressed against the attacker's chest. The attacker applies leverage in opposite directions with each of his arms as shown. Doing this forces the defender's left arm to remain outstretched.

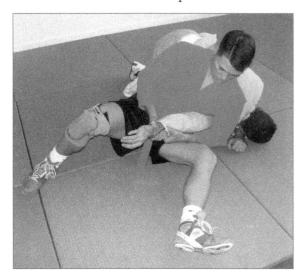

In this armlock, the attacker stretches his opponent's right arm and positions the arm so that its elbow is flat against the attacker's left ribcage or left side of his chest (serving as the fulcrum).

CONTROLLING YOUR OPPONENT IN ORDER TO ARMLOCK HIM

As pointed out in the previous chapter on lower-body submissions, it is vital to control the position in order to get the submission. The attacker's goal is to control as much of the action as possible so that he not only controls what he is doing, but controls what his opponent is doing.

Sometimes, the attacker may have to take some time to set his opponent up and control this position. In some cases, it may be a gradual set of movements that sets an opponent up so that he is susceptible to the armlock. In other cases, the attacker may set a fast pace or initiate a sudden and quickly applied armlock that takes the opponent totally by surprise much like in a throwing technique. In either case, it's most likely that the attacker took the necessary steps to control his opponent and applied the armlock when he sensed his opponent was vulnerable. This is true in applying armlocks as well as in applying leglocks (or anything else). If you don't control your opponent's body and how it moves, you will have to rely on luck to beat him, and luck rarely gets the job done. This is true in any aspect of sambo (or any fighting sport). And while any position that allows you to dominate your opponent's body is a controlling position, there are two specific positions that are common to sambo's approach to armlocks: the leg press and the shoulder sit.

THE LEG PRESS AND THE SHOULDER SIT POSITIONS

In many situations, the attacker will roll or turn his opponent onto the opponent's back and control him in what is called the leg press. Other times, the attacker will follow through from a throw or transition from another attack and control his opponent by pinning him to the mat by sitting or squatting on his head and upper body.

Let's take a look at these two useful controlling positions for armlocks.

LEG PRESS

Any time you roll an opponent over or in any way get him onto his back, and you are (generally) seated at his side with one or both legs pressing him down to the mat, you are in the leg press position. It is commonly used and effective. How long the attacker controls his opponent in the leg press depends on the circumstances. The leg press gives the attacker control over his opponent's body and as a result creates additional time to trap and control his opponent's arm, pry the defender's arm free, and secure the cross-body armlock. Sometimes, the attacker is unable to pry the defender's arms apart and straighten the arm to secure the juji gatame. The attacker can then use the leg press position to switch to another armlock or even control his opponent so he can move into a hold-down or use another variation of the cross-body armlock.

There are a lot of good drills you can do to increase your skill at controlling an opponent using the leg press. Please believe it: I'm not trying to sell books, but the books *Juji Gatame Encyclopedia* and *Conditioning for Combat Sports* have lots of useful and realistic drills for the cross-body armlock, including the leg press. If you study, practice, and drill on the leg press on a regular basis, you will discover that it's an effective position and a vital one in your arsenal of skills.

Leg Press: The Basic Position

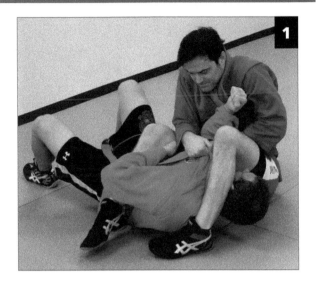

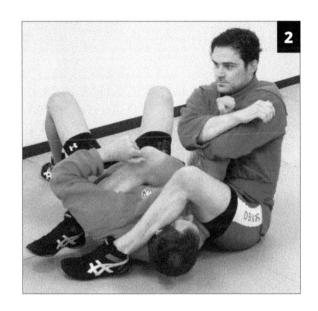

This photo shows the basic application of the leg press. The attacker may keep his opponent on his back in the leg press for a long or short period of time, depending on the situation. The attacker is seated at the side of the defender with one leg over the defender's head, trapping it to the mat. The other leg may be placed over the torso as shown here. In some cases, the leg may be jammed in the side of the defender's body as shown a bit later. The attacker uses this position to "ride," shifting his weight and moving as necessary to control the bottom grappler. This gives the top grappler time to trap the defender's arm and secure further control over him to apply juji gatame. The leg press position also allows the top grappler the opportunity to switch to another position, such as a pin or other submission technique. Many variations of the cross-body armlock in this book will use the leg press position. When in the leg press position, the attacker will "ride" his opponent, shifting his weight and moving as necessary to control the defender and keep him on his back. The attacker will constantly try to assert more control and attempt to lever or pry his opponent's arms apart so he can stretch his opponent's arm and apply the cross-body armlock. The leg press enables the attacker to control his opponent so the attacker can continue on and apply the armlock as shown in the next two photos.

This photo shows how the attacker uses both of his hands and arms to trap and control his opponent's right arm. This trapping action will be analyzed later, but trapping the opponent's arm is a necessary step in applying every armlock, no matter if the armlock is a cross-body armlock, bent armlock, or straight armlock. Now that the attacker has trapped and isolated his opponent's right arm, he will go on to secure the armlock. The attacker uses both of his arms to hug and trap his opponent's right arm to the attacker's chest and torso. Making sure that the defender's right arm is firmly attached to his chest, the attacker will immediately roll back to secure the cross-body armlock using the weight of his body to help straighten the defender's right arm.

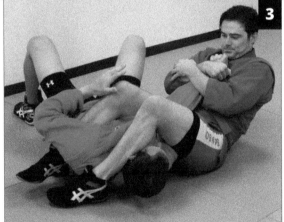

The attacker applies the armlock. The attacker rolls back with the defender's right arm completely straight and secures the armlock. Look at how the attacker keeps his arms hugging tightly to the defender's stretched arm. Doing this, the attacker uses the weight of his body to stretch and lock his opponent's arm rather than relying on his arm strength alone to extend his opponent's arm.

Leg Press: Ride and Control

The guy on the bottom doesn't want to be there. He'll do everything he can to get off of his back. Here are three photos to illustrate some of the many varied and different leg press positions that can (and will) take place. Obviously, not all situations can be presented here, but these three offer a good idea of how the top grappler must ride and control his opponent.

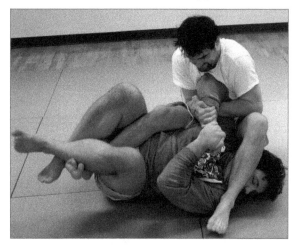

This photo shows how the bottom grappler uses his feet and legs to scissor the top grappler's right leg.

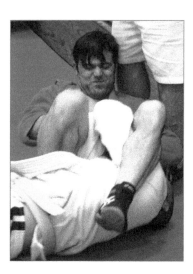

This photo shows the attacker with his left foot and leg positioned over his opponent's head and shoulders and his right leg jammed in his opponent's side. This photo shows that it's not always necessary for the top grappler to have both of his feet and legs over his opponent's head and torso to control him.

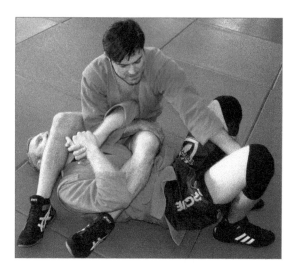

It's often the case that the top grappler will have to use his hands, arms or any part of his body to grab, control, and manipulate his opponent. This photo shows how the top grappler can use his left hand and arm to grab his opponent's right leg in order to prevent him from escaping.

HEAD OR SHOULDER SIT

The "shoulder sit" position is another important position that directly sets your opponent up for both the cross-body armlock and the bent armlock (as well as some applications of the straight armlock). It is a controlling position that is transitional and may not last very long. Think of this as when a vulture traps his prey. The attacker is hovering over his opponent just long enough to establish control and apply his armlock. It is a transitional position that takes place most often from a kneeling or squatting position, a throw (or takedown), or some other dynamic, moving situation. This position gives the attacker time and opportunity to assert more control over his opponent. The attacker may be in this position for a split second, immediately following through after throwing or taking an opponent to the mat or ground, or transitioning from one ground attack to another. The attacker may also be in this position for several seconds in an effort to establish further control of the opponent. The attacker can quickly and effectively use this shoulder sit position to trap his opponent's arm to exert more control and secure just about any armlock or hold-down. While the attacker can often apply the cross-body armlock or bent armlock from the shoulder sit, he can also quickly transition to any groundfighting skill he may choose, according to how the opportunity presents itself. This position also enables the attacker to get lower and closer to his opponent to more effectively trap the defender's arm and get into position to secure an armlock.

Head or Shoulder Sit Position: The Basic Applications

The head- or shoulder sit position is ideal for applying a variety of applications of either the cross-body armlock or the bent armlock. The following photo series shows how these two armlocks can be applied from the head or shoulder sit position.

Head or Shoulder Sit to Cross-Body Armlock

Along with the leg press position, this is one of the most common positions used when applying the cross-body armlock. Basically, the attacker squats directly over his opponent's shoulder and head as shown. This position is momentary and transient. The attacker may not be here very long; just long enough to trap his opponent's arm and secure more control before quickly applying juji gatame.

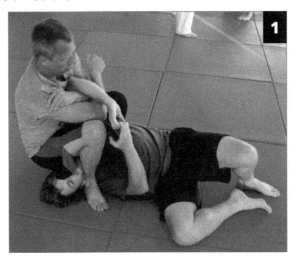

The attacker has just thrown his opponent, turned him over or in some way broken him down, and put him on the mat. The attacker immediately closes as much space as possible between his body and the defender's body by squatting over him as shown. Look at how the attacker has closed all space between himself and his opponent. An important point is that the attacker is squatting at this point and not kneeling. By squatting, the attacker has more mobility and freedom of movement. As the attacker does this, he immediately uses his hands and

arms to trap the defender's left arm (in this photo) to his torso. As he controls his opponent with the head sit, the attacker immediately starts to use his hands and arms to trap his opponent's left arm.

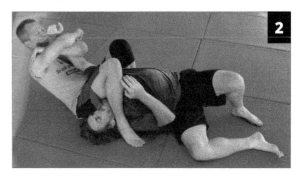

The attacker continues to control his opponent in the head sit and starts to roll back to apply the cross-body armlock from here.

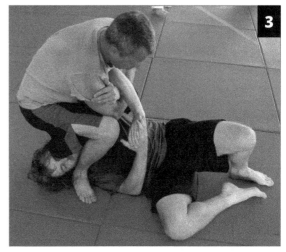

The attacker rolls back and pulls the defender's left arm out straight as he does, securing the cross-body armlock.

Head or Shoulder Sit to Bent Armlock

Not all head-sit positions are from a squat. In many situations, the attacker will sit on his opponent's head or shoulder and use his knees and legs to trap the bottom grappler's head. Doing this limits the movement of the bottom grappler's head and upper body as well as limits his ability to breathe.

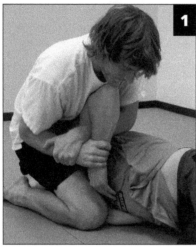

The top grappler sits on his opponent's head and upper body and uses both of his legs and knees to trap and squeeze his opponent's head. Doing this greatly limits the head movement of the bottom grappler and makes the whole situation a bad one for him. Here is a good example of how important it is to make life as bad as possible for your opponent when grappling with him. The less he likes being in this position, the less likely it is that he will attempt an escape or mount an attack of his own.

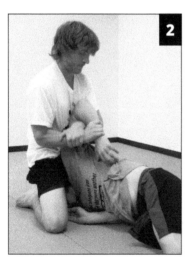

The attacker has used his hands and arms to form a figure-four grip on his opponent's left arm. While continuing to control the bottom grappler with the head sit, the top grappler lifts his body up in order to rotate to secure the bent armlock.

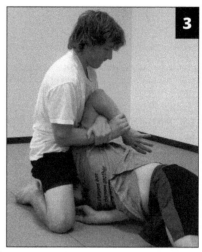

The attacker rotates his body to his left and levers his opponent's left arm, cranking it and getting the tap out. This series illustrates how an effective bent armlock starts from a strong controlling positon with a head or shoulder sit.

Sitting On and Trapping Opponent's Head and Arms

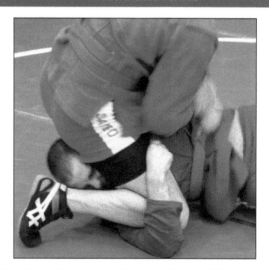

This photo from a match at the Sambo Nationals shows how the top sambo wrestler sits on his opponent's head and shoulders and uses his right knee to trap and control his opponent's right arm. As the top grappler sits and controls his opponent, he is starting to uses both his hands and arms to trap his opponent's left arm in an effort to apply the bent armlock.

TECHNICAL TIP: A good way to think about groundfighting and securing any kind of submission technique is to think of a sequence of three distinct (but interdependent) actions. (1) CONTROL: Control the position (control your opponent's body and limit his movement). (2) TRAP: Trap the appendage (arm or leg) that you intend to attack (or trap any part of your opponent's body that will better enable you to further control him). (3) LEVER: Lever or apply your armlock (or leglock) on your opponent's appendage (arm or leg), securing the armlock or leglock and forcing the opponent to submit.

TRAPPING THE OPPONENT'S ARM

Traps: Control the Opponent's Arm

What we call "trapping" is the action the attacker takes to control his opponent's arm (or leg if doing a leglock) and hugging it to the attacker's torso or chest, or isolating the arm so that the defender no longer has control over it. Doing this controls the opponent's arm and allows the attacker the control necessary to lever the arm free and secure the armlock. In most cross-body and straight armlocks (and in some applications of the bent armlock), the attacker traps and hugs the defender's arm to his chest or torso, and in some applications of the bent armlock, the attacker will trap the defender's arm to the mat or even to some part of the defender's body. An important element when trapping an opponent's arm is that the attacker uses his hands and arms to hook the opponent's arm rather than simply grabbing it with his hands. By hooking the opponent's arm, the attacker can more easily trap the arm to his chest and use the weight of his body to lean, roll, turn, or rotate to isolate and secure the arm for the armlock.

TECHNICAL TIP: Knowing how to trap your opponent's arm is an important skill. It may be boring to practice this phase of armlock training, but it's still a vital aspect to every successful armlock (or leglock, for that matter). The following photos show some of the many ways to trap an opponent's arm.

Trapping with the Arm for Cross-Body Armlock

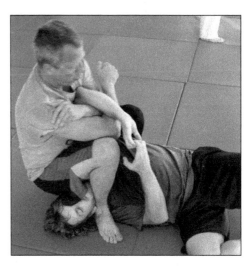

The attacker hooks the defender's arm, latches onto it, and immediately traps it to his chest as shown in this photo. As you can see, the attacker is in the shoulder sit position, and trapping his opponent's left arm is part of the entire controlling position.

Trapping the Arm to Isolate and Immobilize for Control

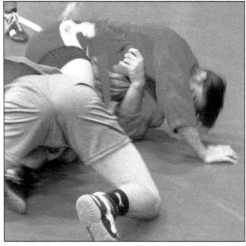

This photo illustrates how the attacker (on top) uses his left hand and arm to hook and trap his opponent's right arm as he turns to attempt either a cross-body armlock or a bent armlock. Often, the attacker may trap his opponent's arm with the intention of attacking it, but the armlock may not develop for some reason. By trapping the defender's arm, the attacker isolates and immobilizes the arm; the attacker can use this to switch to another armlock or use it to control his opponent further. So, even if the trapping action doesn't result in an immediate armlock, the attacker has nonetheless gained more control over his opponent.

Trapping the Arm When Rolling Opponent into Armlock

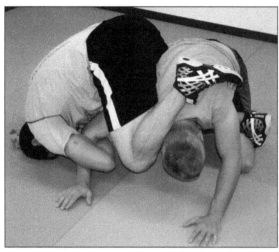

The attacker (on top) uses his left arm to hook and trap his opponent's right arm as the attacker starts his head roll cross-body armlock.

Trapping the Arm to Attacker's Chest or Torso for Bent Armlock

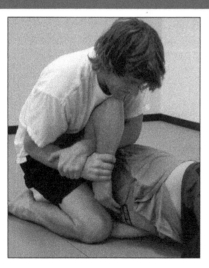

In some applications of the bent armlock, the attacker will trap his opponent's arm to the attacker's chest or torso as shown here. The attacker uses his knees and legs to trap and pin his opponent's head and upper body to the mat as he uses his hands and arms in a figure-four to hug and trap the bottom grappler's left arm to the attacker's chest and torso.

Trapping the Arm to the Mat for Bent Armlock

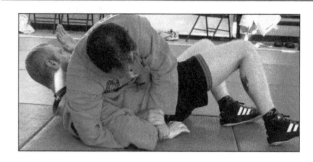

In some applications of the bent armlock, the attacker will trap his opponent's arm to the mat as shown here. By trapping the defender's arm to the mat, the attacker immobilizes and isolates the arm, making it vulnerable.

Trapping Opponent's Arm to Limit His Movement

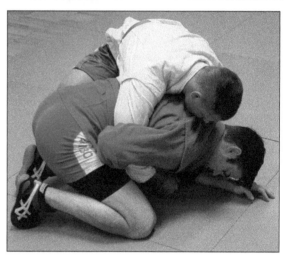

Sometimes, the attacker (in this photo, the bottom grappler) will have to trap his opponent's arm so he can isolate it and continue on with the actual armlock. In this photo, the bottom grappler is using his right arm to trap his opponent's right arm so that the bottom grappler can sit through and apply a straight armlock.

TECHNICAL TIP: You have to trap your opponent's arm before you can lock it. If you don't have control of your opponent's arm, he has a better chance of pulling it free and escaping.

Trapping Opponent's Arm with the Legs

The attacker doesn't just use his arms to trap his opponent's arm. The attacker can use his feet and legs as well.

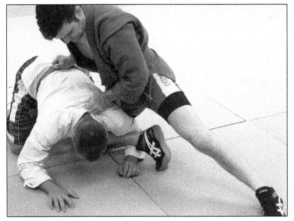

This photo shows a good example of how the attacker uses his (in this photo) right leg to hook and trap his opponent's left arm to start to control him for the armlock attack.

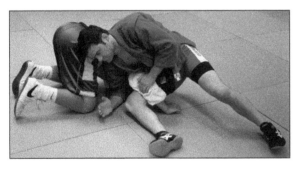

In this photo, the attacker not only uses his leg to trap his opponent's arm, he uses a number of other tools too. The attacker uses his right leg to trap his opponent's right arm as well as his right arm, elbow, and shoulder to assist in the trapping action. The attacker uses his right leg and hip to sit through and trap his opponent's right arm and shoulder

LEVERING THE OPPONENT'S ARM

Levers: Applying Biomechanics to Beat an Opponent

A "lever" is how we refer to the act of the attacker straightening his opponent's arm in order to apply the cross-body armlock or a straight armlock, or how the attacker bends his opponent's arm when applying a bent armlock. Rather than use the words "pry," "pull," or "bend," the term "lever" is a more accurate description. You can still use any of these descriptive words to refer to the act of applying the joint lock, but the word "lever" precisely describes the action of actually applying the joint lock. The opponent's arm serves as the lever as it is placed over the attacker's body part that serves as the fulcrum. From a mechanical point of view, every joint lock is some kind of application of the lever and fulcrum being used to defeat an opponent.

The following photos show the basic ways for the attacker to lever his opponent's arm for the three basic armlocks. While every variation of the three basic armlocks are different in setup and application, the principle of the lever and fulcrum act in the same way for every armlock.

Levering the Arm in a Cross-Body Armlock

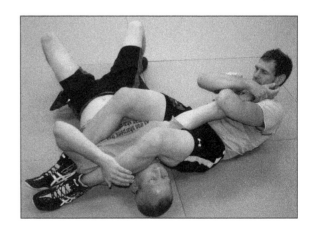

The attacker uses his hands and arms to trap the defender's right arm. The attacker stretches the defender's extended and straight right arm (the lever) across the attacker's pubic bone (the fulcrum).

Levering the Arm in a Bent Armlock (Upward Direction)

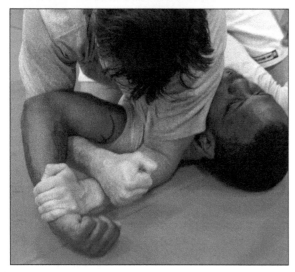

The attacker (top) uses his left hand to trap and anchor the defender's left wrist to the mat. As he does this, the attacker slides his right hand and forearm under the defender's elbow. Doing this places the fulcrum (the attacker's right forearm) directly under the lever (the defender's right elbow joint).

Levering the Arm in a Straight Armlock

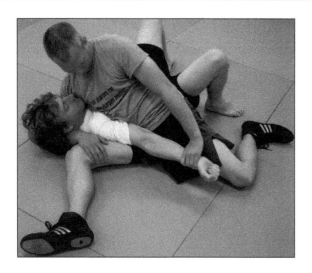

The attacker uses his left hand to grab and control his opponent's extended right arm as shown. As he does this, the attacker maneuvers the defender's right elbow (the lever) so that it is positioned directly over the attacker's upper leg (the fulcrum).

TECHNICAL TIP: By using the term "lever" to describe how you pry, bend, crank, manipulate, pull, or push your opponent's arm, you are accurately describing the action you take to make the armlock work whether you straighten or bend the elbow joint.

PROTECTING YOUR ARM AND ESCAPING FROM THE CROSS-BODY ARMLOCK

One of the worst positons to be in during a sambo match (or in any type of combat sport) is to be on the bottom in the leg press position with your opponent working to secure a cross-body armlock. So, if you are caught on the bottom in the leg press or the cross-body armlock, there are some logical steps to take in order to escape. First, "steal" your shoulder and arm back from his control. Your opponent stole your arm from you, and it's your job to steal it back. In other words, you must (first and foremost) do what is necessary to prevent your opponent from applying the armlock, so you must bend your elbow as you pull your shoulder and arm back into you so that your elbow is no longer situated on the attacker's pubic bone area. It's best to position your arm so that it is below your opponent's crotch or pubic bone so he can't lever your arm against it. The defender can do this regardless of the position. The defender may be flat on his back with the attacker controlling him in a leg press, or the defender may be on his knees with the attacker applying a cross-body armlock from a variety of positions. No matter how the cross-body armlock is applied, the concept is the same; steal your arm back so your opponent can't lock it.

Second, get to a stable base if at all possible. The odds are good that if you are in a defensive position with the attacker attempting a cross-body armlock, you are positioned mostly on your back or backside and not situated in a stable position. If you are on your back, immediately shrimp (or curl up), turning into the attacker. From this position, plant one or both of your feet on the mat for stability (never swing your legs up in the air; it is important to plant them firmly on the mat) and bridge into your opponent so that you are better able to sit up and get to a position on your knees. As you get to a more stable position, continue to steal your arm and shoulder back away from the attacker.

Third, the odds are that if you are able to do steps one and two, you and your opponent are scrambling for the superior position at this time. This is the time to try to control the position and gain the advantage.

Protect Your Arm and Get Off of Your Back, Steal Your Arm and Shoulder Back if You Are the Defender

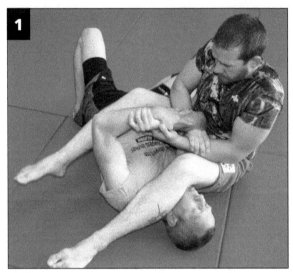

If the attacker has the defender on his back and in the leg press, the defender is in real trouble. While it may seem obvious, it is vital that the defender gets off of his back and, if possible, gets to a stable base and position. The defender's first task is to grab his arms together as tightly as possible and give the attacker as little room as possible to slide his hands and arms in to hook and trap the defender's arms.

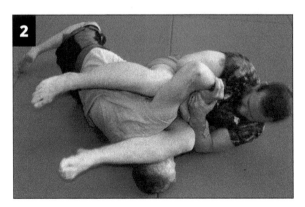

This photo shows how the defender shrimps or curls his body and turns into the attacker in order to get off of his back from the leg press position and initiate an escape.

Look at how the defender uses his feet to push off from the mat. Realize that defending and escaping from a bad position often happens in incremental steps. The defender doesn't jump up and escape from a leg press or other bad position in one big move. Be methodical, and realize that the only way you will get out of this predicament is to keep your cool and take care of things in order of importance. The defender must shrimp into the attacker as he steals his right arm and shoulder back as shown in this photo and not try to turn away; turning away may be a natural instinct, but it will only allow the attacker to control your arm better.

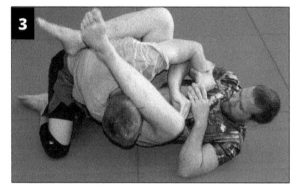

As the defender turns into the attacker and steals his right arm away, the defender makes sure to keep his right arm bent (that's the arm the attacker is trying to trap and lever). The defender makes sure to position his bent right elbow below the attacker's pubic bone (the attacker's crotch). The defender should jam his bent right elbow into his opponent's crotch to prevent the arm from being further straightened. As the defender does this, he continues to turn into the attacker and gets to a more stable position (on both knees for a good base).

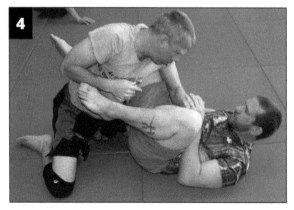

As the defender gets to his knees and a good base, he will be better able to pull his right arm free (the arm the attacker was trying to trap and lever) as shown in this photo.

BACK ROLL CROSS-BODY ARMLOCK

TECHNICAL TIP: Before you can counter (or even mount an effective escape) it is vital that you first protect your arm and get out of trouble. The previous series of photos illustrates the importance of doing everything possible to keep from getting your arm trapped and levered. For more information on defense and escapes, refer to the books *Armlock Encyclopedia* published by Turtle Press **and** *Juji Gatame Encyclopedia* **published by YMAA Publication Center.**

We're starting off with the fundamentals. And make no mistake about it: good fundamentals are the key to success. World-class skills are really nothing more than fundamentals applied to their full potential. This basic back-roll application of the cross-body armlock works for all levels of sambo wrestlers, from novices to masters.

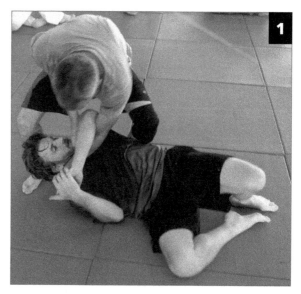

The attacker (standing) stands over his opponent, who is lying on his right side as shown.

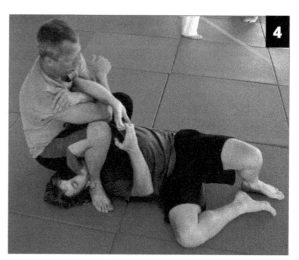

The attacker is squatting low and allows no room for the defender's upper body to move.

BACK ROLL CROSS-BODY ARMLOCK

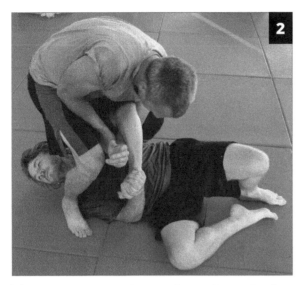

The attacker squats low and uses his right foot to step over his opponent's head, making sure to drive his right heel onto the bottom grappler's head, trapping it. As he does this, the attacker starts to use both hands and arms to trap the defender's left arm to the attacker's chest. The attacker places his left foot under the defender's left shoulder blade area.

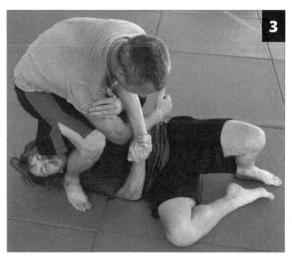

The attacker does a head sit on his opponent's left shoulder, and as he does, the attacker uses both hands to hook and trap the defender's left arm to the attacker's torso.

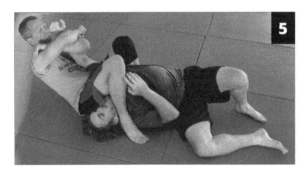

The attacker rolls back, using both of his hands and arms to trap and start to lever the defender's left arm out straight.

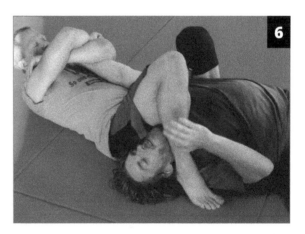

As the attacker rolls back, he uses both of his hands and arms to trap the defender's left arm to the attacker's chest and uses the weight of his body to straighten and extend the defender's left arm. The attacker arches his hips upward as he rolls back to create the joint lock on the defender's elbow.

SPINNING CROSS-BODY ARMLOCK

This is one of the most practical applications of the cross-body armlock used in any fighting sport, including sambo. From a sambo perspective, this application is ideal for the bottom grappler as he is working to get out of a front chest hold-down and apply an armlock as an effective counter. From a coaching perspective, if there is one move that is most recommended as the first thing to teach a novice, the spinning cross-body armlock is it. This movement teaches many important things about groundfighting, including an excellent and aggressive variation of the cross-body armlock.

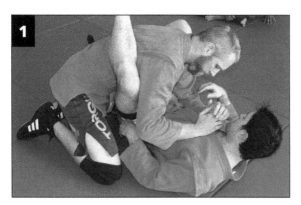

The attacker (on bottom) fights off his opponent's attempt to hold him with a front chest hold-down.

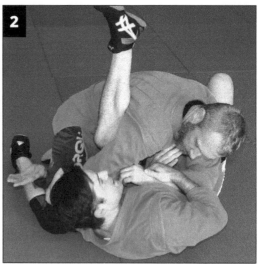

The attacker curls his body and spins to his left. As he does this, he places his left leg across the right side of the opponent's rib care area. The attacker uses his right hand to start to trap his opponent's left arm to the attacker's chest. The attacker uses his left hand to slide under the top grappler's right leg and hook it.

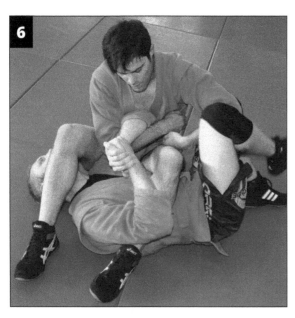

The attacker moves his left hand and arm to start to further trap and lever his opponent's left arm.

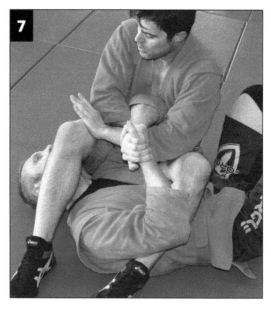

The attacker moves his left hand and arm under his opponent's left arm as shown. Look at how the attacker maintains control over his opponent with the leg press.

SPINNING CROSS-BODY ARMLOCK

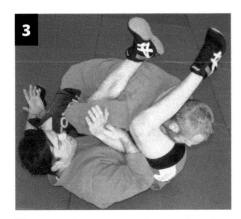

The attacker moves his right foot and leg over the top grappler's head. The attacker makes it a point to hook his right foot and leg tightly over his opponent's head to control it. As the attacker does this, he uses his right hand to further trap his opponent's left arm to the attacker's chest. The attacker doesn't "make a big deal" about trapping the defender's left arm in this way. Be sneaky about it.

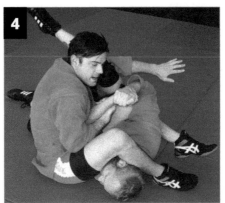

The attacker rolls his opponent over onto his back as shown. As he does this, the attacker makes sure to sit on his buttocks. The attacker's hips, crotch, and buttock are tight against the defender's left shoulder area. Look at how the attacker uses his left hand and arm to hook under his opponent's right leg as the attacker rolls him onto his back. It is essential that the attacker roll up and sit onto his buttocks to gain as much control as possible over his opponent.

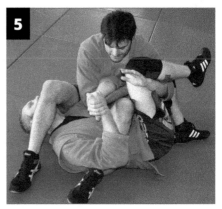

The attacker has his opponent on his back and is controlling him with a leg press. Look at how the attacker uses his right hand and arm to hook and trap the defender's left arm to the attacker's chest. At this point, the attacker still uses his left hand and arm to hook and control his opponent's right leg.

TECHNICAL TIP: When groundfighting, it is vital to "stay round." The spinning cross-body armlock is an excellent example of why staying round is important. Fighting on the ground or mat isn't a static thing. Movement is vital. By staying round, the attacker has more freedom of movement and can spin, shift the weight of his body more easily and generally have more freedom of movement, which translates into being able to exert more control over an opponent's body as well as your own.

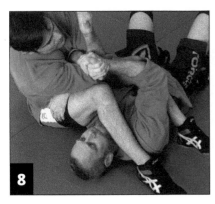

The attacker uses his left hand to grab his right thigh and slides his right hand (palm up) under his opponent's left forearm very near his wrist.

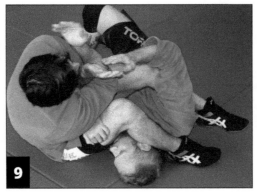

The attacker leans to his right (in the direction of the defender's head). As he does this, the attacker levers the defender's left arm free as shown.

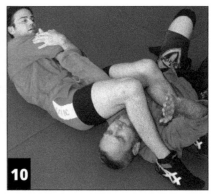

The attacker levers and straightens the defender's left arm and secures the cross-body armlock.

SPINNING CROSS-BODY ARMLOCK FROM A STANDING POSITION

This is one of the most useful and effective applications of the spinning cross-body armlock.

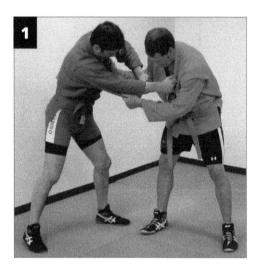

The attacker (left) stands so his left foot is near and slightly outside of his opponent's right foot. The attacker uses his right hand to grip his opponent's left lapel (this is important as an anchor for the attacker). The attacker uses his left hand and arm to grip on the top of his opponent's right sleeve to trap it.

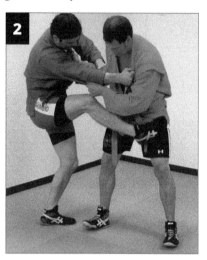

The attacker places his right foot on his opponent's left hip or upper leg area.

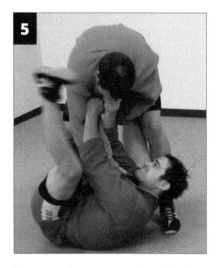

The attacker swings his left foot and leg over his opponent's head.

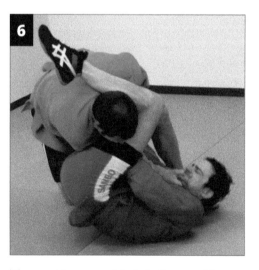

The attacker uses his left foot and leg to hook and control his opponent's head. The momentum of the attacker's spinning action and the attacker's hooking with his left foot and leg force the defender to roll forward as shown.

SPINNING CROSS-BODY ARMLOCK FROM A STANDING POSITION

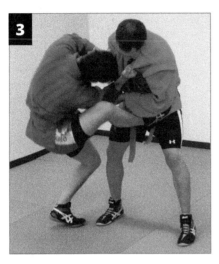

The attacker curls his body to his right and dips and spins under his opponent.

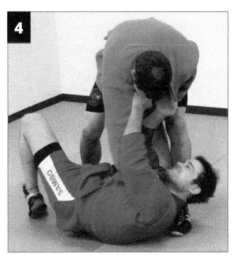

The attacker spins under his opponent, maintaining his right foot on his opponent's left hip area. The attacker is positioned sideways to his opponent as shown. The attacker forces his opponent to bend forward as shown. This is caused by the attacker using both his hands and arms to pull his opponent forward and down. The spin-under action of the attacker creates momentum, forcing the defender to bend over forward.

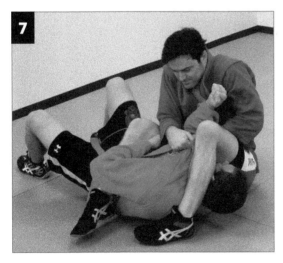

The attacker rolls his opponent over the defender's right shoulder, and the attacker sits up in a leg press position as shown. Look at how the attacker continues to trap and control his opponent's right arm.

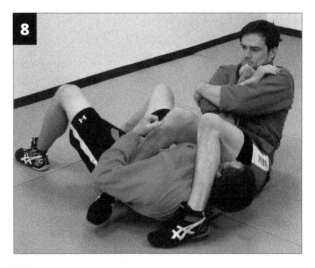

The attacker uses both hands and arms to trap and lever his opponent's right arm. The attacker rolls back and applies the cross-body armlock.

FOOT PROP TO BELLY-DOWN CROSS-BODY ARMLOCK

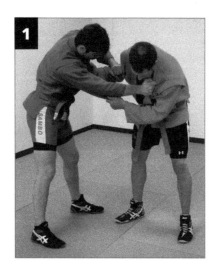

The attacker (left) stands so his left foot is slightly to the outside of the defender's right foot. He uses his right hand to grip his opponent's left lapel and his left hand to grab on top of his opponent's right sleeve or arm.

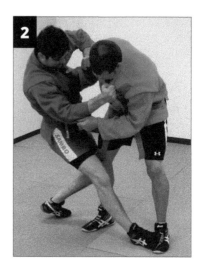

The attacker slides his right foot in front of his opponent and places it so that it blocks or props the defender's left foot as shown. As he does this, the attacker uses his right hand and arm to pull his opponent forward and down.

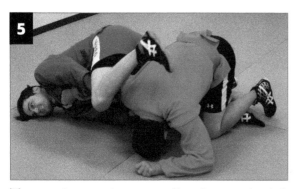

The attacker continues to roll and moves his left foot and leg over his opponent's head.

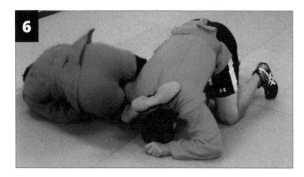

The attacker places his right foot so that the attacker's instep (the laces of his shoes) are placed on the back of his opponent's neck. Look at how the attacker's right knee is bent and how the attacker traps his opponent with his feet and legs. Note how the attacker is positioned so that he is lying on his left hip and side.

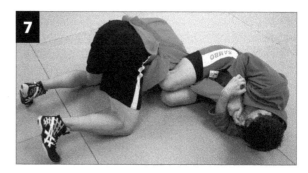

This view shows how the attacker is positioned on his left side and using his knees and legs to trap his opponent's outstretched right arm. Look at how the attacker uses both of his hands and arms to trap and lever the defender's right arm. The attacker can finish the armlock from this position if he chooses or if he is unable to force his opponent to roll.

FOOT PROP TO BELLY-DOWN CROSS-BODY ARMLOCK

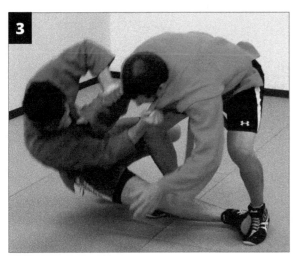

The attacker slides under his opponent as shown and forces the defender forward. Look at how the attacker uses his right foot to prop or block his opponent's left foot.

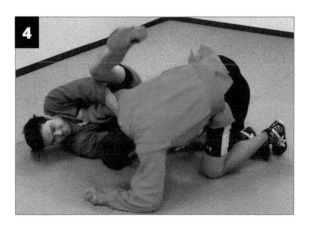

The attacker forces his opponent to fall forward so that the defender lands on his hands and knees as shown. The attacker rolls over his right side and swings his left foot and leg over his opponent's upper body as shown.

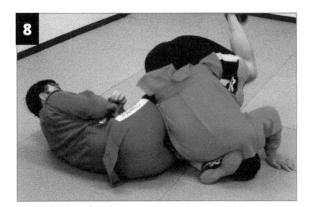

If the attacker chooses to roll his opponent, the attacker uses his right foot that is placed on the back of his opponent's neck to push into the opponent's head. As he does this, the attacker uses his right foot and leg to lift his opponent at the mid-section as shown. This action of the attacker's legs forces a whipping action and causes the defender to roll over his head as shown.

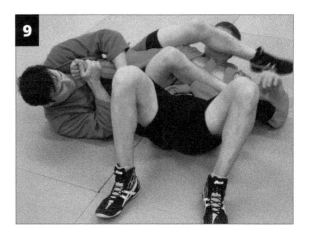

The attacker rolls his opponent over the defender's head so that the defender ends up on his back. The attacker moves his left foot and leg over his opponent's head to prevent him from sitting up and secures the armlock.

LEG DRAG TO CROSS-BODY ARMLOCK

If your opponent comes up on one knee in an attempt to stabilize his position, get past your leg, or to stand up, this leg-drag attack works well. This happens fairly often, so you might want to add this attack to your arsenal of skills.

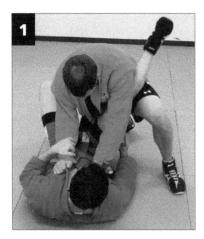

The attacker (on bottom) confronts his opponent who steps up so that his left foot is placed on the mat as shown.

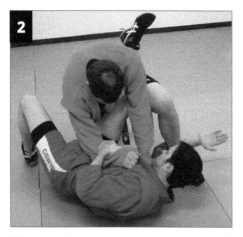

The attacker spins to his right and uses his right hand and arm to hook under his opponent's left lower leg. The attacker's right leg is placed across the left side of the defender's body as shown.

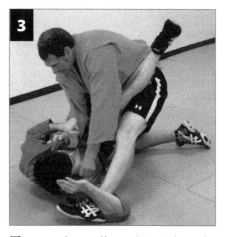

The attacker rolls to his right side, and as he does, he uses his right hand and arm to hook his opponent's left foot as shown. The attacker uses his right hand and arm to hook and pull the top grappler's left leg straight.

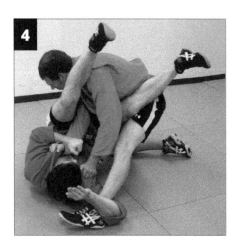

The attacker moves his left foot and leg over his opponent's head as he continues to pull the top grappler's left foot and leg out straight.

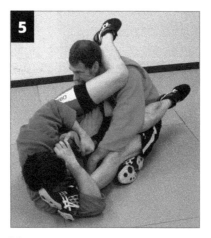

The attacker rolls to his right as he moves his left foot and leg over his opponent's head, hooking and controlling it. He continues to use his right hand to hook and pull the top grappler's left leg out straight. This forces the defender onto his buttocks. Note how the attacker uses his left hand and arm to trap the defender's extended right arm to the attacker's torso.

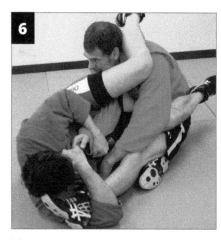

The attacker uses his right hand to grip his left lapel. Doing this firmly traps the defender's left foot, keeping the left leg straightened. As the attacker does this, he arches his hips and applies the cross-body armlock on his opponent's extended right arm as shown.

LEG DRAG TO BELLY-DOWN CROSS-BODY ARMLOCK

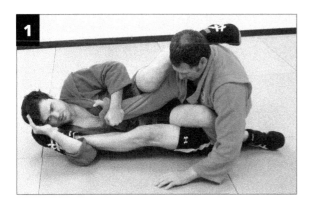

This photo picks up where the attacker has used the leg drag and forced his opponent onto his buttocks. The attacker places his left shin on the left side of his opponent's head so that the attacker's left instep will be placed on the back of the defender's head as shown.

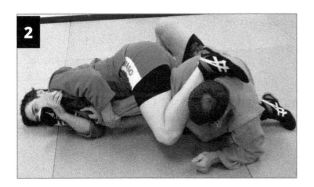

The attacker rolls to his right and as he does, he uses his left hand and arm to grab, hook and trap his opponent's extended right arm. The attacker also uses his right hand and arm to hook and trap his opponent's left extended leg as show. Look at how the attacker jams his left shin and instep on the back on his opponent's head and neck.

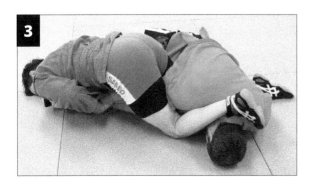

The attacker continues to roll and as he does, he arches his hips creating pressure on the defender's straight and stretched right arm.

LEG DRAG HEAD ROLL CROSS-BODY ARMLOCK

This application is similar to the previous leg-drag applications, but the major difference is that the attacker continues to roll and forces the defender to roll over his head with the attacker continuing on to apply the cross-body armlock.

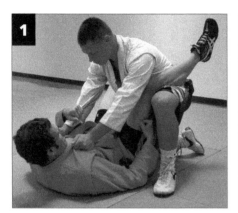

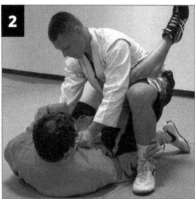

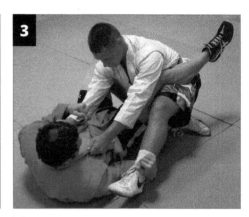

The defender (on top) steps so that his left foot is on the mat and his left knee is bent as shown. The attacker positions his right leg across the defender's left upper leg.

The attacker uses his right hand and arm to reach under and grab the top grappler's left lower leg or ankle as shown.

The attacker uses his right hand to pull and drag his opponent's left foot out straight as shown. The attacker uses his left hand to start to trap the defender's right arm.

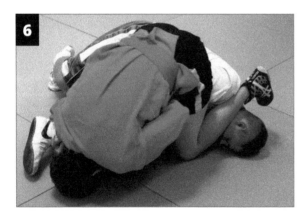

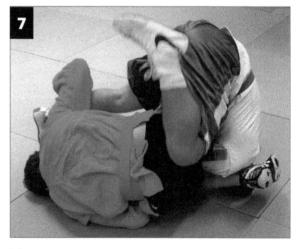

As the attacker rolls to his left, he makes sure to be positioned so that he is posted on the top of his head on the mat as shown. Doing this allows the attacker to roll more freely. Look at how the attacker's left shin is placed on the defender's head as the roll takes place. This forces the defender to roll over his head.

The attacker uses his right hand that is holding onto the defender's left lower leg to drag or pull the defender's left leg over, making for a smoother roll. Look at how the attacker uses his left foot and leg to push onto the defender's head and neck, forcing the defender to roll over his head.

LEG DRAG HEAD ROLL CROSS-BODY ARMLOCK

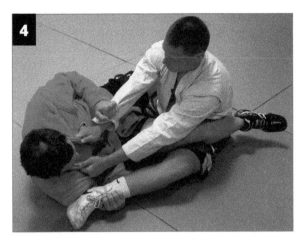

The attacker starts to roll to his right as he uses his left hand to continue to trap his opponent's right arm as shown.

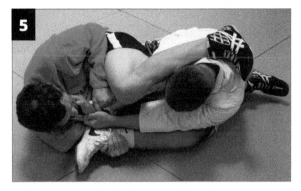

As he rolls to his right, the attacker moves his left bent knee so that his lower left leg (shin) and instep are placed on the back side of the defender's head as shown.

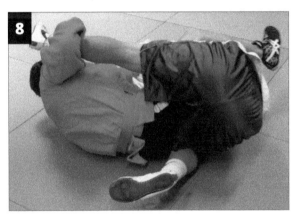

As the attacker rolls, he makes sure to swing the defender's left leg over. While not shown in the photo, the attacker continues to uses his left hand and arm to trap the defender's right arm.

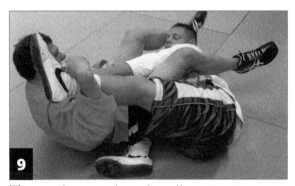

The attacker completes the roll, continuing to use his right hand to hold and control his opponent's lower left leg.

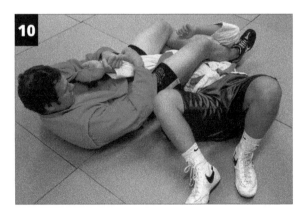

At the completion of the roll, the attacker immediately moves his left foot and leg over the defender's head to control it. The attacker releases his opponent's left lower leg with his right hand and uses both hands to secure the lever and apply the cross-body armlock.

VERTICAL FRONT CHEST HOLD TO HEAD ROLL CROSS-BODY ARMLOCK

This move is useful in both sambo and MMA.

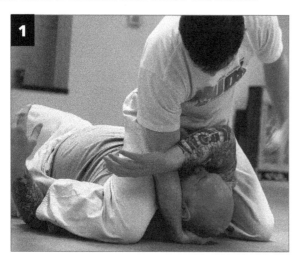

The attacker is holding his opponent with the vertical front chest hold (or mount in MMA). The attacker (on top) has positioned his body so that his knees are positioned high on each side of the bottom grappler's chest under his opponent's arms. The attacker has used his left hand to grab and move the bottom grappler's arm across his face and uses his right hand to hook under the bottom grappler's head as shown.

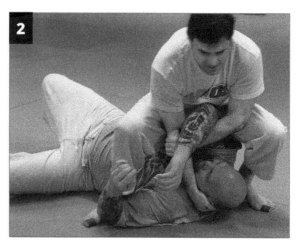

The top grappler springs up onto his feet and as he does, he uses his left hand and arm to hook under his opponent's right arm. Look at how the attacker's left foot in near the back of his opponent's head.

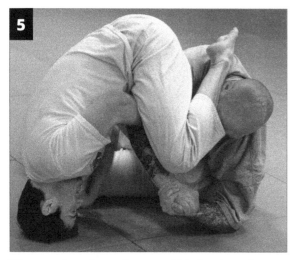

The attacker places the top of his head on the mat and has his left shin and instep firmly planted on his opponent's head as shown.

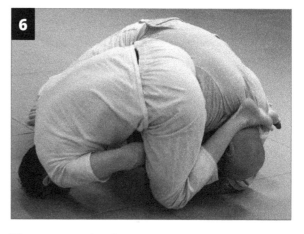

The top grappler drives his left knee to his left (in the direction of the bottom grappler's feet). Look at how the attacker has his left shin and instep firmly trapping the defender's head.

VERTICAL FRONT CHEST HOLD TO HEAD ROLL CROSS-BODY ARMLOCK

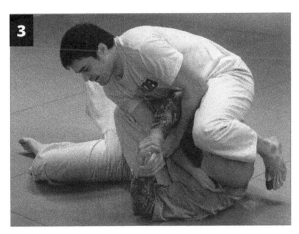

The attacker spins to his right. As he does, he moves his left foot and leg up as shown.

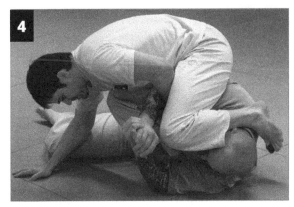

The top grappler continues to turn to his right and places his left shin on the back and side of his opponent's head. The top grappler uses his left hand and arm to continue to hook and trap the bottom grappler's right arm. Look at how the attacker places his right hand on the mat for stability.

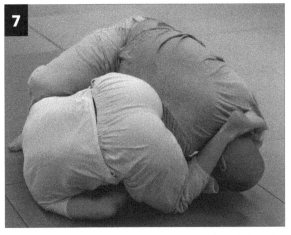

The attacker continues to roll onto his left side. The momentum of this action forces the bottom grappler to roll over his head.

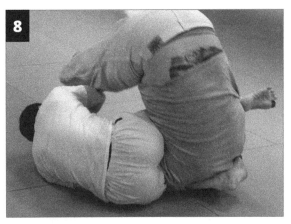

The bottom grappler is forced to roll over his head. Look at how the attacker uses his left foot (placed on the back of the defender's head) to push the defender's head and uses his right foot to push on the defender's torso. Doing this creates a whipping action that forces the defender to roll over his head as shown.

The attacker rolls his opponent over and secures the cross-body armlock.

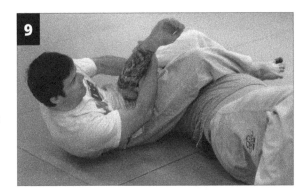

SPINNING CROSS-BODY ARMLOCK TO PREVENT OPPONENT FROM STANDING

This is a common situation where the top grappler attempts to stand and lift the bottom grappler off the mat as a defensive move to escape an armlock. To prevent the top sambo wrestler from standing and lifting him off the mat to negate the armlock, the bottom grappler can use this move. This particular variation of the technique is a fairly basic one, but it is highly effective.

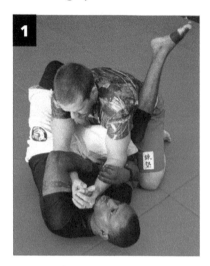

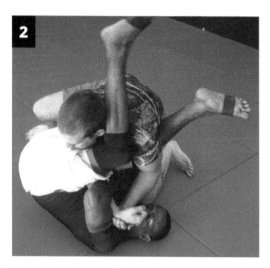

The attacker (on bottom) is attempting a spinning cross-body armlock, and the top grappler starts to get to his knees in an attempt to stand. The attacker uses his left hand and arm to trap the defender's right arm as shown.

As the top grappler attempts to stand, the attacker spins to his right and moves his left foot and leg over the top grappler's head. The attacker makes sure to use his left leg to hook and control his opponent's head. Look at how the spinning action of the attacker helps him to use his left hand and arm to further trap the defender's right arm.

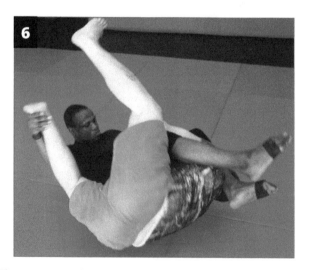

As the bottom grappler continues to spin under his opponent, he forces the top grappler to topple forward as shown.

The top grappler rolls forward over his right shoulder because of the momentum created by the spinning action of the attacker. Look at how the attacker can use his right hand to grab his opponent's right ankle in order to lift the right leg and help force the top grappler to roll over onto his back.

SPINNING CROSS-BODY ARMLOCK TO PREVENT OPPONENT FROM STANDING

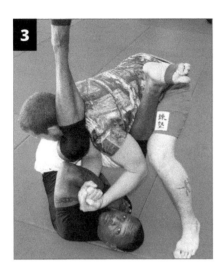

As the defender stands, the attacker continues to spin to his right. The attacker uses his left leg to hook over the defender's head and neck. Doing this prevents the defender from standing upright.

IMPORTANT: Sometimes, as the standing defender attempts to lift the bottom grappler off the mat, the bottom grappler can stretch his opponent's right arm and apply the cross-body armlock from this position.

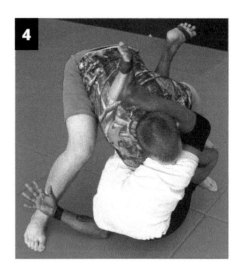

The attacker continues to spin under his standing opponent, making sure to use his left leg to hook over the defender's head as shown. Doing this prevents the top grappler from standing upright and forces him to bend over forward. Look at how the attacker uses his right hand to prop on the standing defender's right leg near the ankle. All the while, the bottom grappler spins under the top grappler.

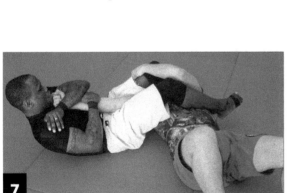

The attacker spins under his opponent and rolls him over onto his back as shown. The attacker applies the cross-body armlock.

KNEE JAM OR BELT LINE SPINNING CROSS-BODY ARMLOCK

The top sambo wrestler has attempted to hold his opponent with a front chest hold-down. The grappler on the bottom has managed to wedge or jam his right foot across the top sambo grappler's midsection or belt line in an effort to break the torso contact and escape from the hold-down.

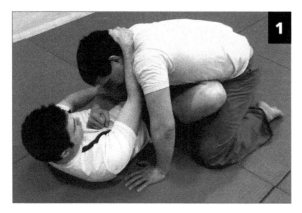

The bottom grappler (the attacker) positions his right bent knee so that his right lower leg is jammed across the midsection or belt line of the top grappler. The bottom grappler's right knee is pointed to his right, and his right foot is pointed to the bottom man's left. Doing this creates space between the bottom grappler and his opponent.

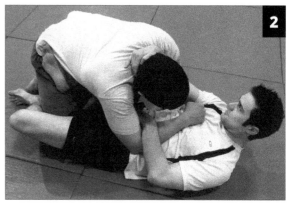

The bottom grappler's right foot is anchored at the top grappler's right hip as shown. Look at how the bottom grappler uses his right lower leg to create space between his body and the top grappler's body. The bottom grappler (the attacker) uses his left hand and arm to trap the top grappler's right arm to the bottom grappler's torso as shown.

TECHNICAL TIP: You don't always have to finish the cross-body armlock with both legs positioned across the defender's torso. Look at how the attacker has his right leg bent with his right foot jammed in the defender's back and right side as he uses his left foot and leg to trap his opponent's head. The important thing is for the attacker to pinch his knees and legs tightly together to trap his opponent's extended and straightened arm.

KNEE JAM OR BELT LINE SPINNING CROSS-BODY ARMLOCK

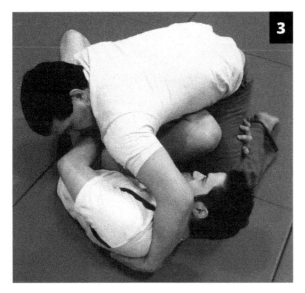

The bottom grappler spins to his right and uses his right hand and arm to hook under the top grappler's left upper leg. Look how close the bottom grappler's head is to his opponent's right knee and leg.

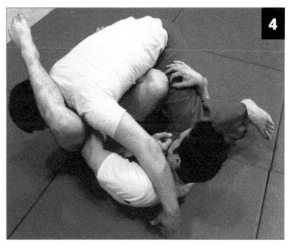

The bottom grappler moves his left foot and leg over his opponent's head and neck, hooking and controlling the head. Doing this forces the top grappler's head down. The bottom grappler continues to spin under his opponent and starts to roll the top grappler over. Look at how the bottom grappler's right knee and lower leg are positioned across the midsection of the top grappler's body. The bottom grappler uses his right leg to help push his opponent over.

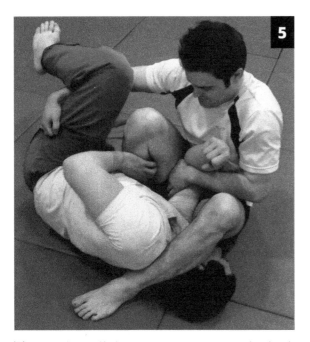

The attacker rolls his opponent over onto his back as shown. Look at how the attacker continues to use his left hand and arm to trap his opponent's right arm to the attacker's torso. The attacker makes sure to use his right foot and leg to hook and control his opponent's head, trapping it to the mat.

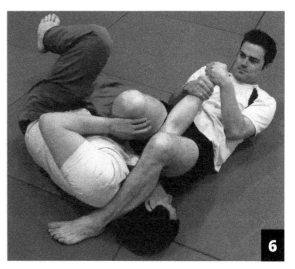

The attacker rolls his opponent onto his back, pinches his knees and legs together to trap the defender's right extended arm, and applies the armlock.

SPIN-AND-STRETCH TRANSITION TO CROSS-BODY ARMLOCK

This is a good example of how to transition from a standing position to an armlock. This is also a good drill that teaches how to throw an opponent and immediately transition to a cross-body armlock.

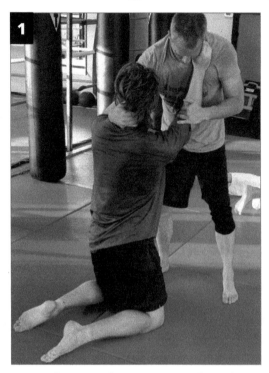

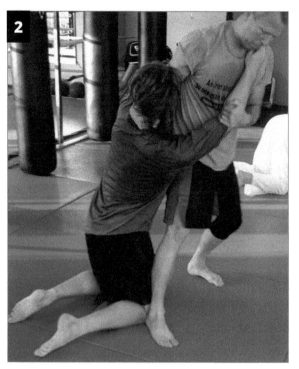

Sometimes, there may be a situation where the attacker (standing) may encounter his opponent who is kneeling. The attacker uses his left hand and arm to grab his opponent's right elbow. The attacker uses his right hand to hook around his opponent's head. When sambo jackets are worn, the attacker will use his right hand to grab his opponent's jacket between the shoulders.

The attacker moves his right foot and leg across the kneeling opponent's body and places his right heel at the right and outside of the kneeling opponent's right knee as shown.

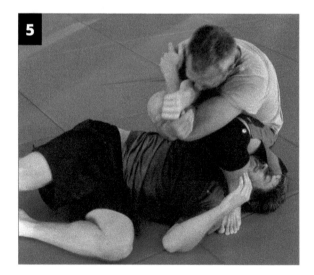

This view shows how the attacker uses his hands and arms to trap the defender's right arm to the attacker's chest as he does a shoulder or head sit. Doing this traps and isolates the defender and makes him vulnerable to the armlock that will follow.

SPIN AND STRETCH TRANSITION TO CROSS-BODY ARMLOCK

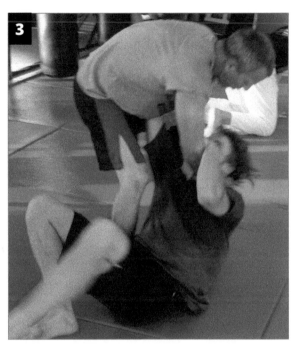

The attacker uses his hands and arms to pull and spin his opponent over as shown.

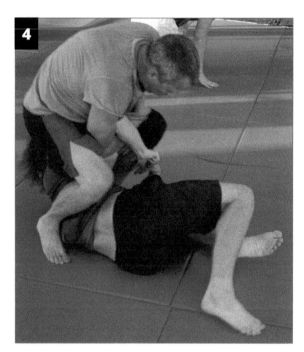

The attacker spins his opponent over and onto his right side as shown. As he does this, the attacker immediately uses his left foot and leg to step over the defender's head and places his right foot and leg at the defender's back as shown. The attacker immediately starts to squat and uses both his hands and arms to hook and trap the defender's right arm to the attacker's torso.

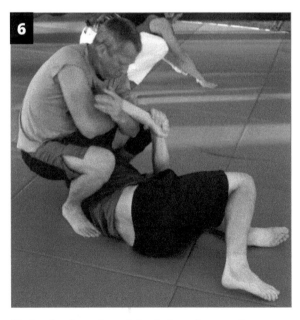

Going back to the original view, the attacker starts to roll back to apply the cross-body armlock.

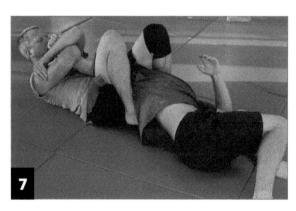

The attacker rolls back, stretching and extending his opponent's right arm, and applies the cross-body armlock.

HEAD ROLL CROSS-BODY ARMLOCK

This is one of the most effective (and as a result, one of the most popular) applications of the cross-body armlock. In this application, the attacker rolls the defender over the defender's head and onto his back. There are numerous variations of this head-roll application.

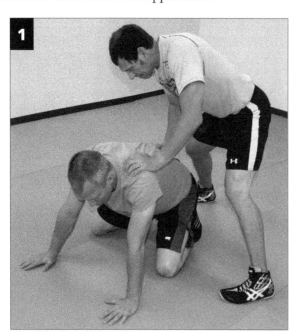

The attacker stands slightly to the left and behind his opponent who is positioned on the mat on his hands and knees as shown.

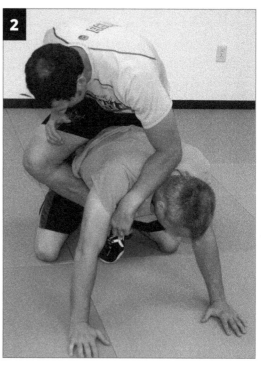

The attacker moves his right foot and leg over the defender's right hip.

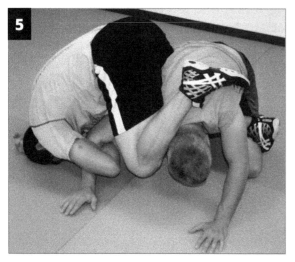

The attacker moves his left foot and leg so that his left shin is placed on the back of his opponent's head. Look at how the attacker is posted on the top of his head and how he uses his left hand and arm to trap his opponent's right arm. The attacker uses his right foot to hook and anchor the bottom grappler's left upper leg near the hip. All of these actions give the attacker excellent control over his opponent.

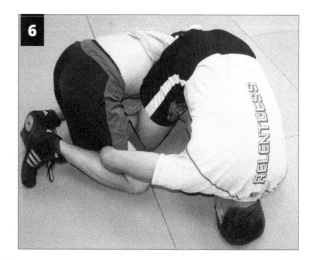

This view shows how the attacker is posting on the top of his head on the mat for maximum stability. Look at how the attacker uses his right hand and arm to hook and trap his opponent's right upper leg near the knee. The attacker's head and body are positioned so that the attacker's body is in a direct line from the defender's right shoulder.

HEAD ROLL CROSS-BODY ARMLOCK

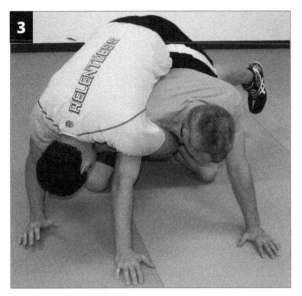

The attacker moves forward over his opponent's back. As he does this, the attacker uses his right hand and arm to hook and trap his opponent's right arm. Look at how the attacker uses his right hand to post onto the mat for stability at this point.

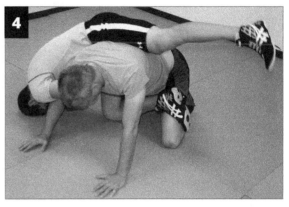

The attacker places his head on the mat so that the top of his head is on the mat (and not the side or front of his head—being on the top of the head is important since it allows the attacker better vision of what he is doing, good stability, and more freedom of movement).

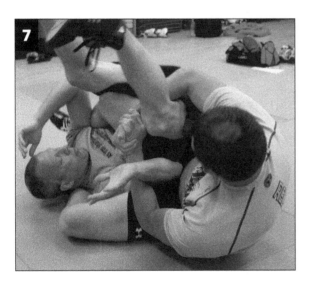

This view shows how the attacker rolls to his left side and rolls his opponent over his head. Look at the attacker's left lower leg on the back of his opponent's head at this mid-point of the roll. Also, look at how the attacker grasps his hands together, trapping the defender's right arm and right leg.

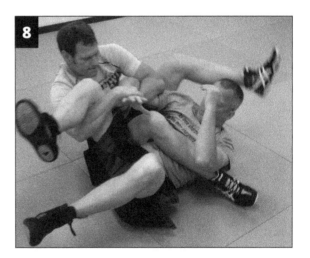

This photo shows how the attacker starts the finish of this attack from a different view. The attacker keeps good control with his right hand and arm to hook and trap his opponent's right leg as shown. The attacker uses his left hand and arm to trap his opponent's right arm as shown. Look at how the attacker moves his left foot and leg over his opponent's head to trap and control it. Notice how the attacker's right leg is positioned over his opponent's torso.

HEAD ROLL CROSS-BODY ARMLOCK

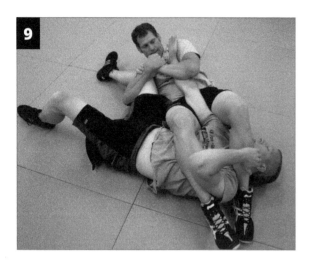

The attacker finishes the armlock by grasping his hands together as shown. By doing this, the attacker completely traps both the right arm and right leg of the defender. Look at how the attacker's body is angled, with the attacker's head close to the defender's right leg. This is a tight and effective finish to the cross-body armlock.

ALTERNATIVE FINISH

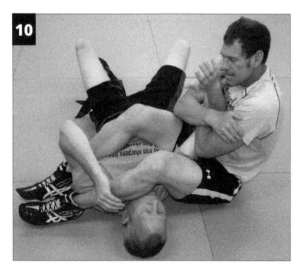

The attacker rolls his opponent over onto his back as shown. The attacker has released his hook and control with his right hand and arm on his opponent's right leg and uses both hands to hook and trap the defender's right arm to the attacker's chest.

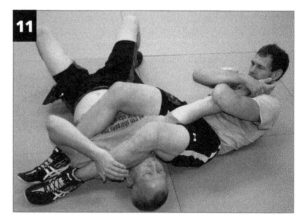

The attacker uses both his hands and arms to trap and lever his opponent's right arm out straight and applies the cross-body armlock.

HIP ROLL CROSS-BODY ARMLOCK

The attacker rolls his opponent in the direction of the opponent's hip in this application of the cross-body armlock.

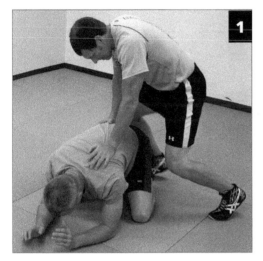

The attacker stands above his opponent, who is on all fours.

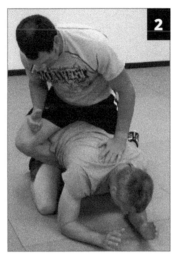

The attacker drives his right foot and leg over his opponent's back and under his body as shown.

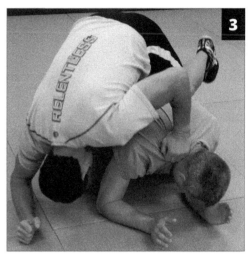

The attacker moves forward and places his right hand on the mat for stability. The attacker will put the top of his head on the mat.

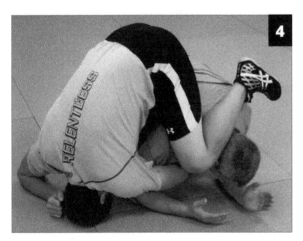

The attacker posts the top of his head on the mat for stability as he uses his left hand and arm to hook and trap his opponent's right arm. The attacker moves his left bent leg over his opponent's upper body and head as shown. So far, this application looks like the head-roll application of the cross-body armlock.

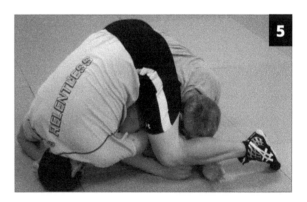

The attacker slides his left foot and leg so that his leg will be positioned under the defender's head. The attacker may choose to do this rather than the head-roll application.

HIP ROLL CROSS-BODY ARMLOCK

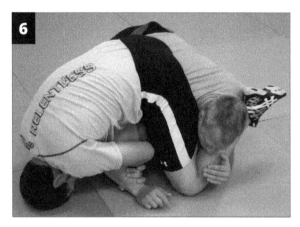

The attacker moves his left leg under his opponent's head as shown. Look at how the attacker uses his left bent leg to trap and control the defender's head. The attacker now uses both hands and arms to trap his opponent's right arm to the attacker's chest.

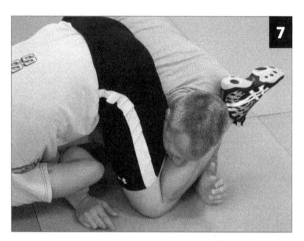

This close view shows how the attacker's left leg traps his opponent's head in this hooking action. Doing this will help control the defender in the rolling action to come.

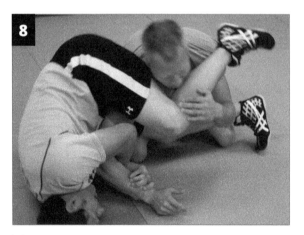

The attacker rolls over his right shoulder in the direction of the bottom grappler's right hip.

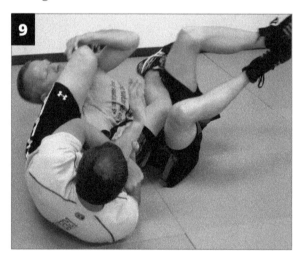

The attacker rolls over his right shoulder and forces his opponent to roll over as well. Look at how the attacker uses his left leg to hook his opponent's head and force it over. As he rolls, the attacker makes sure to use both hands to trap and start to lever the defender's right arm to the attacker's chest.

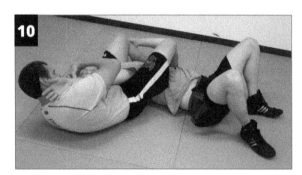

The attacker completes the hip-roll action and secures the cross-body armlock.

ADAMS TURN TO CROSS-BODY ARMLOCK

The author learned this application of the cross-body armlock from World Judo Champion Neil Adams.

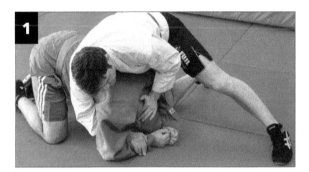

The attacker (top) rides his opponent and uses his right hand and arm to trap his opponent's right forearm as shown.

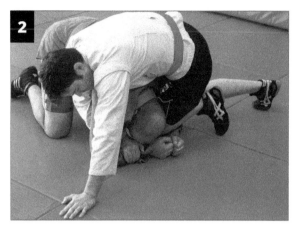

This view shows how the attacker places his left knee on his opponent's left forearm, trapping it. The attacker places his left hand on the mat for stability.

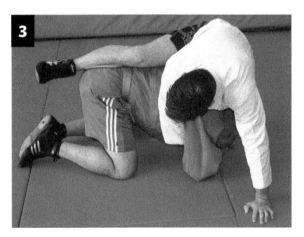

The attacker moves his right foot and leg over his opponent's back and hip as shown.

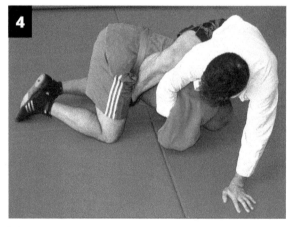

The attacker moves his right foot over his opponent's hip and jams it under the bottom grappler's right hip and upper leg area as shown.

ADAMS TURN TO CROSS-BODY ARMLOCK

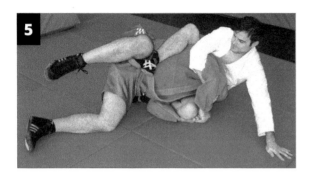

The attacker rolls back onto his left hips and buttocks as he uses his right foot to hook and pull his opponent's right upper leg in an upward direction. Doing this forces the bottom grappler to turn onto his left shoulder.

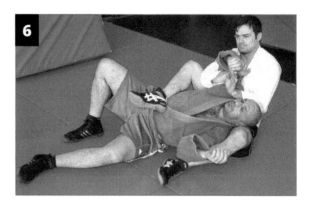

The attacker sits on his buttocks as he turns his opponent. The attacker now has his right foot and leg over his opponent's torso. The attacker's left leg is now positioned under the defender's head. The attacker starts to use both hands and arms to hook and trap the defender's right arm to the attacker's chest.

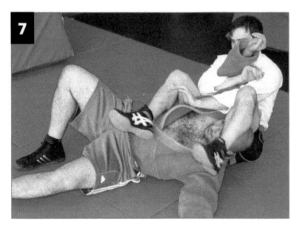

The attacker moves his left foot and leg over his opponent's head.

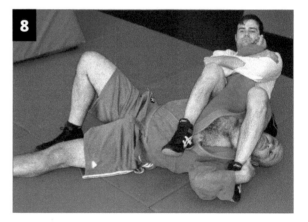

The attacker rolls back and uses both of his hands and arms to trap and lever his opponent's right arm out straight to apply the armlock.

LEG SCISSORS BACK ROLL CROSS-BODY ARMLOCK

Sambo hold-downs can be done when one sambo wrestler holds his opponent to the mat mostly on his back and with torso-to-torso contact. Unlike judo, a sambo hold-down can be applied even if the bottom grappler wraps or scissors his legs around the attacker's body or legs. In sambo, after one grappler holds his opponent down for twenty seconds, the referee will award four points for the hold-down and instruct the sambo wrestler to "go for the submission." This application of the cross-body armlock is a good example of this situation.

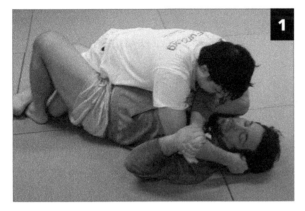

The top grappler (the attacker) holds his opponent with a side chest-hold variation. As he does this, the attacker uses his left hand and arm to hook his opponent's left arm.

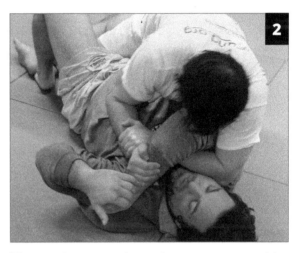

The attacker uses a figure-four grip to control his opponent's right arm as shown.

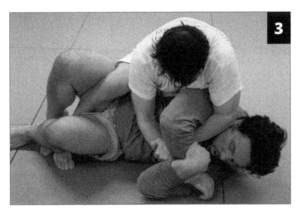

The attacker moves his body to his left (and toward his opponent's head). As he does this, the attacker slides his right foot and leg as loose as possible from his opponent's scissored legs.

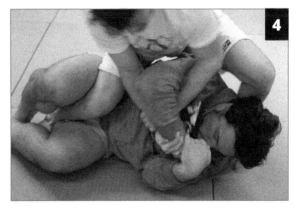

The attacker moves up off of his left knee so he is now squatting with his left shin behind his opponent's head.

LEG SCISSORS BACK ROLL CROSS-BODY ARMLOCK

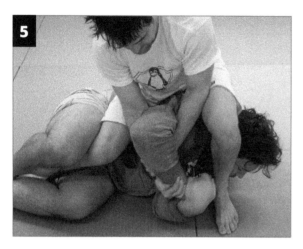

The attacker moves his left foot and leg over his opponent's head. As he does this, the attacker uses both hands and arms to further trap his opponent's right arm.

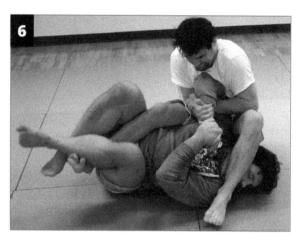

The attacker now has his opponent in the leg press and controls the situation as shown. The attacker continues to trap and lever his opponent's right arm as shown.

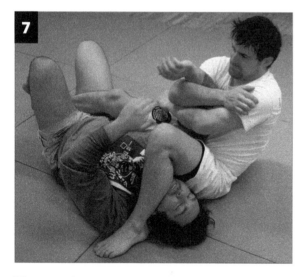

The attacker rolls back to lever the defender's right arm out straight. Look at how the attacker's right leg is still being scissored by his opponent.

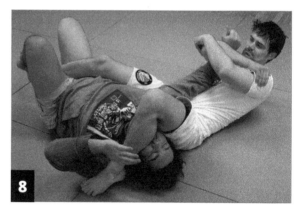

The attacker rolls back, arches his hips, and applies the cross-body armlock.

BELT-AND-NELSON TO CROSS-BODY ARMLOCK

This is a useful application of the cross-body armlock when an opponent is lying flat on his front. There are several belt-and-nelson applications, and this is a good example of one with a high rate of success.

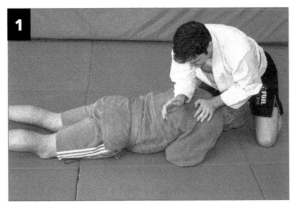

The attacker is positioned at the top of his opponent near his head.

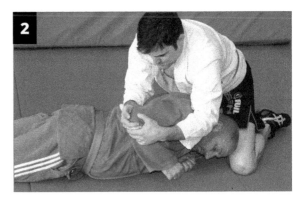

The attacker moves his body so he is positioned at his opponent's left shoulder area. The attacker uses both of his hands to scoop and pull upward on his opponent's right elbow.

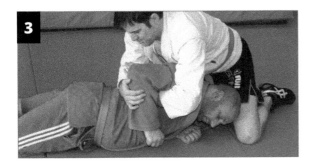

The attacker slides his left hand and arm under his opponent's right upper arm as shown.

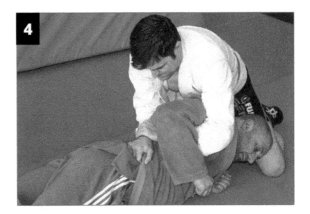

The attacker uses his right hand to grab his opponent's belt (palm down). The attacker then uses his left hand to grab onto his right wrist. This forms the "belt and nelson" hold. Look at how the attacker's body is still positioned at the bottom grappler's left shoulder area.

BELT AND NELSON TO CROSS-BODY ARMLOCK

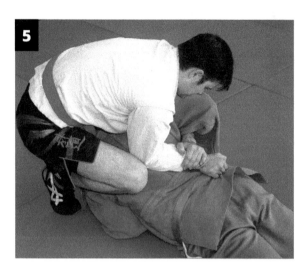

This view shows how the attacker moves up so he is squatting and has his right shin placed on the bottom grappler's back.

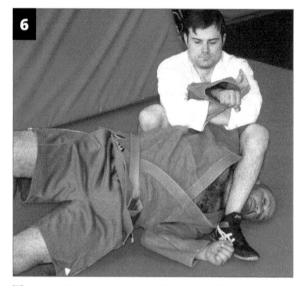

The attacker moves his left foot and leg over his opponent's head, trapping the bottom grappler's head. As he does this, the attacker rolls back onto his buttocks. The attacker uses both hands and arms to trap his opponent's right arm to the attacker's chest.

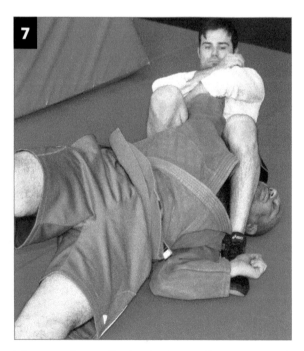

The attacker rolls back, levers his opponent's right arm straight, arches his hips, and applies the cross-body armlock.

HUNGARIAN ROLL TO CROSS-BODY ARMLOCK

This is a popular and effective roll. The first time the author saw this roll, a Hungarian athlete did it, and this is how it got its name.

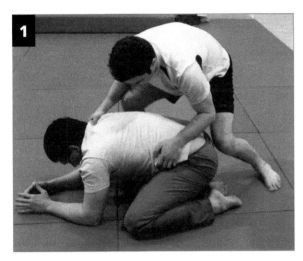

The attacker (top) stands behind his opponent's right hip as shown.

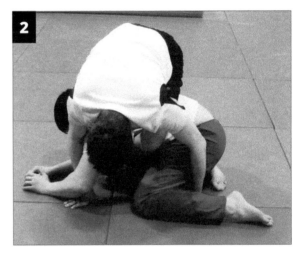

The attacker steps over his opponent's back with his left foot and leg. As he does this, the attacker uses his right hand and arm to hook his opponent's left arm and uses his left hand and arm to hook his opponent's left leg as shown. Look at how the attacker starts to roll forward.

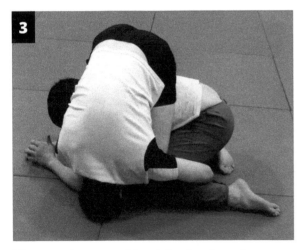

The attacker uses his right hand and arm to securely hook the bottom grappler's left arm and uses his left hand to securely hook the bottom grappler's left leg. The attacker is now positioned so he is on top of his head as shown.

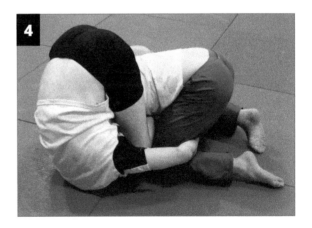

The attacker rolls over in a somersault.

HUNGARIAN ROLL TO CROSS-BODY ARMLOCK

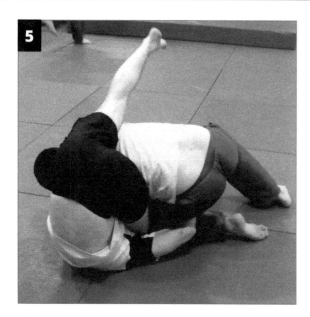

The attacker continues to roll. Often the attacker's back leg (in this case, his right leg) will whip over as shown, creating more momentum in the roll.

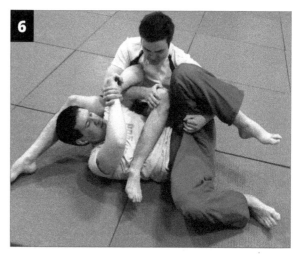

The attacker rolls his opponent over onto his back as shown. The attacker will quickly move his right foot and leg over his opponent's head to trap it.

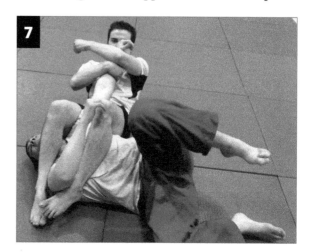

The attacker uses both hands and arms to trap his opponent's left arm to the attacker's chest. As he does this, the attacker rolls back and applies the cross-body armlock.

LEVERS: PRYING AND STRETCHING THE OPPONENT'S ARM

Rolling, turning, or otherwise breaking an opponent down so that he is vulnerable to a cross-body armlock are vital skills. Another vital skill is levering your opponent's arm out straight. As mentioned earlier in this chapter, a "lever" is the act of prying, pulling, or straightening an opponent's arm and immediately securing the cross-body armlock. No opponent will ever give you his arm, so it is important to learn many effective levers and practice them on a regular basis. Levers are often applied from a leg press or shoulder sit position, but can be applied from any position. Presented here are a few levers that have a high rate of success.

ARM-AND-LEG LEVER

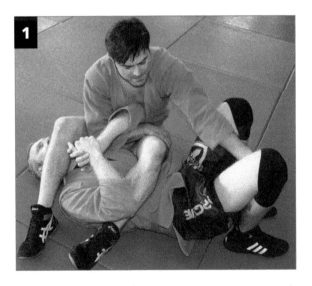

The attacker (on top) controls his opponent with a leg press.

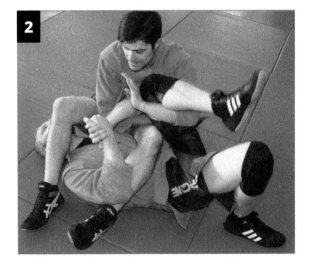

The attacker uses his left hand and arm to hook under his opponent's near leg (left leg) as shown. As he does this, the attacker uses his right hand and arm to trap his opponent's left arm to the attacker's chest.

ARM AND LEG LEVER

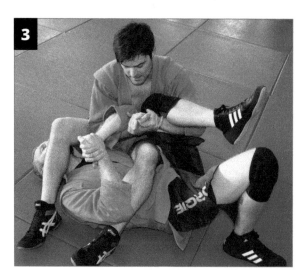

The attacker grasps his hands together firmly in a square grip. Doing this traps the bottom grappler's left knee and left arm firmly to the attacker's chest.

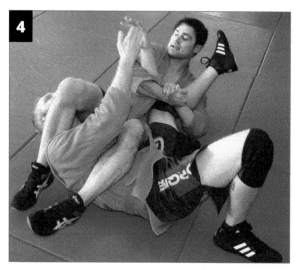

The attacker rolls back onto his left hip and buttocks area. Doing this starts to straighten the bottom grappler's left arm and left leg.

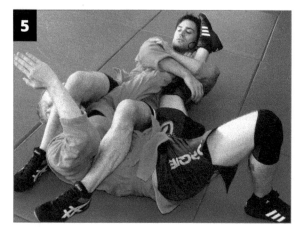

The attacker rolls back, trapping the bottom grappler's left arm and left leg and levering them out straight. The attacker arches his hips and applies the armlock.

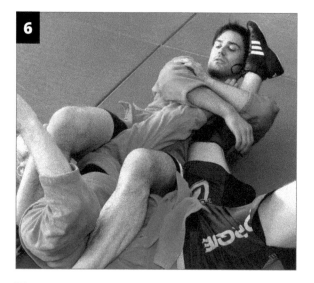

This close view shows how the attacker straightens out his opponent's left arm and left leg. This is a bad position for the bottom grapple to be in!

ARM-AND-LEG LEVER IF OPPONENT SITS UP

Sometimes the bottom grappler will try to sit up in an effort to escape from the leg press. When he does, this is a useful and effective variation of the arm-and-leg lever.

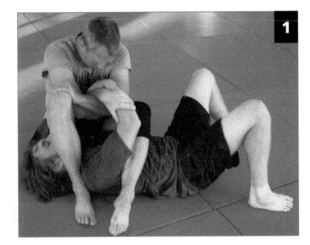

The top grappler controls his opponent with a leg press.

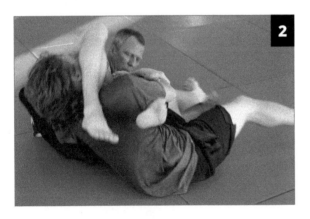

In an effort to escape, the bottom grappler attempts to sit up. As he does this, the top grappler rolls to his left hip (in the direction of the bottom grappler's feet). The top grappler uses his bent right leg to hook his opponent's head and force it back down to the mat. As he does this, the top grappler uses his left hand and arm to hook around the bottom grappler's left leg at about the knee.

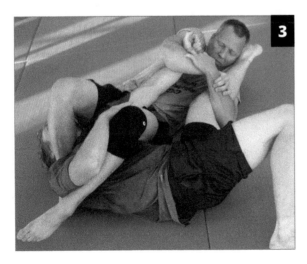

The top grappler uses his right leg to force his opponent's head back down to the mat. As he does this, the top grappler grasps his hands together in a square grip and applies the cross-body armlock as shown in this photo.

THIGH TRAP AND UPPERCUT LEVER

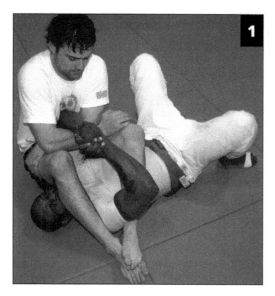

The top grappler controls his opponent with the leg press. As he does this, the top grappler slides his left hand under his opponent's left arm and grabs his right thigh with his left hand as shown. The top grappler uses his right hand and arm to also slide under the bottom grappler's left arm to trap it.

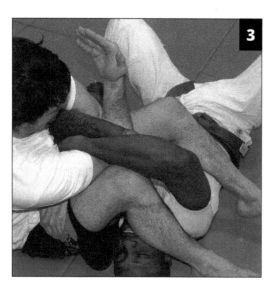

The top grappler's left hand is firmly grabbing his left upper leg and thigh. Doing this securely traps the bottom grappler's left arm and isolates it. The top grappler turns his right hand over so that it will be palm up.

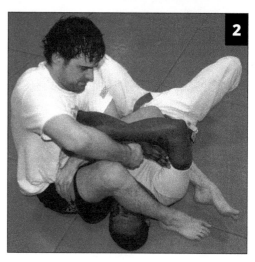

The top grappler slides his right hand (palm up) under his opponent's left forearm close to his wrist. The top grappler now has firm control of his opponent, with the attacker's left arm trapping the defender's left upper arm to the attacker's chest. The attacker uses his right arm to trap the defender's left arm near his wrist. This "high and low" control of the defender's arm really traps it and makes it vulnerable to the lever.

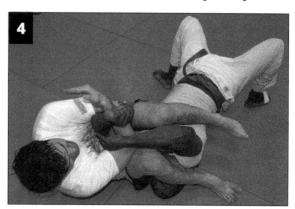

The attacker rolls to his right hip and side with his opponent's left arm trapped to the attacker's chest. The weight of the attacker's body will pry the defender's hands apart and straighten the defender's left arm.

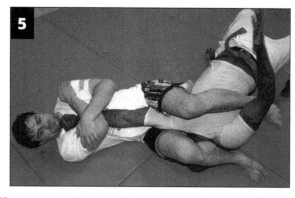

The top grappler uses both hands and arms to hook and trap the bottom grappler's left arm, and the top grappler rolls to his right side, levering the bottom grappler's arm straight.

BENT ARM LEVER TO CROSS-BODY ARMLOCK

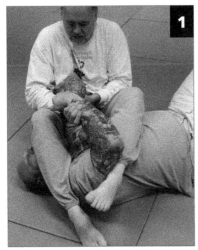

The attacker controls his opponent with the leg press.

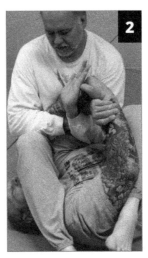

The attacker slides his left hand under his opponent's left upper arm as shown. As he does this, the attacker uses his right hand and arm to trap the defender's left arm to the attacker's chest.

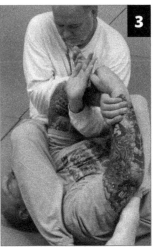

The attacker moves his right arm out and slides his right forearm between his chest and the defender's left forearm.

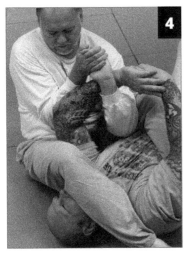

The attacker grasps his hands together in a square grip as shown. Look at how the attacker has his right elbow placed on his opponent's left elbow and how the attacker has his left forearm trapping his opponent's left forearm near his wrist.

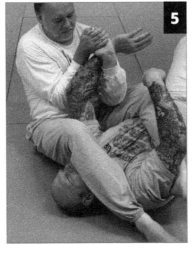

The attacker rotates his bent arms so that the defender's left elbow is cranked outward as shown. Look at how the defender has released his grip. This is a good armlock, but if the defender doesn't submit, the attacker will go on to the cross-body armlock.

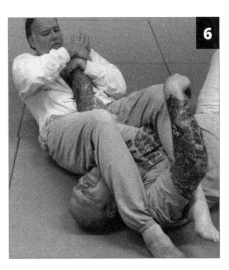

The attacker has levered his opponent's left arm straight and rolls back, applying the cross-body armlock.

FOOT KICK OR FOOT PUSH LEVER TO CROSS-BODY ARMLOCK

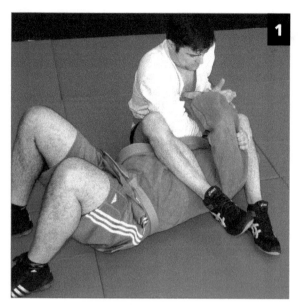

The attacker controls his opponent with the leg press and uses both hands and arms to trap the bottom grappler's right arm.

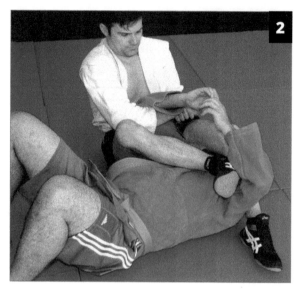

The attacker uses his right foot to push or kick the bottom grappler's left arm as shown.

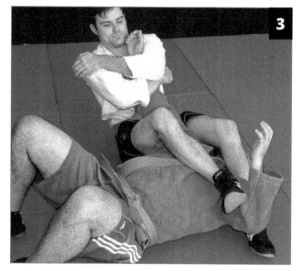

The defender releases his grip and the attacker rolls back to apply the armlock.

BOTH ARM HUG TO CROSS-BODY ARMLOCK

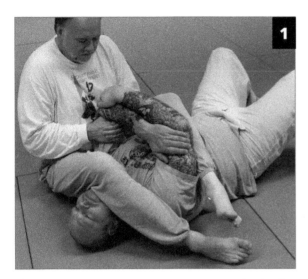

The attacker controls his opponent with the leg press.

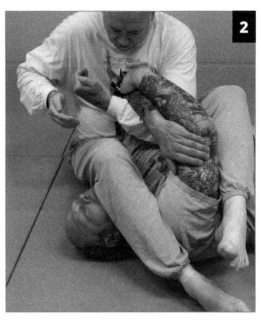

The attacker drives his right hand and arm (palm up) in a scooping or uppercut motion under his opponent's left wrist area. All the while, the attacker hugs and traps the bottom grappler's left arm tightly to the attacker's chest.

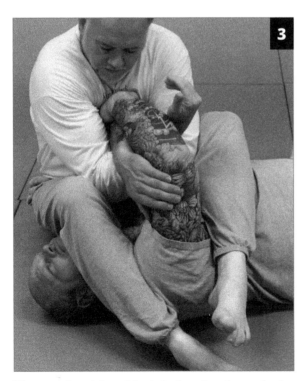

The attacker forcefully drives his left hand and arm in a scooping or uppercut motion under his opponent's left arm near the bottom grappler's elbow. Look at how the attacker's left hand is palm up. Doing this gives the movement more power.

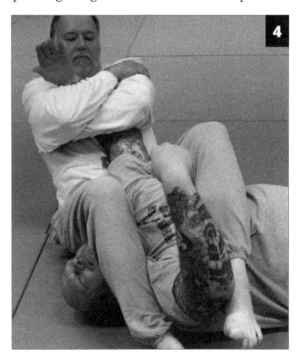

The attacker uses both hands and arms to hug his shoulders as shown, trapping and levering the defender's left arm straight. The attacker rolls back and applies the cross-body armlock.

HEAD SIDE LEG TRIANGLE COMPRESSION BENT ARMLOCK FROM THE LEG PRESS

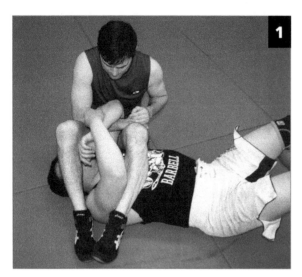

The attacker controls his opponent with the leg press. The attacker uses his right hand and arm to hook under his opponent's left arm. The attacker places his right hand on his left thigh to trap the bottom grappler's left forearm as shown.

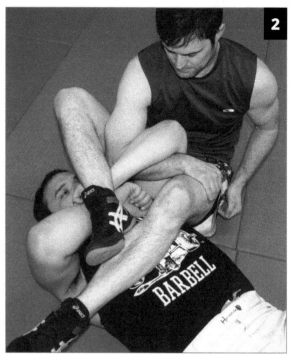

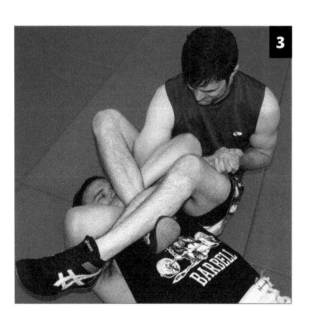

The attacker moves his right foot and leg over his opponent's left forearm near the wrist.

The attacker forms a triangle with his feet and legs as shown and uses this to apply pressure to his opponent's left bent elbow. As he does this, the attacker drives his right forearm in deeper and grasps his hands together in a square grip as shown. The combined action of the attacker's triangle pressure and the arm pressure makes for a nasty compression bent armlock.

HIP SIDE TRIANGLE TO COMPRESSION BENT ARMLOCK FROM THE LEG PRESS

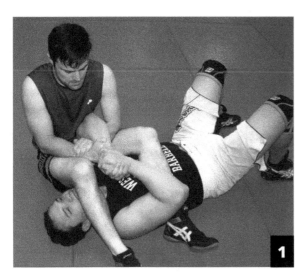

The attacker controls his opponent with the leg press. The attacker drives his left forearm under his opponent's left forearm. The attacker uses his right hand to grab his right wrist.

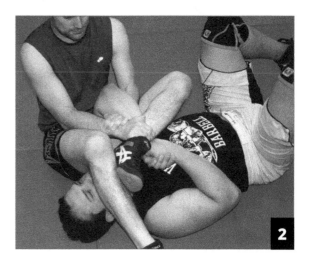

The attacker moves his right foot and leg up and over the attacker's left ankle, forming a strong triangle with the legs. As he does this, the attacker applies pressure with the leg triangle to the defender's left forearm. Look at how the attacker uses his left forearm as a wedge, creating a tight compression bent armlock.

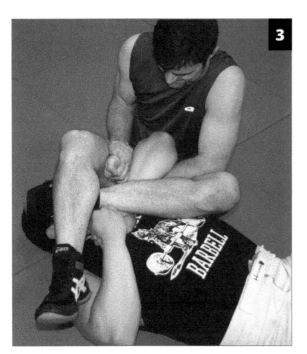

The attacker moves his left foot and leg up and over the bottom grappler's left forearm. At this point, the top grappler can create a nasty compression bent armlock using his left leg by grabbing and pushing down on his left ankle with his right hand as shown. If the bottom grappler doesn't tap out at this point, the top grappler can go on to apply the leg triangle.

PRETZEL COMPRESSION BENT ARMLOCK

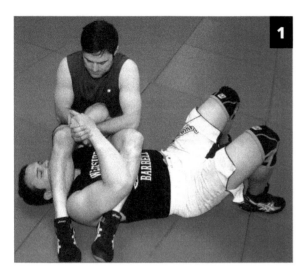

The attacker controls his opponent with the leg press. The attacker moves his left hand and arm under his opponent's left arm.

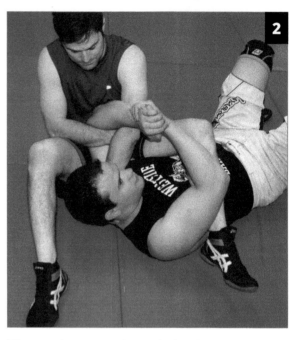

The attacker moves his right leg from the bottom grappler's head as shown. As he does this, the attacker uses his left hand (palm) to hook on the back of the bottom grappler's head as shown.

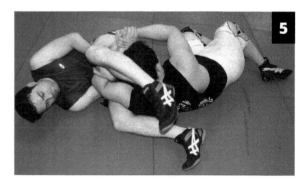

The attacker is now positioned on his right side. He moves his left foot and leg over his opponent's arms and head as shown.

PRETZEL COMPRESSION BENT ARMLOCK

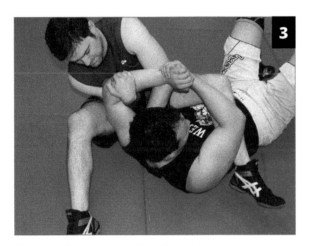

The attacker uses his right hand (palm up) to grab the bottom grappler's left forearm as shown. As he does this, the attacker starts to turn to his right and uses his right hand to push on the back of his opponent's head.

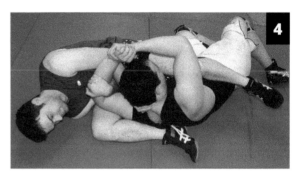

The attacker turns and leans to his right side and continues the pressure using both of his hands as shown.

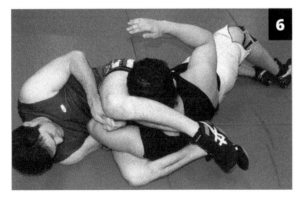

The attacker hooks his left leg over his opponent's head and neck and arches with his hips. As he does this, the attacker grabs his hands together, forming a square grip and creating a wedge in the defender's bent left arm with the attacker's right forearm. Combining all of these actions creates a nasty compression bent armlock

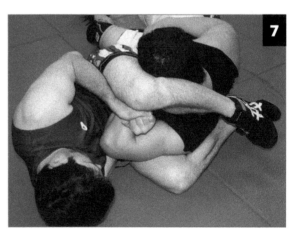

This view shows how the attacker uses his hands and arms to create the compression bent armlock and how the attacker uses his feet and legs to hook the defender's head and neck, creating the compression bent armlock.

BENT ARMLOCK (UPWARD DIRECTION) FROM A SIDE CHEST HOLD

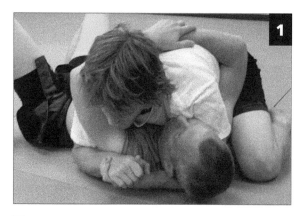

The top grappler controls his opponent with a side chest hold as shown.

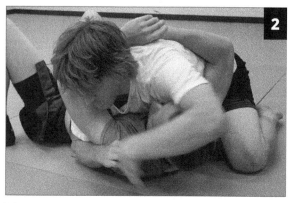

The top grappler moves his left hand and arm over his opponent's head.

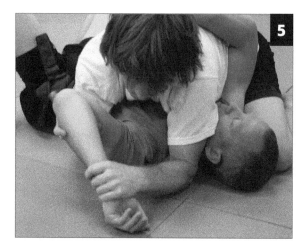

The attacker uses his left hand to grab his opponent's left wrist. As he does this, the attacker uses his right hand to push upward on his opponent's bent left elbow.

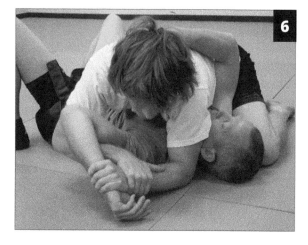

The attacker uses his right hand to grab his left wrist as shown. The attacker lifts his right elbow upward, forcing the bottom grappler's left elbow to raise as well. Doing this creates the bent armlock.

BENT ARMLOCK (UPWARD DIRECTION) FROM A SIDE CHEST HOLD

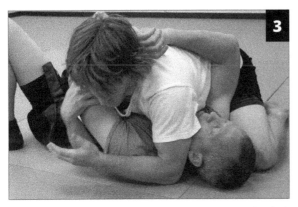

The top grappler jams his left elbow in the left side of his opponent's neck.

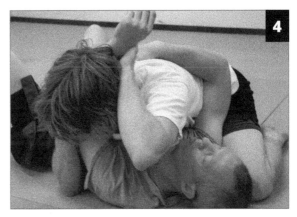

The attacker uses both hands to grab the bottom grappler's left forearm and wrist.

ALTERNATIVE FINISH: TWO-ON-ONE WRIST GRIP

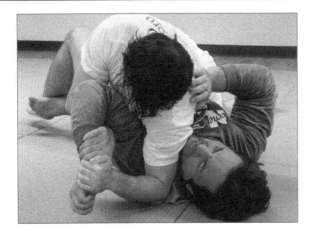

The attacker uses both hands to grab his opponent's left wrist and forearm as shown.

ALTERNATIVE FINISH—ELBOW SCOOP

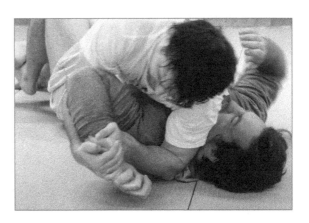

The attacker uses his right hand to grab (palm up) his opponent's left wrist as the attacker slides his right forearm under the bottom grappler's left elbow. As he does this, the attacker uses his left hand to grab (palm up) the bottom grappler's left wrist. The attacker cranks the defender's left elbow upward as shown.

BENT ARMLOCK (DOWNWARD DIRECTION) FROM THE SIDE CHEST HOLD

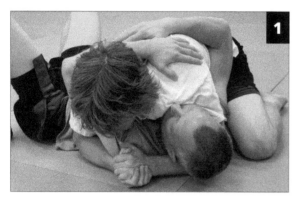

The top grappler controls his opponent with a side chest hold.

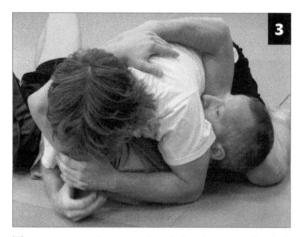

The attacker moves his left arm over his opponent's head as shown.

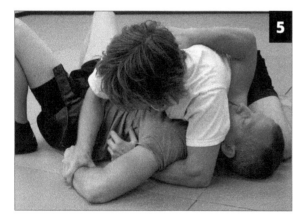

The top grappler jams his left elbow in the left side of the bottom grappler's neck.

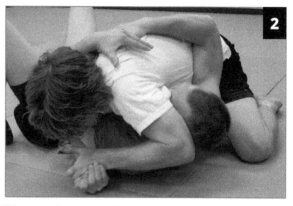

The top grappler uses his left hand to grab and push up on the bottom grappler's left upper arm. As he does this, the top grappler uses his left hand to grab his opponent's left wrist.

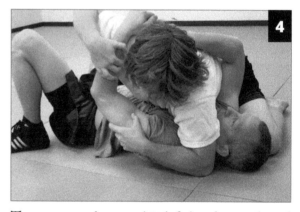

The top grappler uses his left hand to grab and pin the bottom grappler's left hand to the mat as shown. As he does this, the top grappler slides his left hand and arm under the left shoulder and upper arm of the bottom grappler.

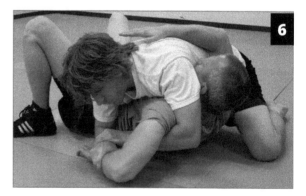

The top grappler uses his left hand to grab his right wrist, forming a figure-four grip. Look at how the attacker uses this grip to pin the bottom grappler's left hand to the mat. As he does this, the attacker raises or lifts his left elbow and forearm. Doing this creates a nasty bent armlock.

BOTH KNEES AND NEAR NELSON BREAKDOWN TO BENT ARMLOCK

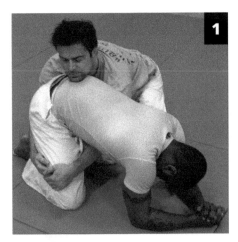

The attacker (right) uses both hands and arms to reach and grab his opponent's right knee.

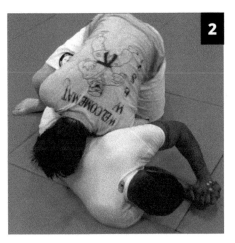

The attacker drives his upper chest and body into his opponent's left side as the attacker scoops in with his hands and arms to break his opponent down as shown.

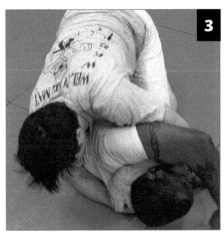

The attacker drives his left hand and arm under his opponent's left shoulder and places his left palm on the back of his opponent's head and neck. As he does this, the attacker uses his left hand to pry his opponent over onto his back.

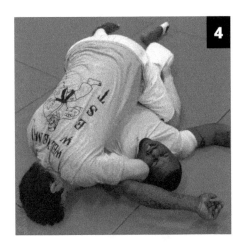

The attacker breaks his opponent down as shown.

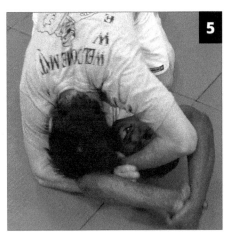

The attacker uses his forehead to pin his opponent's left upper arm to the mat. As he does this, the attacker moves his left hand and arm free.

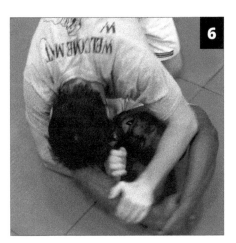

The attacker uses his left hand to grab and hold his opponent's left wrist. As he does this, the attacker slides his right hand and arm under his opponent's left upper arm.

BOTH KNEES AND NEAR NELSON BREAKDOWN TO BENT ARMLOCK

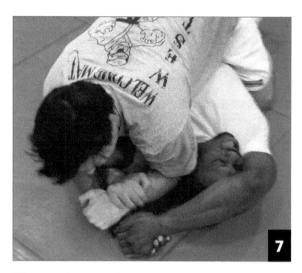

The attacker uses his right hand to grab his left wrist, forming a figure-four grip. As he does this, the attacker drives his left elbow into the left side of the bottom grappler's neck.

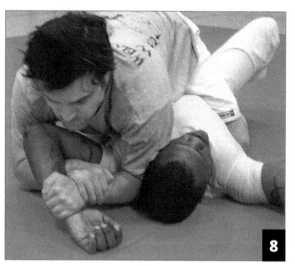

The attacker forms a strong bent armlock and applies pressure to get the tap out.

ALTERNATIVE FINISH—HAMMER BENT ARMLOCK

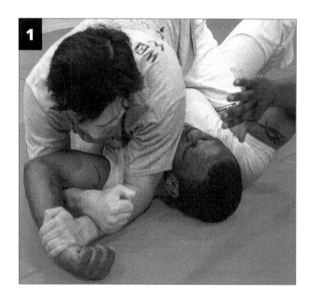

The attacker makes a fist with his right hand and turns his right forearm so the bottom of the attacker's fist is placed on his left forearm as shown.

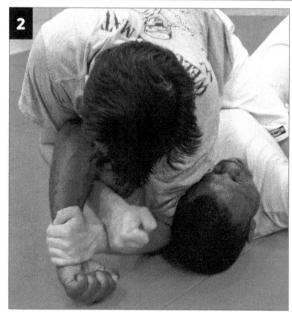

The attacker drives his right elbow up as he uses his left hand to lift his opponent's left wrist off of the mat. As he does this, the attacker cranks the bottom grappler's left arm with this nasty variation of the bent armlock.

UPPER CHEST HOLD TO BENT ARMLOCK (UPWARD DIRECTION)

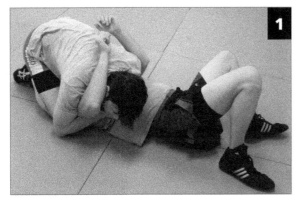

The attacker holds his opponent with an upper chest hold.

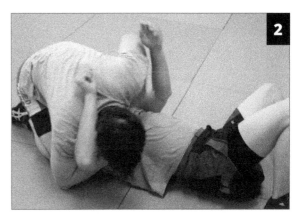

The attacker has already used his right hand and arm to trap and hold the bottom grappler. As he does this, the attacker starts to shift his body position, moving his hips and lower body to his left.

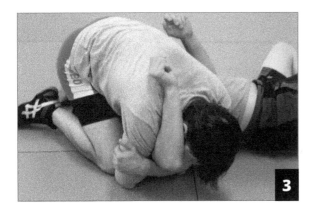

The attacker uses both hands and arms to hug and trap his opponent's right arm as shown.

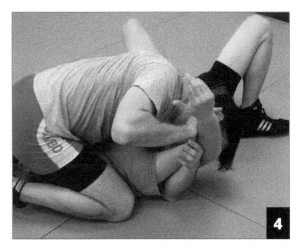

The attacker uses his right hand to grab his opponent's right forearm near the wrist and push it downward to the mat. Look at how the attacker uses his left hand and arm to trap and control the defender's right upper arm.

UPPER CHEST HOLD TO BENT ARMLOCK (UPWARD DIRECTION)

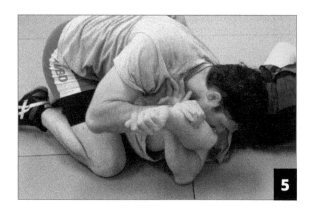

This view shows how the attacker places his left elbow on the mat as a base and uses his left hand to reach up and grab his right hand that he has already used to grab his opponent's right wrist.

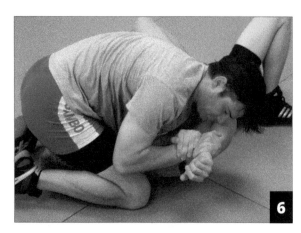

The attacker uses his hands and arms to form a figure-four grip on his opponent's bent right arm. Look at the angle of the top grappler's body, allowing for the top grappler to exert more pressure on the armlock.

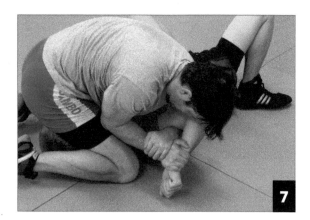

The attacker uses his left arm to lift upward on the bottom grappler's bent right upper arm. As he does this, the attacker uses his right hand to push on the bottom grappler's right wrist. Doing this creates a cranking action making this a painful application of the bent armlock.

UPPER CHEST HOLD TO BENT ARMLOCK (DOWNWARD DIRECTION)

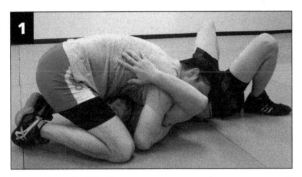

The attacker holds his opponent with an upper chest hold.

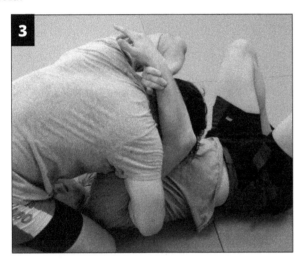

The attacker uses his arms to force the bottom grappler to roll to the bottom grappler's left a bit. As he does this, the top grappler uses his right arm to lift the bottom grappler's right arm and shoulder up and off the mat.

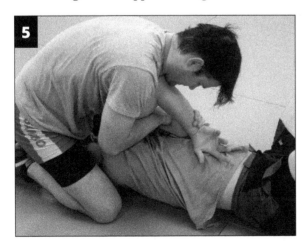

The attacker reaches over his head with his left hand and arm and grabs his opponent's right wrist as shown.

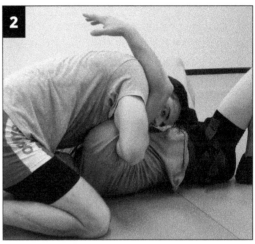

The top grappler uses his left hand to push the bottom grappler's right wrist and arm over his head and down to the belly area of the bottom grappler.

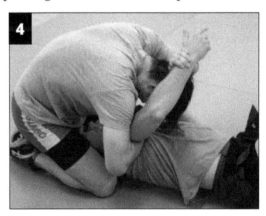

The top grappler continues to roll the bottom grappler onto his left side. The top grappler uses his left hand to pull the bottom grappler's right wrist to the bottom man's torso. As he does this, he uses his right hand to grab his left hand, forming a figure-four grip. The top grappler makes sure to jam his opponent's right upper arm to the attacker's chest, trapping and controlling it.

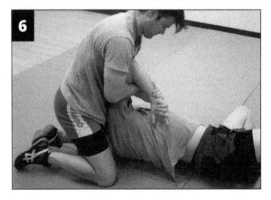

The attacker sits upright and pulls his opponent's arm up. Look at how the opponent's right upper arm is pressed firmly on the attacker's chest. The attacker rotates to his right and cranks the bottom grappler's bent right arm with the bent armlock.

HEAD-AND-ARM SIDE CHEST HOLD TO BENT ARMLOCK WITH A HEAD TRAP

This series shows two armlocks that start from the same hold-down and are similar in that the attacker can use either one by choice or opportunity.

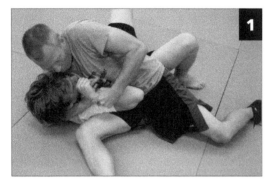

The attacker holds his opponent with a head-and-arm side chest hold. The attacker uses his right hand to grab his opponent's right wrist and push it down to the mat.

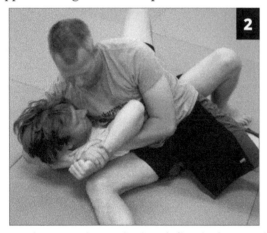

The attacker uses his right hand (hooked around the bottom grappler's head) to grab the bottom grappler's right wrist. He also uses his left hand to grab his right wrist forming a figure-four grip. Now the attacker can apply a bent armlock from this position, trapping his opponent's head as he does so.

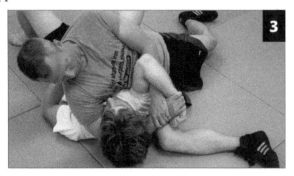

This view shows how the attacker applies the bent armlock with a head trap.

HEAD-AND-ARM SIDE CHEST HOLD TO BENT ARMLOCK

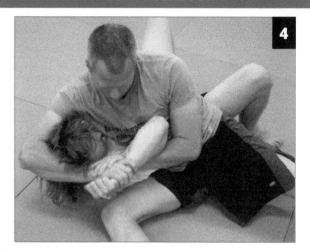

The attacker slides his right arm over his opponent's head.

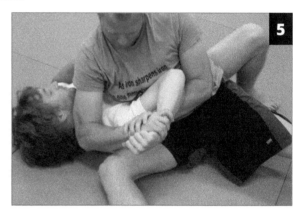

The attacker drives his right elbow directly in the right side of the bottom grappler's neck. As he does this, he lifts his left arm up, cranking the bottom grappler's right elbow higher, and uses his hands to push downward and in the direction of the attacker's legs. This creates a nasty cranking action on the defender's bent right arm.

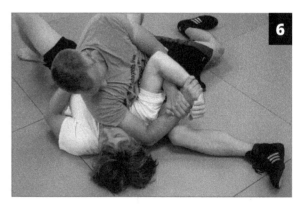

This view shows how the attacker bends the bottom grappler's right arm and exerts tremendous torque. Doing this creates a nasty bent armlock.

HEAD-AND-ARM SIDE CHEST HOLD TO LEG TRAP BENT ARMLOCK

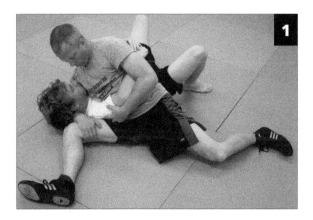

The attacker holds his opponent with a head-and-arm side chest hold.

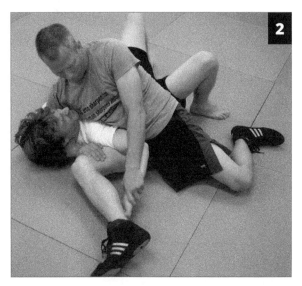

The attacker uses his right hand to grab his opponent's right wrist and push it down to the mat. As he does this, the attacker moves his right foot and lower leg so that he can push the defender's right hand and wrist under the attacker's right ankle area.

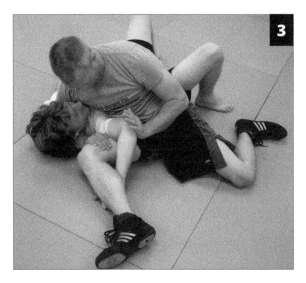

The attacker can force his right leg downward and apply a great deal of pressure, forcing the bottom grappler to tap out. The attacker can also use his left hand to push up and forward on the defender's right bent elbow and create pressure as well.

FRONT CHEST HOLD TO THE BENT ARMLOCK FROM A TRIPOD

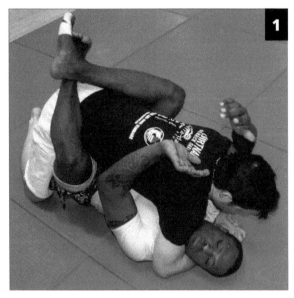

The attacker holds his opponent with a front chest hold-down. The attacker has his right arm hooked around his opponent's head. This will come into play later.

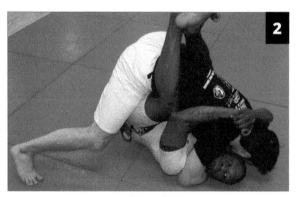

The attacker quickly pops up with his feet wide on the mat, forming a tripod and a strong base. Look at how the attacker leans forward and forces the bottom grappler to roll back high on his shoulders.

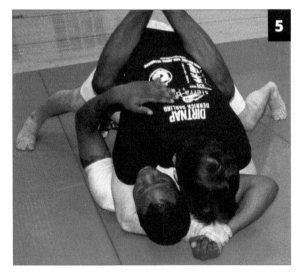

The attacker uses his head to trap his opponent's right upper arm to the mat and as he does this, the attacker uses his right hand to grab his opponent's right wrist. At this point, the attacker uses his left hand to grab his right wrist, forming a figure-four grip.

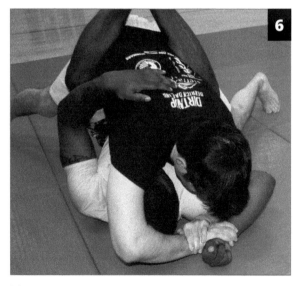

The attacker slides his right arm over his opponent's head.

FRONT CHEST HOLD TO THE BENT ARMLOCK FROM A TRIPOD

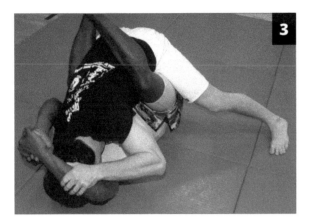

The attacker uses his left hand to grab his opponent's right forearm to "peel" it up and over his head as shown.

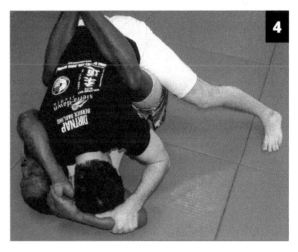

The attacker uses his head to trap his opponent's right upper arm to the mat.

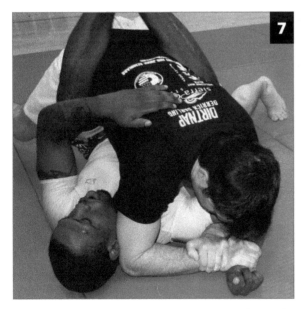

The attacker jams his right elbow into the right side of his opponent's neck.

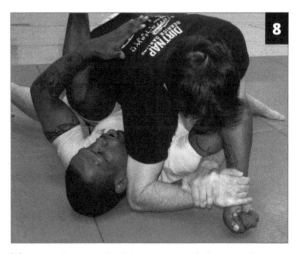

The attacker cranks his opponent's bent right arm to get the tap out.

DOWNWARD BENT ARMLOCK FROM THE HEAD SIT

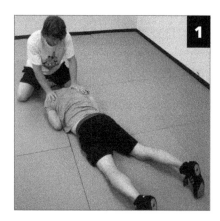

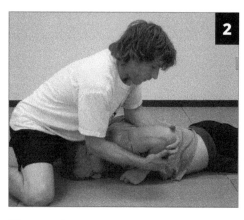

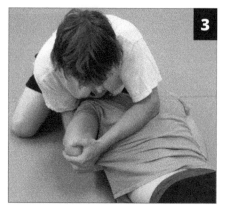

The attacker (kneeling) is positioned at the head of his opponent, who is lying on his front in a defensive position.

The attacker uses both hands to grab and scoop under the defender's left elbow.

This view shows how the attacker places his left elbow on his opponent's back as the attacker uses his hands and arms to scoop and lift the bottom grappler's left elbow. The attacker's left elbow exerts a great deal of pressure on his opponent's back, making this situation uncomfortable for the bottom grappler.

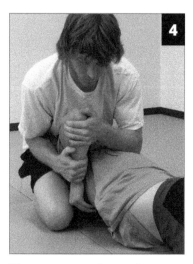

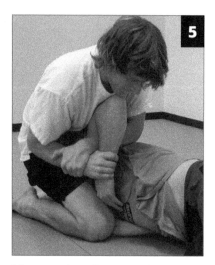

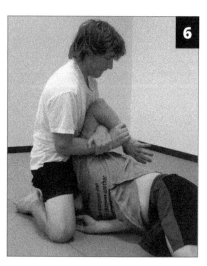

The top grappler makes sure to pin the bottom grappler's head by squeezing his knees together. As he does this, the attacker continues to pull up on his opponent's left elbow, pulling the elbow to the attacker's chest.

The attacker forms a figure-four grip with his hands and arms on his opponent's left bent arm. As he does this, the top grappler starts to sit upright and makes sure to keep the bottom grappler's left upper arm hugged and trapped to his chest.

The top grappler turns his body to his left, creating a tight bent armlock and a lot of pain for the bottom grappler.

BENT ARMLOCK FROM THE BOTTOM

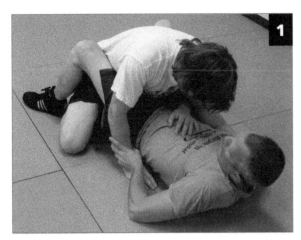

The attacker (on bottom) is fighting off his opponent and attempting to prevent the top grappler from securing a front chest hold-down. The attacker uses his left hand to grab his opponent's right forearm or wrist.

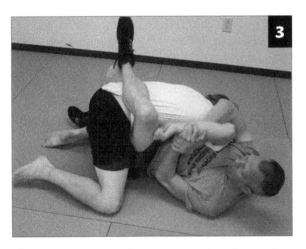

The bottom grappler turns to his left and moves his right hand and arm over his opponent's right shoulder and upper arm as shown. The bottom grappler will use his right hand to grab his left wrist to start to form a figure-four grip.

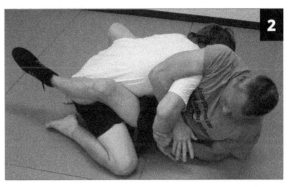

The bottom grappler secures the figure-four grip on his opponent's right elbow (now bent downward). As he does this, he spins to his left. The bottom grappler moves his left foot and leg over his opponent's hip and low back area.

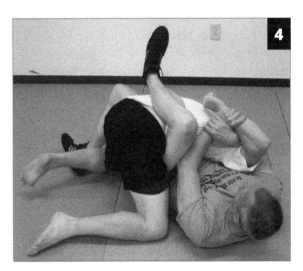

The bottom grappler spins to his left and uses his left foot and leg to push down on his opponent's low back. As he does this, he uses his left hand to push his opponent's right wrist and uses his left elbow to pull and draw down, creating a cranking action on the top grappler's bent right arm.

This view shows how the attacker places his right foot on the mat with his right knee bent. As he does this, the bottom grappler uses his left foot and leg to push down on the top grappler's back. By doing this, the bottom grappler traps the top grappler's body with his feet and legs and allows for the bottom grappler to apply more pressure to the bent armlock.

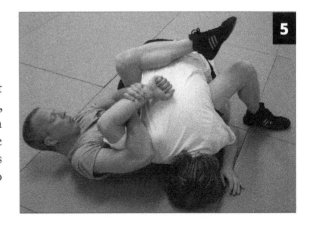

KICK OVER BENT ARMLOCK

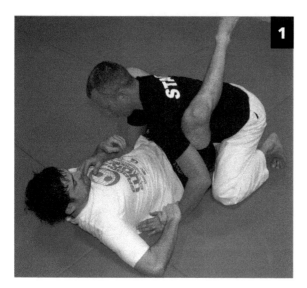

The attacker (on bottom) fights off his opponent from this bottom position. As he does, the attacker uses his right hand to grab his opponent's left wrist. The attacker moves his right foot and leg up against the top grappler's left side.

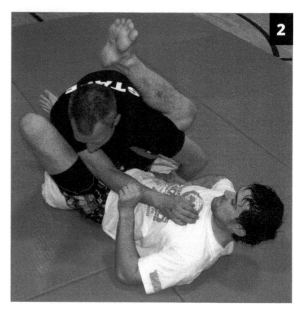

The bottom grappler spins to his right, and as he does, he moves his right foot and leg over the top grappler's left side and arm as shown. At this point, the attacker uses his right hand to hold and trap the top grappler's left wrist to the mat.

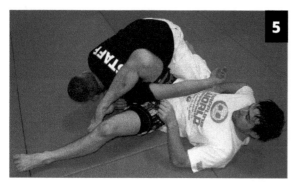

The bottom grappler continues to spin to his right and uses his right foot and leg to hook and trap his opponent's left upper arm.

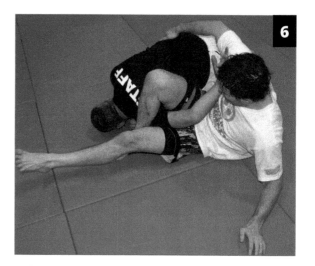

The attacker completes his spinning movement to his right and now has his opponent's left upper arm trapped completely with his left foot and leg. The attacker uses his right hand and arm to reach over his opponent's lower back and grabs the top grappler's right hip. Doing this adds pressure to the bent armlock and, more importantly at this point, allows the bottom grappler to start to sit up.

KICK OVER BENT ARMLOCK

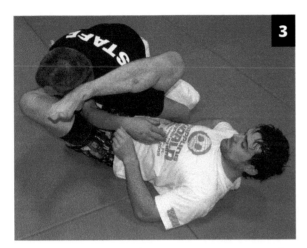

As the bottom grappler continues to spin to his right, he further moves his right foot and leg over his opponent's left arm and shoulder.

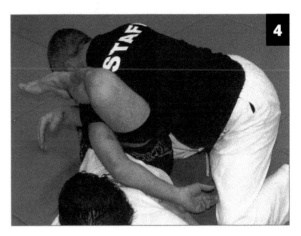

The bottom grappler uses his right foot and leg to hook and control his opponent's right shoulder as shown. At this point, the attacker no longer holds his opponent's left wrist.

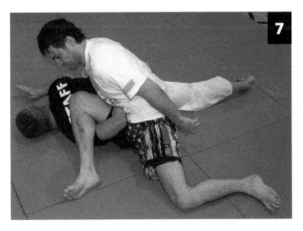

The attacker sits up onto his right buttocks and leans forward. The defender's left arm is trapped between the attacker's right upper leg and his right side of his torso. Doing this creates pressure on the defender's left shoulder and elbow. At this point, the defender will tap out.

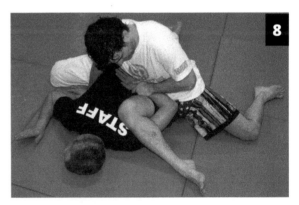

If the defender's right arm isn't trapped, the attacker can use his left hand to grab his opponent's left wrist or forearm and pin it to his back. As he does this, the attacker leans forward to create pressure.

ALTERNATIVE FINISH

The attacker can lean forward and use his left hand and arm to hook under his opponent's neck, pulling up on it as he leans into the bottom grappler. This is painful to the bottom grappler.

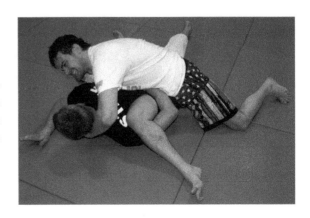

ROLLING BENT ARMLOCK

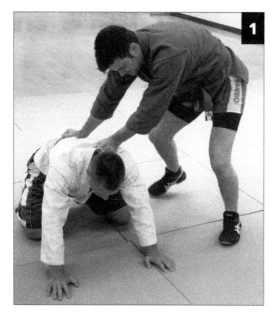

The attacker (standing) is positioned at the left side of his opponent.

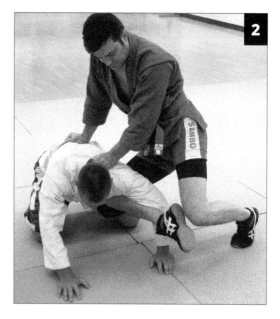

The attacker uses his right foot and leg to hook his opponent's left arm from behind.

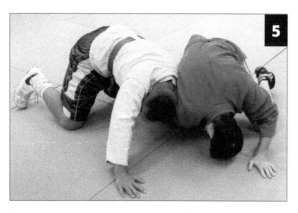

The attacker uses his right hand and arm to reach through and grab his opponent's left leg.

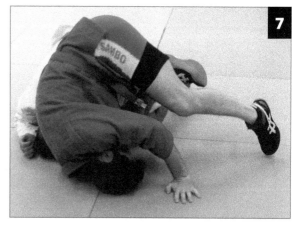

This view shows how the attacker rolls over his right shoulder.

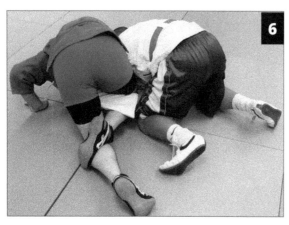

This view shows how the attacker uses his right leg to hook and trap his opponent's left arm. The attacker places his right foot in the back of his knee to further trap his opponent's left arm.

ROLLING BENT ARMLOCK

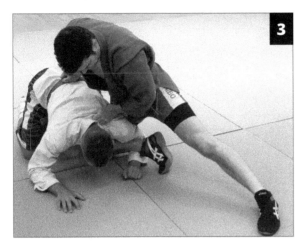

The attacker drives forward, using his right leg to hook even harder so that the bottom grappler's left arm is bent. Doing this traps the defender's left arm firmly.

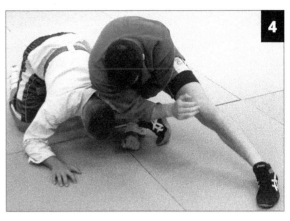

The attacker leans forward in the direction of his opponent's head. As he does this, the attacker moves his right hand and arm over the bottom grappler's left shoulder.

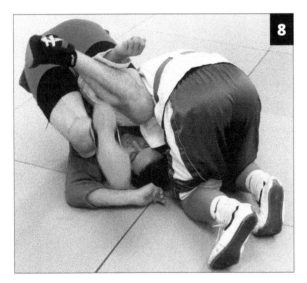

This view shows the attacker rolling over his right shoulder and head. Look at how the attacker uses his right leg to continue to hook and control the defender's left arm. The attacker still holds (with his right hand) his opponent's left leg.

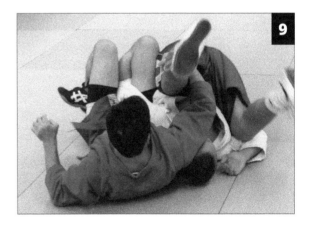

As the attacker rolls, he uses his right hand to lift his opponent's left leg. The attacker makes sure to forcefully use his legs to control his opponent during the roll.

ROLLING BENT ARMLOCK

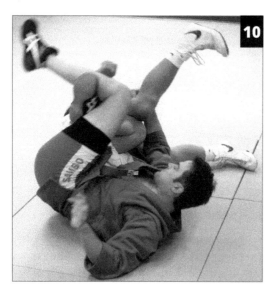

This view shows how the attacker rolls and uses his legs (which have formed a triangle) to control his opponent's left bent arm. Look at how the defender is being forced to roll. This is because of the momentum of the attacker's roll and the pressure the attacker places on his opponent's left shoulder with his legs.

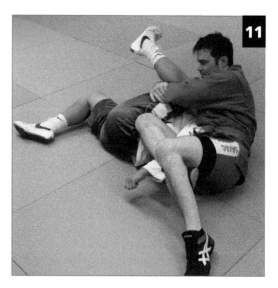

As the attacker completes the roll, he uses both hands to grab and control his opponent's left leg. The attacker continues to use his feet and legs formed in the triangle to trap the defender's left bent arm.

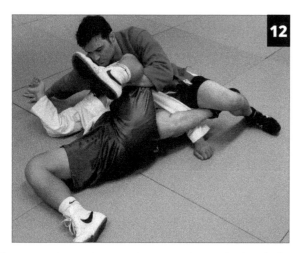

This view shows the attacker using his right hand placed on the mat to stabilize his position as he leans to his right. Doing this starts to add pressure on the bottom grappler's left shoulder and elbow.

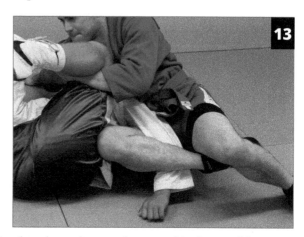

Look at how the attacker uses his feet and legs to trap and lock his opponent's left arm and shoulder.

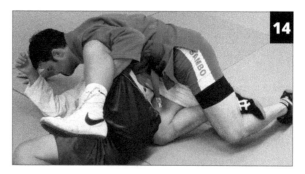

The attacker turns his body to his right. Doing this adds tremendous pressure on the bottom grappler's left shoulder and arm, creating a nasty bent armlock.

SODEN ROLL TO BENT ARMLOCK

If you get stuck on the bottom, this is a good move to get out from a bad situation and turn it into an effective armlock.

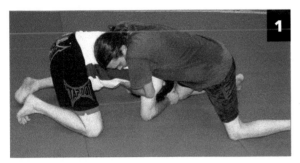

The attacker (on bottom) is on his hands and knees with his opponent riding him from the top.

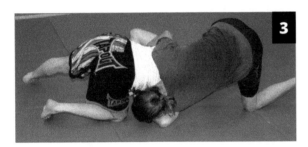

The attacker uses his right arm to hook around his opponent's left upper arm and uses his left arm to hook around his opponent's right upper arm. Doing this traps the top grappler's arms to the bottom grappler's sides. As he does this, the attacker places his left foot out to his side for stability and comes up on his right knee as shown.

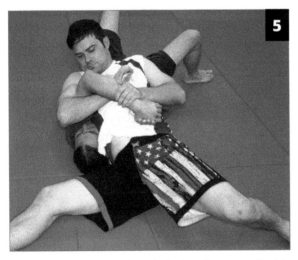

The top grappler moves his head to his left as he forcefully rolls to his right, causing the top grappler to roll with him.

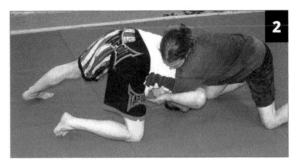

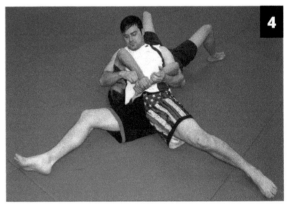

The attacker uses his left hand to grab his opponent's left wrist. As he does this, the attacker starts to slide his right hand and arm under his opponent's left elbow and forearm.

The forceful rolling action by the bottom grappler rolls the top grappler over and onto his back as shown. The attacker ends up with his right hip wedged at the right side of his opponent's head as shown. It is important that the attacker roll over and end up on his right hip and buttocks. Look at how the attacker's legs are positioned for maximum control. The top grappler uses both arms to hook his opponent's arms. This is an effective hold-down, and if the attacker wishes, he can hold his opponent for time and score points. When the mat official scores the points and signals the top grappler to go for the submission, the attacker can go on to the next step.

SODEN ROLL TO BENT ARMLOCK

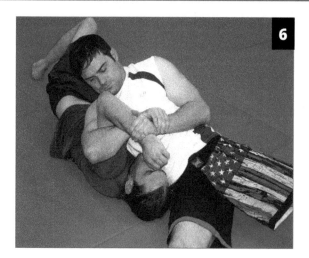

The attacker uses his right hand to grab his left wrist, forming a figure-four grip to control his opponent's left bent arm as shown.

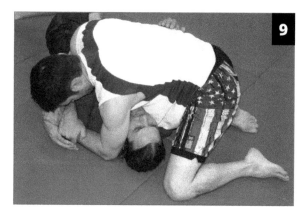

The attacker rolls to his right and leans forward so that pressure in created on his opponent's left arm and shoulder.

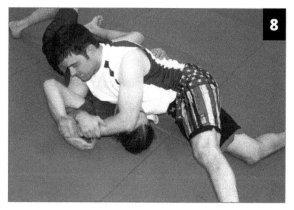

As the attacker turns to his right, he slides his right foot and leg back as shown. At this point, the defender may tap out from the armlock, but if he doesn't, go on to the next step.

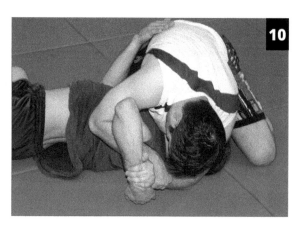

The attacker moves to his knees (but stays low to the mat) and controls his opponent as shown. At this point, the attacker has the position and leverage necessary to apply a strong bent armlock.

This view shows how the attacker is able to apply a strong bent armlock to finish his opponent.

NEAR ARM SIT BACK COMPRESSION BENT ARMLOCK

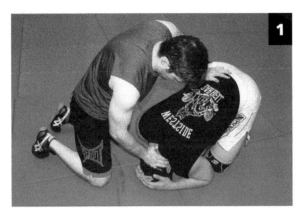

The attacker (on the left) controls his opponent as shown with the attacker using his right hand to push down on the back of his opponent's head.

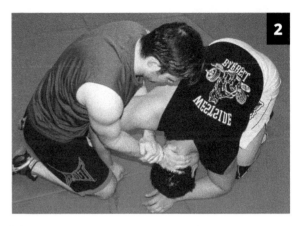

The attacker moves his left hand and arm under his opponent's left upper arm as shown. As he does this, the attacker uses his right hand to grab his left wrist and forms a figure-four grip. The attacker makes sure that the bottom grappler's right upper arm is trapped to the attacker's torso.

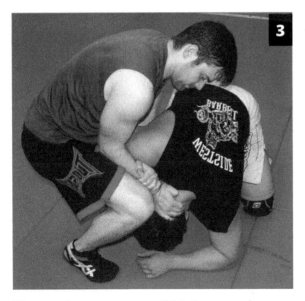

The attacker comes up off his knees and moves up into a squatting position as shown. Doing this, he positions his feet so he is able to go to the next step.

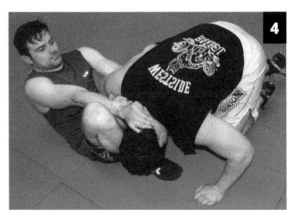

The attacker squats and rolls back onto his buttocks, and as he does this, he jams his right shin in the right side of the defender's head as shown. The next photo shows a top view of this.

NEAR ARM SIT BACK COMPRESSION BENT ARMLOCK

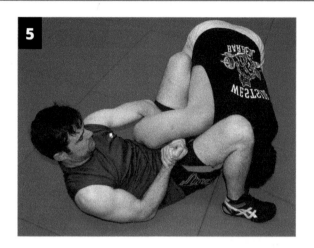

This view shows how the attacker rolls back onto his buttocks and jams his right shin against the right side of his opponent's head. The attacker's left shin is jammed against the defender's right side or hip.

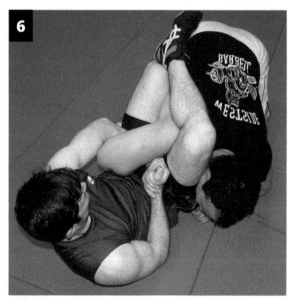

The attacker moves his right foot and leg over his opponent's right shoulder as shown. It is important to point out that the defender's right lower arm has been trapped between the attacker's legs from the start of this move. By doing this, the attacker has his opponent's right arm trapped in a strong compression bent armlock.

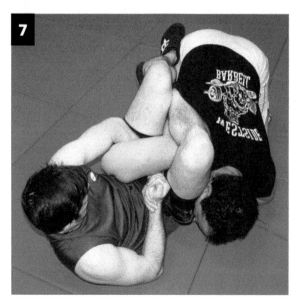

The attacker places the top of his right foot (his instep or the laces of his shoes) in the back of his left knee, forming a triangle with his legs. The attacker applies pressure with his legs and arches his hips, creating a strong compression bent armlock.

VERTICAL FRONT CHEST HOLD TO PRETZEL COMPRESSION BENT ARMLOCK

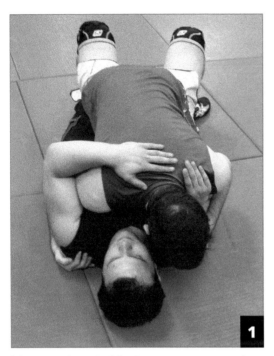

The attacker holds his opponent with a vertical front chest hold and will go on to apply the armlock from this position.

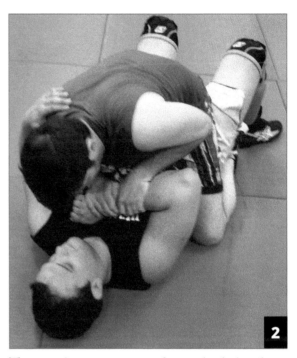

The attacker raises up and uses both hands to grab onto his opponent's right forearm and wrist as shown.

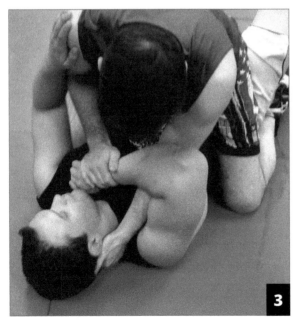

The attacker continues to use his right hand to hold his opponent's right wrist as he moves his left hand between the bottom grappler's right upper arm and neck as shown.

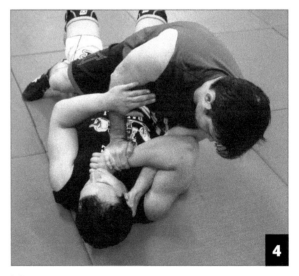

The top grappler leans forward and to his left as he uses his right foot and leg to push off the mat. The top grappler will move his right leg up and over the bottom grappler's head

VERTICAL FRONT CHEST HOLD TO PRETZEL COMPRESSINO BENT ARMLOCK

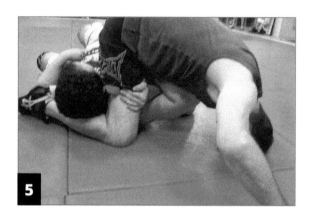

The top grappler moves his right foot and leg over his opponent's head and jams it under the bottom grappler's neck as shown. Doing this traps the bottom grappler's right forearm between the top grappler's legs, creating the start of a compression bent armlock. The top grappler uses his right hand and arm to post for stability.

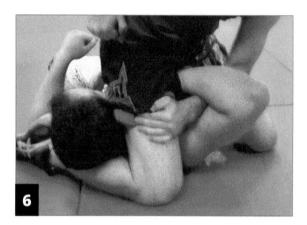

This photo shows how the attacker sits up (for a better view) to illustrate how he traps his opponent's bent right forearm between the attacker's legs. Look at how the attacker has placed his left forearm between his opponent's right forearm and right upper arm and places his left hand on his right upper leg for control and leverage. This is the compression bent armlock that will be applied.

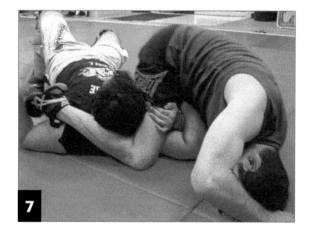

The attacker leans forward and uses his right foot and leg to hook his opponent's head. Doing this creates a strong compression bent armlock.

STRAIGHT ARMLOCK FROM THE HEAD-AND-ARM SIDE CHEST HOLD-DOWN

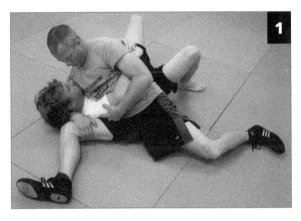

The attacker (on top) controls his opponent with a head-and-arm side chest hold-down.

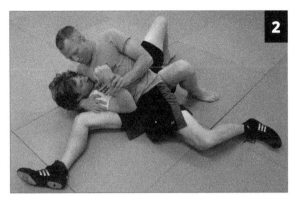

The attacker uses his left hand to grab his opponent's right wrist or forearm and start to push it down toward the mat.

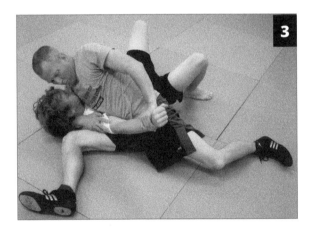

The attacker makes sure to use his left hand to grab low on his opponent's right arm at his opponent's right wrist. Doing this helps control the bottom grappler's right arm better.

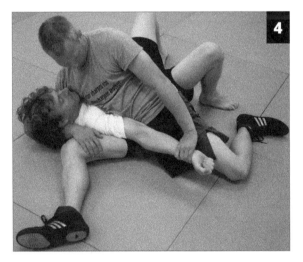

The attacker straightens his opponent's right arm so that the bottom grappler's right elbow is stretched and levered over the attacker's right hip as shown.

IMPORTANT: This may be a simple and basic move, but it's worked for a long time for a lot of sambo wrestlers and will continue to work for a long time for a lot more sambo wrestlers.

STRAIGHT ARMLOCK WITH FOOT PUSH FROM HEAD-AND-ARM SIDE CHEST HOLD-DOWN

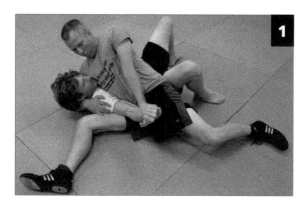

The top grappler holds his opponent with a head-and-arm side chest hold-down and uses his left hand to push his opponent's right arm down toward the mat.

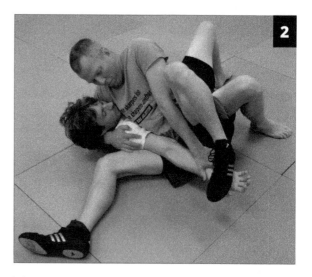

The top grappler moves his left foot and leg up and places his left foot on his opponent's forearm and wrist. The attacker pushes down with his left foot, barring the bottom grappler's extended right arm.

STRAIGHT ARMLOCK WITH KNEE FROM HEAD-AND-ARM SIDE CHEST HOLD-DOWN

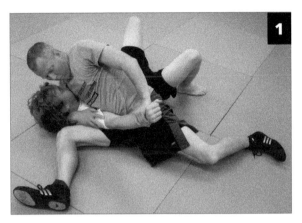

The attacker holds his opponent with a head-and-arm side chest hold-down. As he does this, the attacker uses his left hand to grab and push his opponent's right forearm and wrist down toward the mat.

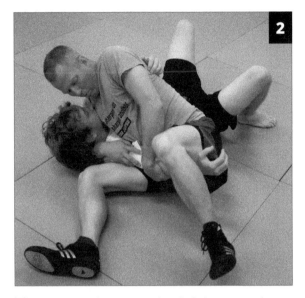

The top grappler swings his left leg up and over the bottom grappler's extended right arm as shown.

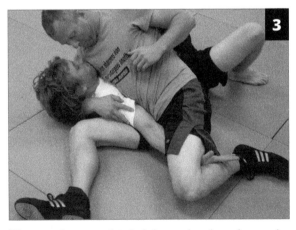

The attacker uses his left leg to hook and trap the bottom grappler's right extended arm, levering it over the attacker's right upper leg.

ALTERNATIVE FINISH

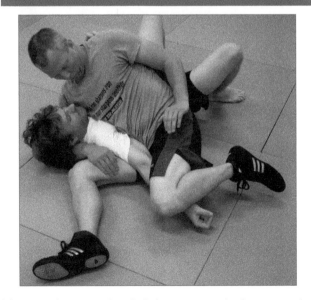

The attacker uses his left knee to push down on the extended right arm of the bottom grappler, creating a straight armlock.

SAMBO ENCYCLOPEDIA

FRONT SIT-THROUGH STRAIGHT ARMLOCK

This armlock is useful if the bottom grappler grabs the top grappler's leg. This is common if a sambo wrestler attempts a single leg takedown or otherwise grabs his opponent's leg during groundfighting.

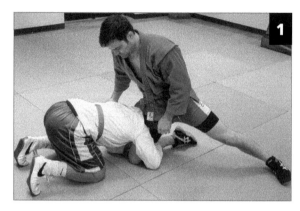

The attacker (top) is positioned at the head of his opponent. The bottom grappler has used both of his hands and arms to grab the top grappler's right upper leg. The attacker moves his left foot to his left side for stability.

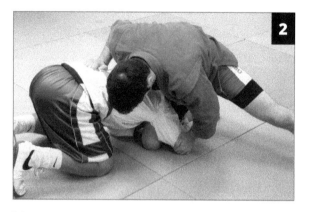

The attacker uses his left hand to grab and trap the bottom grappler's right elbow. As he does this, the attacker drives his right knee forward.

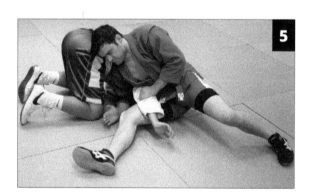

The attacker continues to sit through with his right foot and leg as shown.

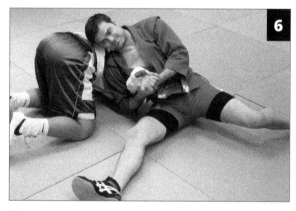

The attacker immediately uses both hands and arms to grab onto the defender's right forearm. It is important that the attacker grab with his palms up.

FRONT SIT THROUGH STRAIGHT ARMLOCK

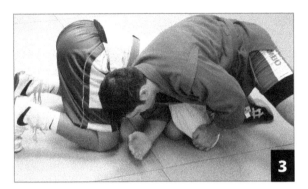

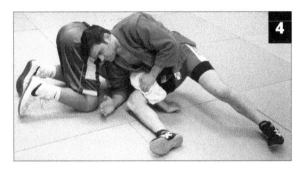

The attacker leans forward and jams his right elbow in the bottom grappler's right armpit area as shown. Doing this traps the bottom grappler's right arm more securely.

The attacker slides his right leg forward and sits through. Doing this starts to straighten the bottom grappler's right arm as shown. Look at how the top grappler continues to lean forward so that he uses the right side of his body to trap the bottom grappler's right arm.

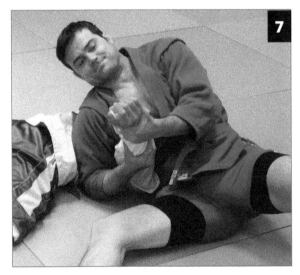

By grabbing palm up with his hands, the attacker has more leverage when applying the armlock. Sometimes the defender may collapse on his belly, and sometimes the defender may stay on his knees. Either way, this armlock is effective.

SIT-THROUGH STRAIGHT ARMLOCK

This is a pretty standard approach to doing this armlock, but it really works.

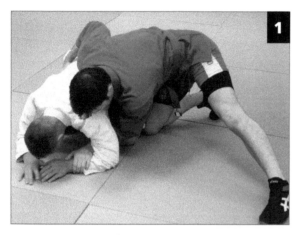

The attacker rides his opponent from the side and uses his left hand to grab his opponent's left wrist.

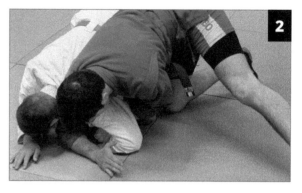

The attacker reaches over the bottom grappler's left shoulder as he leans forward.

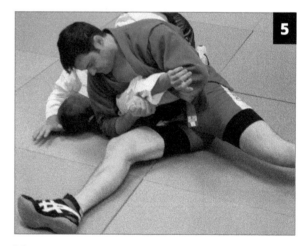

The attacker sits through with his right foot and leg as shown. As he does this, he drives his body so that his right side is pressed hard on the bottom grappler's left side and shoulder blade area. The attacker continues to use both of his hands and arms to lift and straighten the defender's left arm. Look at how the attacker's right upper arm is positioned on the bottom grappler's left upper arm and how the attacker's left forearm is positioned under the bottom grappler's left forearm. The attacker uses his left forearm to lift upward on his opponent's left forearm and uses his right upper arm to trap the defender's left upper arm as he uses the weight of his body to apply a downward pressure. Doing this creates a strong armlock.

SIT-THROUGH STRAIGHT ARMLOCK

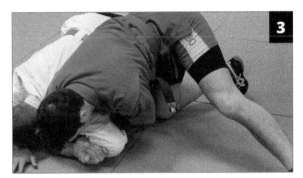

The attacker grasps his hands together in a square grip, trapping the bottom grappler's left arm.

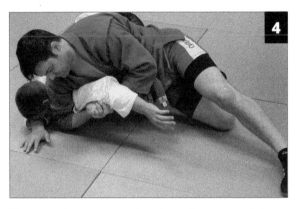

The attacker uses his hands and arms to lift his opponent's left arm off of the mat and starts to move his right leg forward.

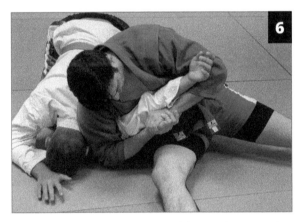

This close view shows how the attacker uses his hands and arms to trap and lever his opponent's straight left arm.

TRANSITION TO STRAIGHT ARMLOCK FROM A STANDING POSITION

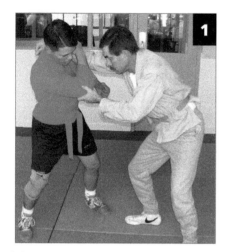

The attacker (on the left) uses his left hand to push off his opponent's right-hand grip as shown.

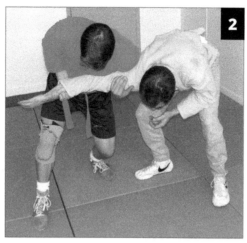

The attacker does an arm drag and secures a two-on-one grip on his opponent's right arm.

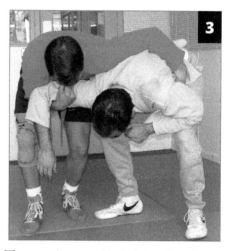

The attacker uses his left hand and arm to reach around his opponent's low back area and secure a tightwaist. As he does this, the attacker uses his right arm to hook and trap his opponent's right arm to the attacker's chest.

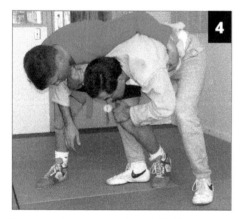

The attacker moves his left foot in so that it is placed on the inside of his opponent's right foot and leg as shown. Look at how the attacker has turned so he is facing the same direction as his opponent.

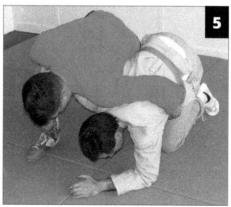

The attacker drives his opponent forward to the mat.

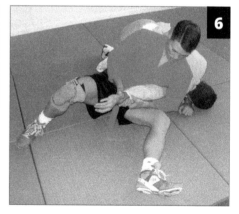

As he drives his opponent to the mat, the attacker quickly sits through with his left foot and leg and traps his opponent's right arm as shown. As the attacker continues to drive forward and down, he places a great deal of his body weight directly on the defender's right arm and elbow (as well as his right shoulder). Doing this creates a powerful straight armlock.

ALLAN SIT-THROUGH TO THE STRAIGHT ARMLOCK

This move is named for World Sambo Champion Maurice Allan who first taught it to the author in the 1970s.

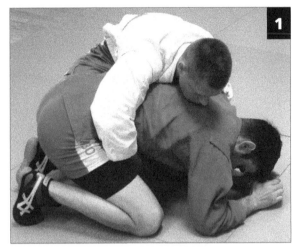

The attacker (bottom) is on all fours with his opponent riding him with his right arm around the bottom grappler's waist.

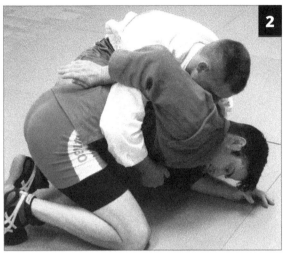

The bottom grappler uses his right hand and arm to grab and hook the top grappler's right upper arm (grab between his elbow and shoulder).

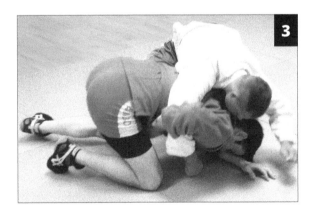

The bottom grappler uses his right hand to hook and trap his opponent's right arm. As he does this, the bottom grappler moves his lower body to his right so that the top grappler now is positioned higher up on the bottom grappler's back as shown. As he does this, the attacker moves his left foot and leg out straight.

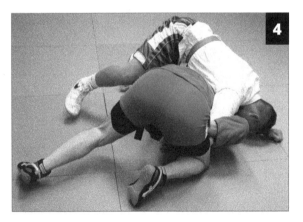

The bottom grappler continues to move his lower body to his right so that he is now starting to duck under the top grappler's right side as shown.

ALLAN SIT THROUGH TO THE STRAIGHT ARMLOCK

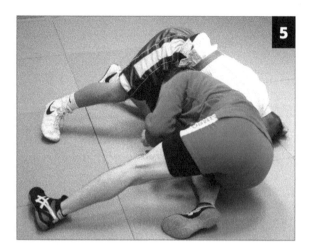

The bottom grappler continues to move his lower body to his right and moves his head out from under his opponent's body as shown.

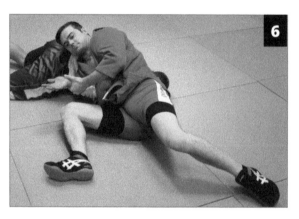

As the bottom grappler continues to move backward and to his right, he kicks his left foot and leg back so that his left foot is placed on the mat as shown, and he is now positioned on his right hip. As he does this, the attacker uses both hands to pull his opponent's right arm out straight.

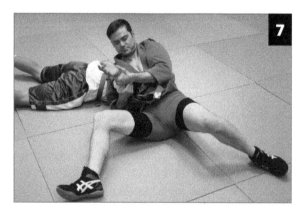

The attacker leans back and uses both hands (palms up) to pull and stretch his opponent's extended right arm, securing a strong straight armlock.

SQUARE GRIP TRAP STRAIGHT ARMLOCK

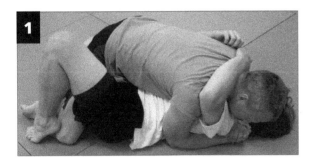

The attacker (on top) holds his opponent with a side chest hold-down.

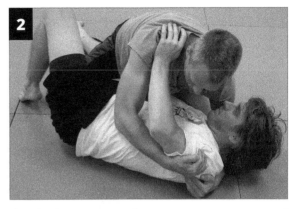

The top grappler uses his right hand and arm to hook and trap his opponent's left upper arm as shown. As he does this, the attacker uses his right arm to pull the bottom grappler up and off the mat and close to him.

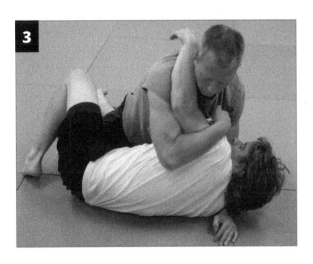

As the bottom grappler attempts to escape and make space between the two bodies, the attacker will focus on the bottom grappler's right arm and hand, which is pushing on the top grappler's shoulder.

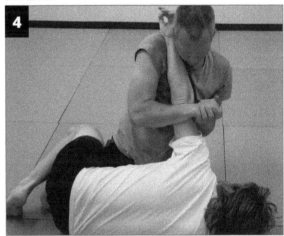

The attacker pulls his opponent's left arm up and cradles or traps the bottom grappler's left wrist and forearm between his right shoulder and head. As he does this, the attacker uses his right forearm and hand (palm down) to trap the defender's left elbow and uses his left hand to grab his right hand and form a square grip. The attacker pulls the defender's extended and straight left arm into the attacker's chest and applies the straight armlock.

Sambo has a rich history and tradition of innovative, functional and realistic armlocks. What's been presented in this chapter on upper body submissions is a sample of the many, varied, and effective armlocks practiced and used in the sport of sambo. Let's now turn our attention to the hold-downs of sambo and what makes make them work.

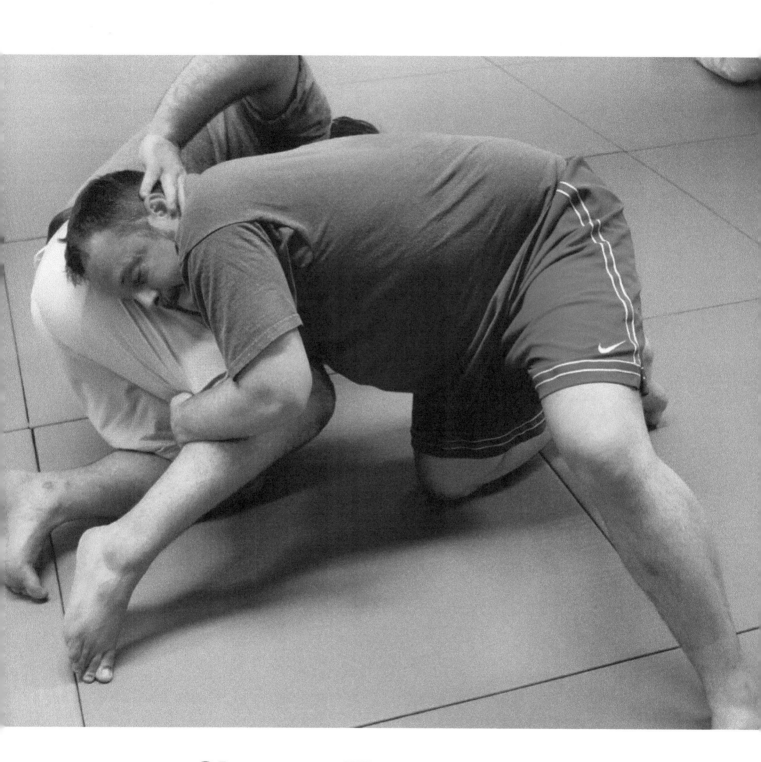

Chapter Five: The Holds and Breakdowns of Sambo

"Park him there until he quits."

SAMBO'S HOLD-DOWNS

This chapter examines the hold-downs and breakdowns used in the sport of sambo. Hold-downs and breakdowns are the "bread and butter" of sambo, a mainstay of good, effective grappling. Hold-downs have two primary purposes in sambo. First, hold-downs score points. Second, hold-downs are used to control an opponent long enough to secure a submission technique. Unlike most styles of Western wrestling where a "pin" wins a match when a wrestler's shoulders touch simultaneously or for a short period of time, the hold-downs in sambo place emphasis on controlling an opponent who is largely on his back with his shoulders touching the mat and with the attacker's torso (front, side, or back) maintaining contact with the defender's torso.

As a result of not being able to gain an outright win by holding an opponent to the mat, hold-downs are often used as the basis for transition moves where the attacker holds his opponent for a maximum score of four points and, upon the mat official's signal, will transition to an armlock or leglock.

The hold-downs of sambo appear very similar, if not identical in some cases, to many of the hold-downs used in judo and are based directly on judo's concept of "osaekomi," holding or immobilizing an opponent on the mat. The rules of sport judo evolved so that holding an opponent for a specific period of time will win the match, but the rules of sambo allow for a maximum of four points for a twenty-second hold-down and two points for a hold-down of ten to nineteen seconds. A maximum of four points are permitted for hold-downs in a sambo match.

In addition to holding an opponent for time on the mat, the skills necessary to put him there are called breakdowns, and they are analyzed in this chapter as well. No one is going to lay down and allow you to hold him to the mat on his back, much less armlock or leglock him. The primary purpose of a breakdown is to take an opponent from a stable to an unstable position while in groundfighting and ultimately secure a hold-down or submission technique. The best way to describe a breakdown is that it is a transition from one position to another position to control an opponent and very much like a throwing technique, only done in a groundfighting situation. It's also common to use the term "turnover"

when describing what we call breakdowns. But there is a fundamental difference in these terms that goes to the heart of what sambo is about. A "breakdown" describes what you do to an opponent. You aggressively pursue him, control him, dominate him, and then hold him down long enough to apply a submission technique. You break him down from a stable to an unstable position and may not always turn him over onto his back. In addition to breaking down his body, you are aggressively pursuing your opponent and breaking down his will to fight. The term "turnover" limits the scope of the movement, indicating that the only thing you can do is turn your opponent over. Additionally, the word turnover doesn't convey the aggressive nature of what a sambo wrestler is doing. A turnover is a benign word, and to this author's way of thinking, a turnover is a sweet pastry that is nice to have at breakfast.

Hold-downs and breakdowns may not be flashy or the kind of thing that gets a spectacular tap out, but they are fundamentally important for every sambo wrestler to know and master. A good way to look at hold-downs and breakdowns is to compare them to a good, reliable friend who is always there when you need him.

This chapter will first analyze the key points common to all effective hold-downs and then go on to present some of functional hold-downs used in sambo and key points about each of them. After that, we will analyze several effective breakdowns and controlling skills that are used to secure hold-downs as well as gain further control of an opponent.

TECHNICAL TIP: Hold-downs and breakdowns are important skills. A hold-down serves two primary purposes in sambo. It scores points and it sets an opponent up to apply a submission technique to finish him off. A breakdown takes an opponent from a stable to an unstable position, allowing the attacker to apply a hold-down or even apply a submission technique.

VITAL POINTS COMMON TO ALL HOLD-DOWNS

Effective control over an opponent with hold-downs requires some fundamentally important things to take place. Each is important by itself, but they are dependent on each other for maximum results. Not every situation is the same, but if the top grappler applies these fundamental elements, the bottom grappler's odds of escaping or reversing the position diminish quickly over the period of time the hold is maintained. These basic characteristics of effective control are:

Solid, Yet Mobile Base

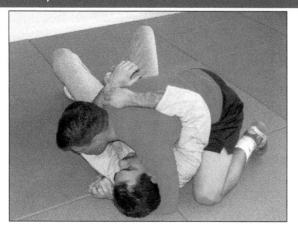

The top grappler's hips are low to the mat, and he keeps a wide base using his legs. Doing this allows the top grappler to shift his body weight as necessary to maintain control of his opponent.

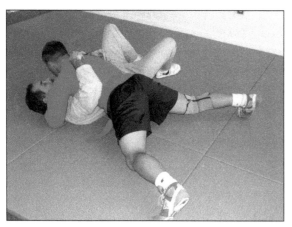

A mobile and strong base is necessary. The top grappler's feet, legs, and hips comprise this base, and this base is mobile. The top grappler is prepared to shift his body weight and move his feet, legs, and hips as necessary to control and ride the bottom grappler, maintaining control. This photo shows how the attacker extends his legs to provide a wider base when holding his opponent.

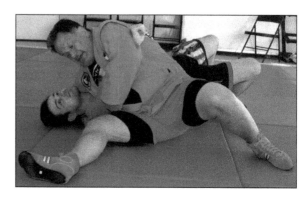

The top grappler uses his feet and legs independently of each other, yet they are interdependent for the success of the hold. This photos shows how the top grappler uses his left leg and foot to push off of the mat and provide stability and uses his right leg and foot to steer where the bottom grappler is allowed to move. A good analogy is how sailors control a ship in the water; the top grappler uses his left leg as the ballast that provides stability for the ship and uses his right leg to serve in the same way a rudder steers the ship.

Hip Control

Attacker Controls His Own Hips

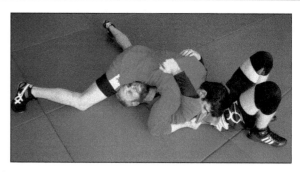

The attacker controls his hips. The top grappler controls his hip movement and (as a result) often controls the hip movement of his opponent. This photo shows how the attacker uses an upper chest hold and keeps his hips low to the mat, pressing his opponent down onto the mat as much as possible. The hips are the center of the human body. A vital element to controlling and holding an opponent to the mat for time is to control his hips and to use your hips effectively. The attacker initiates his control over his opponent by how he moves his hips and shifts the weight of his body as he moves his hips. A fundamental rule to remember when applying a hold-down is "hips on the mat." This means that the top grappler holding his opponent should keep his hips low to the mat for maximum control. But it is also important to remember that while the attacker's hips must be low to the mat, the attacker must also make sure he has the ability to move his hips as necessary to shift the weight of his body to maintain control. By extension, the top grappler controls the legs and feet of his opponent by controlling his hips. Likewise, the top grappler also has better use of his feet and legs if he has good hip placement and control. With this good hip control, the top grappler can better shift from one position to another and use his legs and feet more effectively to maintain control and then go on to gain further control or a finishing hold.

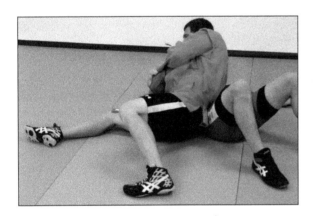

The attacker controls his own hip movement to control his opponent's hips. An experienced athlete develops a "feel" as to when it's the best time to move or shift his body weight to maintain control of his opponent. Moving, shifting, and controlling an opponent using hip movement is a vital skill in holding an opponent to the mat for time. This is a good example of how the top grappler maintains control with a fluid, moving (yet solid) base starting with good hip control. Remember, your legs are an extension of your hips, and it's important to use them to work independently as well as jointly to control your opponent.

Attacker Controls Opponent's Hips

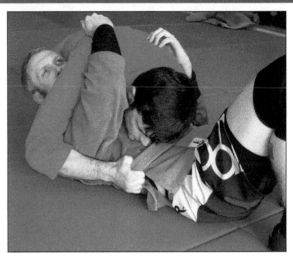

The attacker controls his opponent's hips, with his hands and arms holding his opponent's uniform or belt. This photo shows how the attacker uses his hands to hold onto his opponent's belt and control the bottom grappler's hip movement. The attacker can (and should) use any permitted hold or grip on the opponent's body or uniform to control his opponent. This is a good example of Rene Pommerelle's advice: "Everything is a handle."

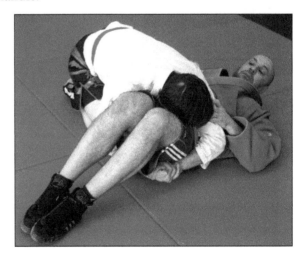

The attacker controls his opponent's hips by actually holding onto the bottom grappler's hips and trapping him to the mat. The attacker makes it direct and effective by controlling his opponent's hips by holding onto them and locking his hands together as shown.

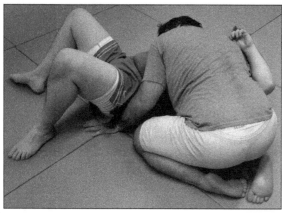

The attacker controls his opponent's hips with a hand check. The top grappler prevents the bottom grappler from shrimping in to initiate an escape by using his left hand to "check" the bottom man's hips. Doing this prevents the bottom man from turning into the top grappler as shown in the photo below.

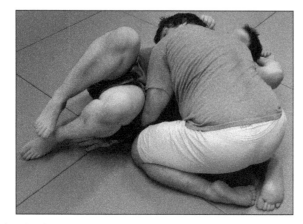

As the bottom man shrimps into the top grappler, the top grappler stops the shrimping action with his hand check.

Control Opponent's Head

The old saying, "Where the head goes, the body follows" is certainly true when using head control while holding an opponent. It's often true that if you control your opponent's head, you control his body.

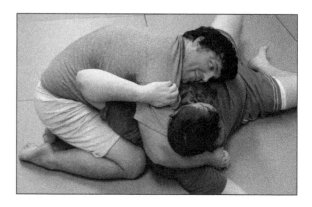

The top grappler controls his opponent's head and shoulders (and as an extension of the shoulders, the opponent's arms as well). The top grappler must prevent his opponent from being able to use his head to bridge off of the mat, and this is why head control is important. The bottom man's shoulders must be controlled so that he is unable to use them to provide a base on the mat to push up and against the top grappler. Think of this as similar to the bench press. If your shoulders are flat and square on the bench, you are better able to press the barbell off of your chest than if your shoulders are lying uneven on the bench or are crunched together. By extension, because the arms are, of course, connected to the shoulders, it is important for the top grappler to control both the shoulders and arms of the bottom grappler to negate their power.

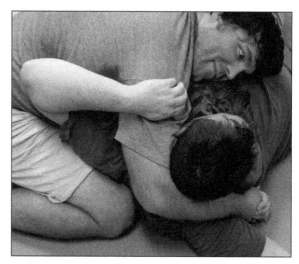

Elbow to Knee for Control: The top grappler positions his right elbow to his right knee in this photo so that the top grappler's right elbow and right knee almost touch. Doing this traps the bottom grappler's head securely. Additionally, the top grappler must see to it that the bottom man's near arm (in this photo, the bottom grappler's left arm) is made useless. If the bottom grappler can get his inside arm free, the bottom man has a better chance of using it to push against the top grappler or sliding it under the top grappler's body to initiate an escape.

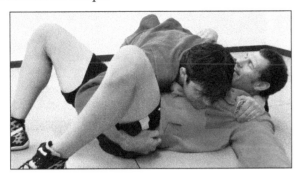

The primary reason the top grappler controls the bottom man's head is to prevent him from bridging and initiating an escape. However, by using his left arm (in this photo) to trap and control his opponent's head, the top grappler also makes the hold an unpleasant and often painful experience. Making the whole thing unpleasant keeps the bottom man's mind more tuned in to survival than to trying to escape. One of my athletes, Shawn Watson, once remarked, "Park him there until he quits. Make it so bad for your opponent that if he doesn't give up from the hold-down, he'll be softened up for an armlock or leglock." This exemplifies sambo's hard-core and aggressive approach to controlling and holding an opponent to the mat.

Control Opponent's Chest and Torso

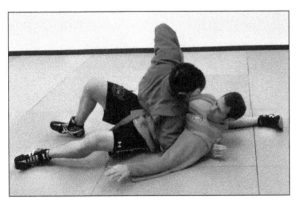

By placing his weight and pressing down, the top grappler forces the bottom man to bear the burden of the top man's weight, pinning him and taking a lot of the fight out of him at the same time. This photo shows how the top sambo wrestler can use his chest to press down on his opponent's chest and torso to maintain control. The top grappler's chest is often the part of his body that does this, but the top grappler may use any part of his body to get the job done.

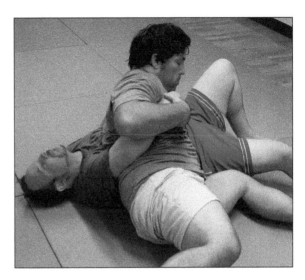

This photo shows how the top grappler distributes the weight of his body and creates a fluid but solid base with his hips and legs to apply pressure to his opponent. Look at how the top grappler uses his right hand and arm to trap and pull up on the bottom grappler's right arm to add pressure to the chest control he already has.

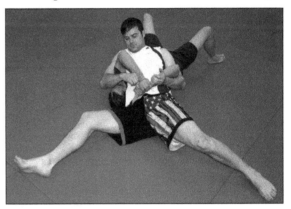

This photo shows the top grappler holding his opponent with the top grappler's back in contact with the bottom grappler's chest. The top grappler is not required to have only "chest to chest" contact but can have his back in contact with the bottom grappler's chest or any variation of torso contact as long as the bottom grappler is on his back and being held under the control of the top grappler.

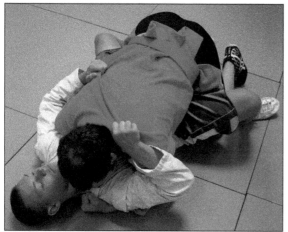

and control his opponent's right upper leg. The most important thing is that the top grappler has his opponent on his back and has torso-to-torso contact, making this an effective hold-down. Another factor to consider is that any number of holds can (and are) combined with each other in actual, competitive situations, providing a wide range of hold-down variations.

The hold-down is effective even if the top grappler is between his opponent's legs or has a leg scissored by the bottom grappler. The top grappler does not have to be clear of his opponent's legs for the hold to be effective. Unlike the sport of judo or some other grappling sports where the hold is considered broken or terminated when the bottom grappler, the rules of sambo allow this.

THE HOLD JUST HAS TO WORK, IT DOESN'T HAVE TO BE PERFECT

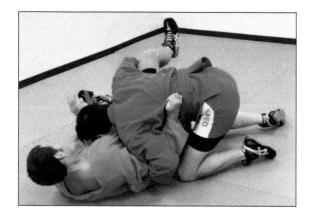

This photo shows what a sambo hold-down can often look like in an actual competitive situation. Holding an opponent to the mat is a fluid, dynamic activity. For this reason, not every effective hold is picture perfect. The idea is for the attacker to hold and control his opponent to the mat to score points and ultimately set him up for a submission technique. As long as the top grappler's hold-down meets the criteria for effectiveness, it doesn't matter what it looks like. This photo show how the top grappler has just taken his opponent to the mat and uses his left hand and arm to trap and control the bottom grappler's right arm. The top grappler gains further control by using his right hand and arm to hook

TRANSITION FROM THROW TO HOLD-DOWN

The sequence of an attacker throwing his opponent to the mat and immediately transitioning to a hold-down is one of the most commonly used skills in the sport of sambo. It's what I call an "eight-point move." The attacker can score a maximum of four points for the throw and immediately apply a hold-down that can earn him another four points for a total of eight points. After gaining his points from his hold-down, the attacker can go on to attempt a submission technique to finish the match.

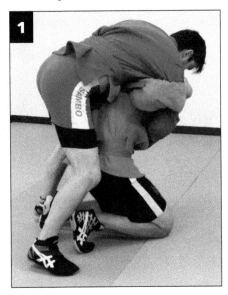

The attacker does a knee-drop back carry throw as shown. Any throw can be used, but this is a good example because the throw is used so often in this situation.

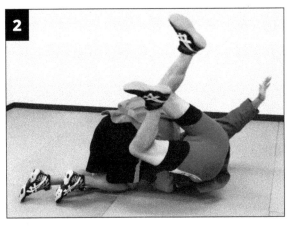

The attacker throws so he can score maximum points. The more points the better for the attacker.

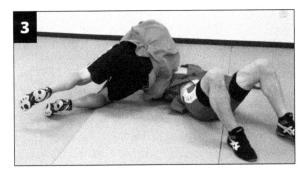

The attacker follows through to ensure that he scores as many points as possible for the throw and that he is in the best position possible as he finishes the throw to secure a hold-down.

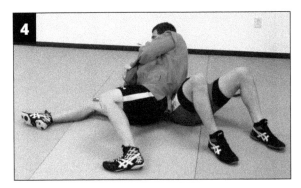

The attacker immediately transitions to a hold-down.

TRANSITION FROM A HOLD-DOWN TO SUBMISSION TECHNIQUE

Transitioning from a hold-down to a submission technique is a vital aspect of sambo. As mentioned throughout this chapter, the two purposes of a hold-down are (1) holding an opponent for time to score points and (2) holding an opponent in order to transition to a submission technique. Presented here is a series of photographs illustrating a typical transition from a hold-down to a submission technique (in this case, a cross-body armlock).

Vertical Hold Transition to Cross-Body Armlock

Here is an example of how the top grappler transitions smoothly and with maximum control to a cross-body armlock.

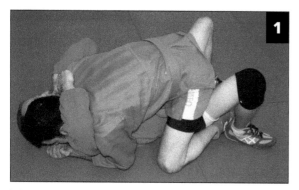

The attacker (on top) holds his opponent with the vertical chest hold as shown.

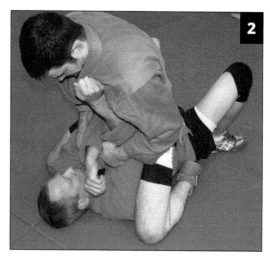

After scoring four points for the hold and on the mat official's signal, the attacker postures up, making sure that his knees and legs are jammed tightly along each side of the bottom grappler's upper torso as shown. As he does this, the attacker uses his left hand and arm to start to trap the bottom grappler's right arm.

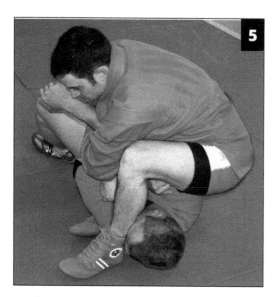

The attacker moves his left foot and leg over the bottom grappler's head. Look at how the top grappler's left heel is jammed on the bottom grappler's head. As he does this, the attacker uses both hands and arms to hug and trap his opponent's right arm to the attacker's chest. At this point, the attacker rolls back onto his buttocks.

TECHNICAL TIP: Make it a regular habit at your workouts on the mat to transition from hold-downs to submission techniques. Everyone has his or her own favorite transitions, but you won't know them or become skilled at them unless you practice this aspect of sambo on a regular basis.

TRANSITION FROM A HOLD-DOWN TO SUBMISSION TECHNIQUE

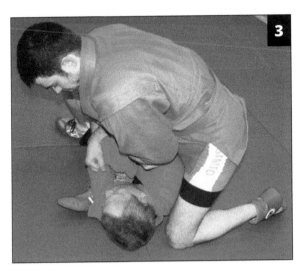

The attacker turns to his right, coming up on his right foot and left knee as shown. As he does this, the attacker uses his left hand and arm to hug and trap the bottom grappler's right arm to the top grappler's chest. The top grappler uses his feet and legs to trap the bottom grappler's body with the top grappler's right foot (heel of his foot) jammed in the bottom man's torso and with the top grappler's left knee jammed in the back of the bottom grappler's upper back as shown.

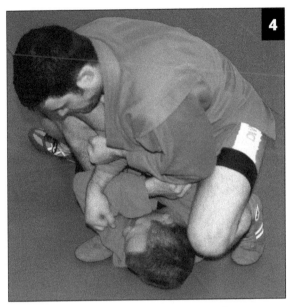

The attacker comes up to his feet and continues to turn to his right, making sure to stay round and compact. Doing this further controls the bottom grappler.

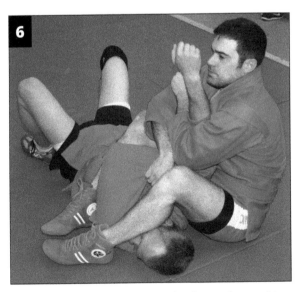

The attacker rolls back onto his buttocks, making sure to control his opponent's body with his feet and legs and use both hands and arms to hug and trap his opponent's right arm.

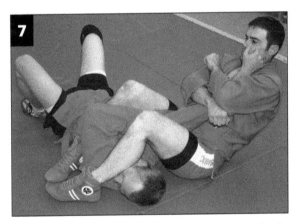

The attacker rolls back and applies the cross-body armlock.

This series of photographs illustrates how an effective hold-down is the basis for an effective submission technique.

THE TOP GRAPPLER ALWAYS MAINTAINS CONTROL OF THE HOLD AND CONTINUALLY ATTEMPTS TO GAIN MORE CONTROL

The sambo wrestler holding his opponent knows that he has to hold the bottom grappler to the mat for twenty seconds in order to secure four points from the referee. The top grappler also knows he wants to control his opponent so he can more easily secure a submission technique from this position. Another thing the top grappler knows is that his opponent won't just lie on his back and let the top grappler win. The bottom man will fight and do everything he can to escape. Because of this, the top grappler may have to switch from one hold or position to another to maintain control over his opponent. In some cases, the top grappler may not initially be in the best of positions as he applies the hold and may not have enough control to hold his opponent for any length of time. In this situation, the top grappler must continually do what he can to gain more control over his opponent so he can hold him for the maximum time. Also, the top grappler may have a solid hold but, by design or opportunity, decide to modify his original hold or switch to another. In any event, the top grappler will continually improve his position of control over his opponent. The top grappler will use any part of his body to shift, move, or switch from one controlling position to another. Presented here are a couple of typical situations where the top grappler does what is necessary to maintain control and gain even more control over his opponent.

Sit Through with Feet and Legs

Here is an example of how the top grappler will continually attempt to improve his position. This series shows a specific situation where the top grappler uses a sit-through with his feet and legs to shift his body weight and control his opponent.

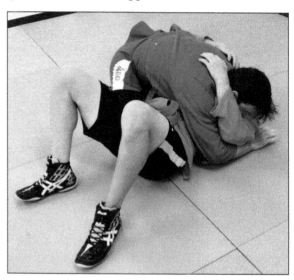

The top grappler holds his opponent with a chest hold.

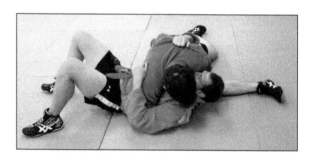

As the bottom grappler struggles to escape, the top grappler shifts his right foot and leg forward and kicks his left leg back, rotating his hips so that the top grappler sits though with his right foot and leg and maintains control over his opponent.

Top Grappler Uses Hand and Arms to Control Opponent

Sometimes, the top grappler may not have as strong of a hold on his opponent as he would like. In this situation, the top grappler can switch to another hold to improve his control over his opponent.

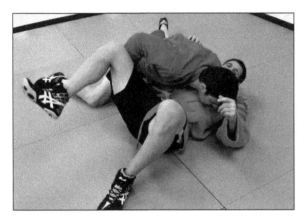

This series of photographs specifically shows how the top grappler will switch from one hold to another by securing control of his opponent's near (right) leg.

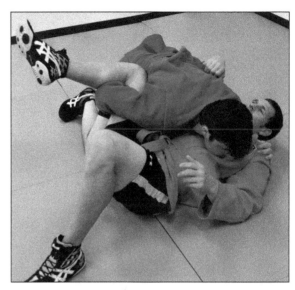

The top grappler quickly uses his right hand and arm to hook over and control his opponent's right upper leg, switching from a chest hold to a side chest hold with near leg control. This series of photographs illustrates a common and effective way to switch from a hold that may not be strong to begin with to a stronger hold.

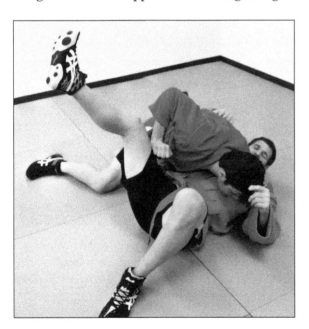

As the bottom grappler attempts to escape, the top grappler looks for anything he can use as a handle to grab, trap, and control his opponent. This photo shows the top grappler moving his right hand to hook over the bottom grappler's right leg.

ESCAPING FROM A HOLD-DOWN

We've all been on the bottom of a hold-down at some time in our careers, and there is no doubt that winning is more fun than losing. For this reason, it's a good idea to regularly practice defense and escapes for hold-downs. Presented here is an effective skill to escape from the most commonly used hold-down in sambo, the chest hold.

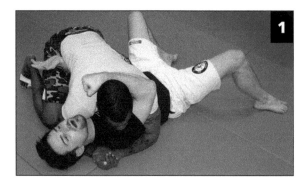

The top grappler holds his opponent with a chest hold.

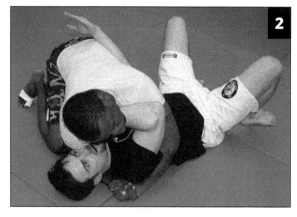

The bottom grappler uses his right forearm to wedge and push up against the top grappler's head. As he does this, the bottom grappler slides his left hand and arm under the top grappler's body as shown.

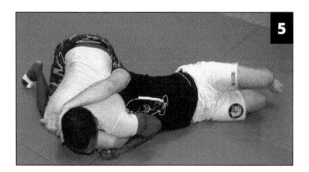

The bottom grappler continues to forcefully turn to his right side, compelling the top grappler to start to roll. As he does this, the bottom grappler uses his left hand to hook the back and side of the top grappler's head and uses his left hand to grab his right hand. Doing this traps the top grappler's head.

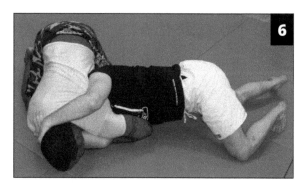

The bottom grappler has control with both of his hands and arms on his opponent's head as the bottom grappler continues to turn to his right forcefully.

ESCAPING FROM A HOLD-DOWN

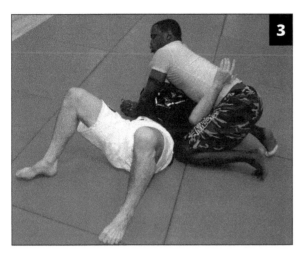

The view shows how the bottom grappler slides his left hand and arm (palm up for maximum power) under his opponent's torso. Look at how the bottom grappler's feet are firmly planted on the mat with his knees bent. The bottom grappler does this for the stability and leverage he will need in the next step of this move.

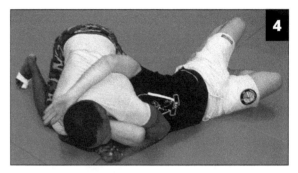

The bottom grappler pushes off of his feet and drives upward and to the right with his body as shown. As he does this, the bottom grappler quickly turns to his right side.

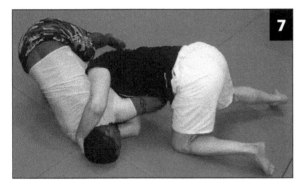

As the bottom grappler turns to his right, he uses both of his hands and arms to roll his opponent over him. The bottom grappler has escaped from the hold-down and will continue on to counter with his own hold-down.

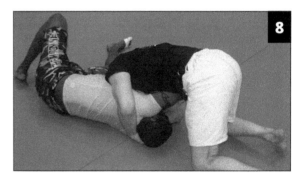

The attacker has escaped and uses an upper chest hold to control his opponent.

SOME OF SAMBO'S BASIC HOLD-DOWNS

Presented here are some of the fundamental hold-downs used in sambo. As with any dynamic and performance-based set of skills, there are many variations of these holds, and the holds shown on the following pages represent some of the most popular holds used in the sport of sambo. Later in this chapter, breakdowns, the skills that put an opponent onto his back and into a hold-down, will be analyzed.

CHEST HOLD

One of the most often-used holds in sambo at all levels of competition is the chest hold.

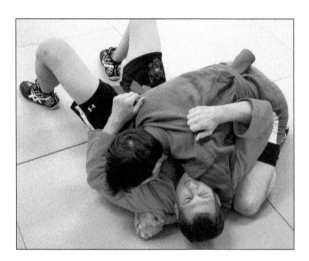

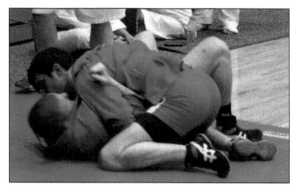

This shows a chest hold with the top grappler not controlling his opponent's head with his left hand and arm. Instead, the top grappler uses his left arm to hook and control his opponent's left arm. The low, wide base that the top grappler uses provides a strong and stable base that will hold the bottom grappler for the maximum time and provide the top grappler a strong position from which to launch a submission technique as well.

The top grappler positions his left arm under his opponent's head, and as he does this, the top grappler uses his right hand and arm to reach over the bottom grappler's chest, forming a square grip with his hands as shown. The top grappler makes sure to use his left elbow and arm to hook and trap the bottom grappler's head and prevent the bottom grappler from bridging in an effort to escape. The top grappler's legs are bent with his hips low to the mat. The top grappler's left knee is nearly touching his left elbow so that the bottom grappler's right shoulder is trapped. Doing this also traps the bottom grappler's right arm and prevents the bottom grappler from using his right hand and arm to push against the top grappler in an effort to escape. The top grappler's right knee is positioned against the bottom grappler's right hip (not shown in this photo). This low, wide position with the top grappler's knees wide and hips low creates a strong yet mobile base and allows the top grappler maximum control over his opponent. Look at how the top grappler's chest is positioned directly on his opponent's chest with the top grappler pressing downward with the weight of his body. All of these actions provide the top grappler a strong, fluid hold that controls the bottom grappler.

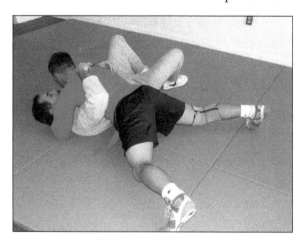

This photo shows a common variation of the chest hold where the top grappler extends his feet and legs, making sure that his hips are low to the mat.

CHEST HOLD

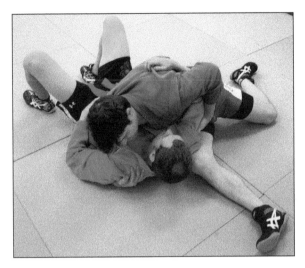

The top grappler started with a standard chest hold and shifted his leg position so that he performed a sit-through with his right foot and leg. Doing this shifted the top grappler's weight and hip position.

The chest hold is a versatile and effective hold with many variations. These photographs show a few of the most common.

TECHNICAL TIP: When holding your opponent, you may have to shift the position of your feet, legs, hips, or upper body in order to maintain control. Don't just lie there thinking the weight of your body will hold him down. React to your opponent's movement and do not hesitate to shift the weight of your body, change your position, or grab and control any part of his body or uniform (or your body or uniform) by using it as a handle to maintain control and hold him down.

FRONT CHEST HOLD

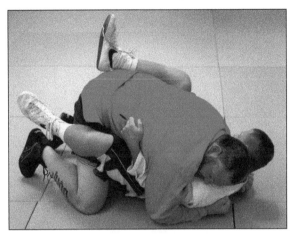

A common and effective hold is the front chest hold. The top grappler is situated between his opponent's legs and makes chest-to-chest contact as shown.

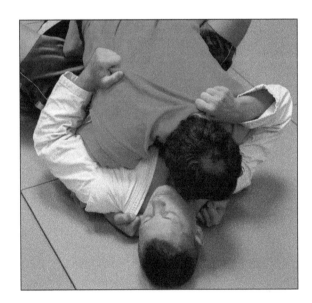

This photo shows how the top grappler uses his hands and arms to reach under the bottom grappler's shoulders and grab his collar to control him.

FRONT CHEST HOLD

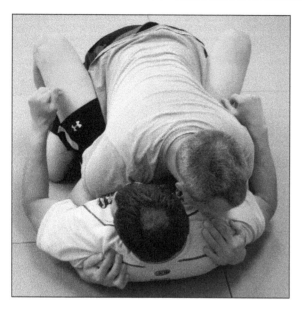

In situations where sambo wrestlers are fighting in sports that don't use sambo jackets, the top grappler uses his hands and arms to reach under his opponent's shoulders and hook with his hands at the bottom grappler's shoulders to control him.

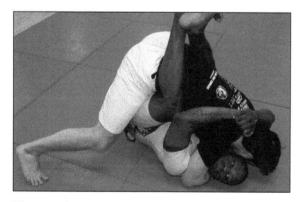

This application is similar to the previous one, but in this variation, the top grappler holds his opponent with a front chest hold with a tripod base. The attacker leans forward and extends his feet and legs out wide, creating the tripod base. As he does this, the top grappler rolls his opponent high onto the bottom grappler's shoulders. This gives the top grappler strong chest-to-chest contact and makes it difficult for the bottom grappler to escape. While using this hold, it is important for the top grappler to maintain his balance to prevent the bottom grappler from rolling over backwards and escaping.

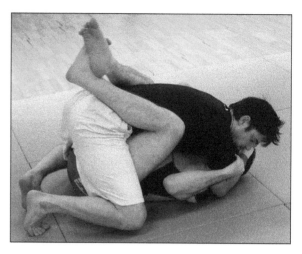

Here is an example of how the top grappler uses his feet and legs to control his opponent. The top grappler jams his knees and upper legs firmly against the bottom grappler's upper legs as shown. Doing this traps the bottom grappler's legs, making them ineffective. The top grappler uses his right arm to hook under the bottom grappler's neck to control it. The attacker drives forward on his feet so that the bottom grappler is rolled onto his upper back, allowing the top grappler more chest-to-chest contact and control in the hold.

SIDE CHEST HOLD

Actually, the side chest hold is the same hold-down as the chest hold with the exception that the top grappler uses (as shown here) his right hand and arm to reach between his opponent's legs and control either of the legs. There are two basic applications of the side chest hold. The first is when the attacker reaches with his hand and arm and controls his opponent's far leg (the bottom grappler's left leg in the first photo). The other basic application is when the attacker controls his opponent's near leg.

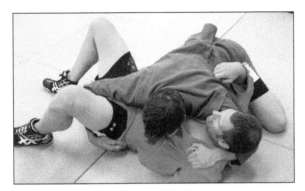

The attacker uses his right hand and arm to reach between his opponent's legs. The attacker uses his right hand to grab onto the bottom grappler's belt or jacket at the area of the bottom grappler's left hip as shown.

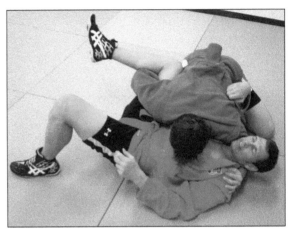

The second basic application of the side chest hold is shown here. The attacker uses his right hand and arm to reach between his opponent's legs. The attacker uses his right hand and arm to hook and trap the bottom grappler's right upper leg.

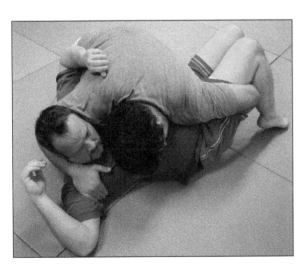

The side hold has numerous variations and here is an example of one. In this photo, the top grappler uses his left hand and arm to hook around his opponent's upper leg area. The top grappler uses his right hand and arm to reach under his opponent's head and neck. As he does this, the attacker uses his right hand to trap on the bottom grappler's right shoulder and armpit. Look at how the top grappler uses his right arm to control the bottom man's head.

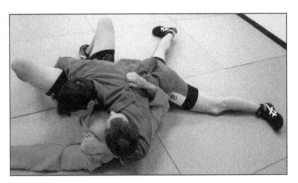

This photo shows the side hold with the top grappler's hips low to the mat and a wide leg base. This is a common and effective variation to give the top grappler a strong and stable base.

CRADLE SIDE CHEST HOLD

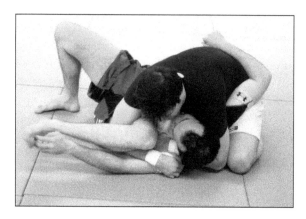

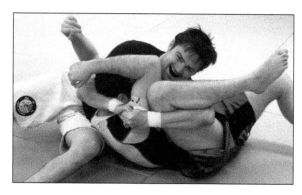

Basically, a cradle hold can be used in most any holding situation and is formed when the attacker grabs or hooks his hands or arms together (or otherwise uses his hands and arms to control his opponent) and forces his opponent to bend, making for an unpleasant, if not downright painful hold.

Cradles can be used along with any number of holds, and as shown here, the top grappler grabs his hands together to form a strong grip as he sits through with his left foot and leg to increase the pressure of the hold-down. Doing this bends the bottom grappler in half, making the whole situation painful and unpleasant for him. Sometimes, the pressure from the cradle is enough to make the bottom grappler tap out.

A cradle is a variation of the side chest hold but can be used in just about any situation. Made popular in freestyle and collegiate wrestling, cradles are effective because they bend the bottom grappler in two and are often extremely uncomfortable. The top grappler wants to make the whole experience of being controlled as unpleasant as possible for his opponent on the bottom. If the bottom guy is bent in half and stuck in a cradle, good for the top guy and bad for the bottom guy. If the bottom fighter is thinking of how much it hurts, he's not thinking of how to beat the top fighter.

HEAD AND ARM SIDE CHEST HOLD

A commonly used and effective application of the chest hold is the head and arm side chest hold. This hold is called kesa gatame (scarf hold) in judo.

The attacker is positioned on his right hip. The top grappler uses his right hand and arm to reach around his opponent's head and neck and grabs the top grappler's right upper leg. The attacker uses his left hand and arm to trap his opponent's arm to the top grappler's left chest area. The top grappler's feet and legs are positioned as shown here for maintaining a wide and fluid base.

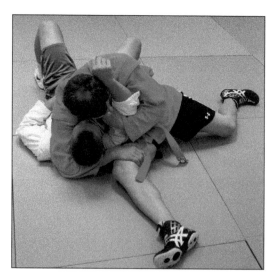

HEAD-AND-ARM SIDE CHEST HOLD

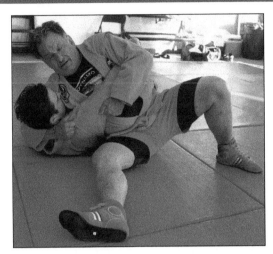

Often, the top grappler will use his right foot and leg as a rudder to steer where the bottom grappler goes. The top grappler places his left foot on the mat as shown in this application of the head-and-arm side chest hold to provide a stable base. In some cases, the top grappler may lean back so that he places a great deal of pressure on the bottom grappler's chest, forcing the bottom grappler to tap out from the pressure.

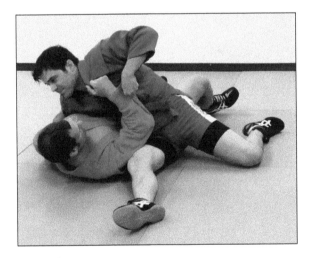

The top grappler uses his left hand to hold low on his opponent's sleeve and pull upward in this application. This illustrates that there are probably as many variations of hold-downs as there are situations in the sport of sambo.

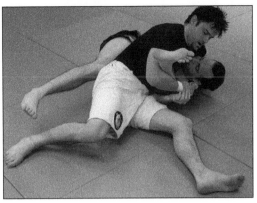

The top grappler uses a cradle hold with the side head-and-arm hold, and in this case the attacker uses his right hand and arm to trap low on his opponent's left leg. Doing this forces the bottom grappler's left leg up very high as shown, making the bottom grappler very weak in this position.

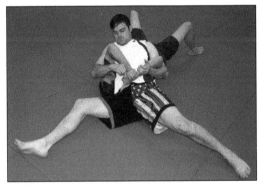

The top grappler may have back-to-chest control using this hold as shown here.

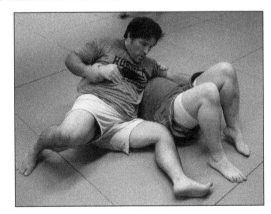

A useful variation of this hold is shown here where the attacker's left side and chest are in contact with the bottom grappler's right side and chest area. The top grappler uses his right hand and arm to trap and control the bottom grappler's right arm. The top grappler is facing his opponent's feet rather than his head as in the other application.

UPPER CHEST HOLD

This is a strong and effective hold-down and is an excellent hold from which to transition to an armlock.

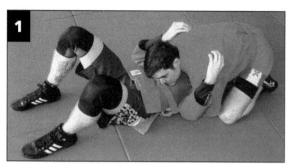

The basic application of the upper chest hold is shown here.

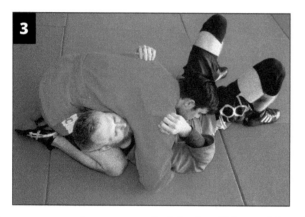

The top grappler uses his hands and arms to reach under his opponent's shoulders and arms and uses his hands to grab the bottom grappler's belt at about the hip area. Doing this creates a strong hold-down.

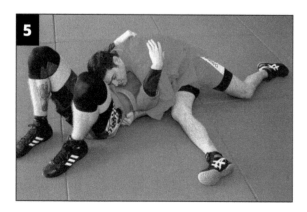

In some cases, the top grappler's body will be positioned as shown here. Doing this allows the top grappler to trap the bottom grappler's head at the top grappler's right hip between the attacker's right armpit and right upper leg and knee. This is a strong application of the upper chest hold.

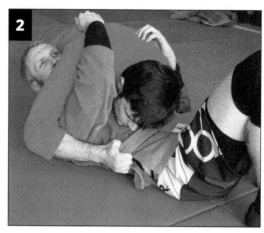

Sometimes, the top grappler will lower his hips to the mat and extend his feet and legs out wide to create a strong and stable base.

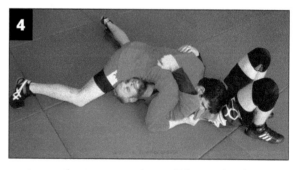

From this wide base, the top grappler can sit through with his right foot and leg, shifting his body weight and hips to maintain the hold if necessary.

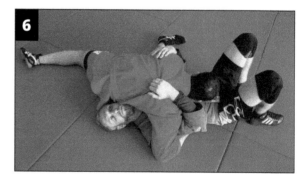

This view from above shows how the top grappler sits through with his right foot and leg to maintain control of the hold.

HIP HOLD-DOWN

The hip hold is an effective hold that allows the top grappler to control the bottom grappler's hips and is often used as an effective transition to lower body submissions.

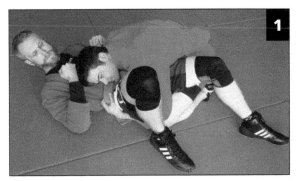

The top grappler uses his left hand and arm to reach between his opponent's legs and grab the bottom grappler's belt as shown. The top grappler's right hand and arm are placed under the bottom grappler's lower back and hip area and the right hand grabs the bottom man's belt.

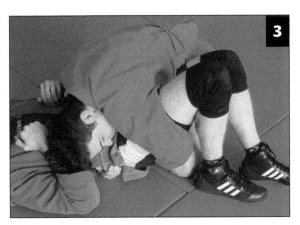

This view shows how the top grappler has excellent control of the bottom grappler's hips and lower torso. Think of a hip hold as a chest hold, only lower down on the opponent's torso.

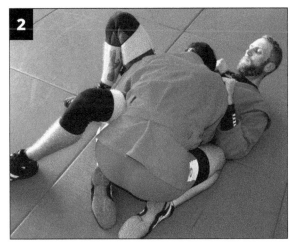

This photo shows how the top grappler uses his left hand and arm to reach over his opponent's far leg (his right leg). Look at how the attacker's right hand and arm are placed under the bottom grappler's hip and holding his belt.

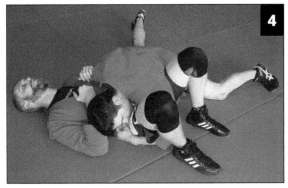

As in other hold-downs, the top grappler may have to lower his hips more to the mat and extend his feet and legs to widen his base to maintain control.

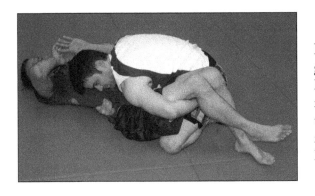

In situations such as MMA or submission grappling, the top grappler can use his left hand and arm to reach over his opponent's right upper leg and hook it for control. The top grappler uses his right hand and arm to reach under his opponent's low back and hook his hip.

VERTICAL CHEST HOLD

The vertical chest hold is similar to the front chest hold except that the top grappler is not situated between his opponent's legs.

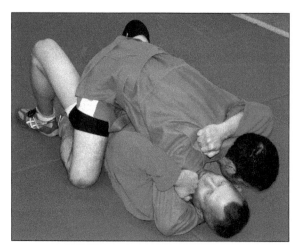

The top grappler straddles the bottom grappler with chest-to-chest contact as shown. There are many variations of how the top grappler uses his hands, arms, head, and shoulders to control his opponent and this photograph shows a common method.

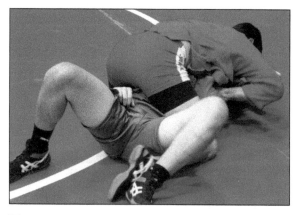

This shows how the top grappler uses his body to trap the bottom grappler's right arm, making it useless.

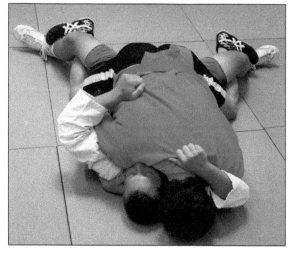

Sometimes, the top grappler will use his feet and legs to grapevine his opponent and spread the bottom grappler's legs as wide as possible, making it as uncomfortable as possible. In some cases, the bottom grappler may tap out from the pain caused by having his legs split far apart.

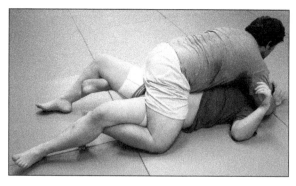

This shows how the top grappler uses his feet and legs to grapevine and control the bottom grappler.

VERTICAL CHEST HOLD

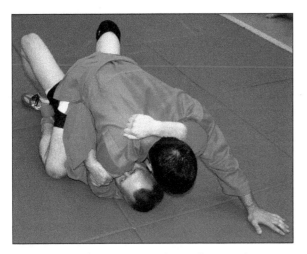

Sometimes, the top grappler will extend an arm or a leg and post a hand or foot on the mat to add stability to the hold as shown here.

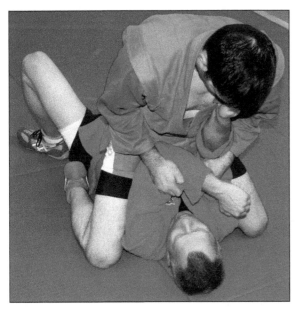

Here is the mount so often seen in MMA. The mount is a variation of the vertical chest hold and is a strong controlling position. There are variations of the mount and this photo shows a high mount where the top grappler is holding his opponent and controlling him with the intention of applying an armlock.

BREAKDOWNS AND TAKING CONTROL

The primary purpose of a breakdown is to take an opponent from a stable to an unstable position in groundfighting and ultimately secure a hold-down or submission technique. The best way to describe a breakdown is that it is very much like a throwing technique, only done in a groundfighting situation.

Breakdowns are considered transitions and can be applied from just about any position on the mat. In both theory and practice, the grappler doing a breakdown on his opponent is making a transition from one position to a more dominant or controlling position. The sambo wrestler doing the breakdown doesn't always have to start from a dominant position. The common theme of all breakdowns is that the sambo wrestler doing them took the initiative and then took control of the match.

THE PURPOSE OF A RIDE

As illustrated in many of the photographs in this book, one sambo wrestler is positioned beside or near his opponent and controlling him. When this takes place, the offensive grappler is riding his opponent. What is called a "ride" is a temporary controlling position used to enable the attacker to gain even more control over his opponent. A ride is part of a chain of events where the attacker wants to gain control over an opponent and maintain control over him as long as possible in order to break him down so he can apply a submission technique or finishing hold. And, in reality, a hold-down is actually also considered a ride because the attacker controls his opponent for a period of time and works to further control his opponent in order to secure a submission technique to finish him off.

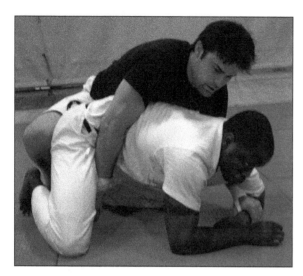

This photograph shows a typical spiral ride used in all forms of grappling, wrestling, or fighting sports. There are many ways to ride an opponent, and the spiral ride is one of the most basic (and effective). Unlike collegiate, folkstyle, or freestyle wrestling, a ride in sambo does not score points. The purpose of a ride in sambo is to give the offensive grappler time and opportunity to gain further control of his opponent, which leads to a hold-down or submission technique. Often, a ride leads to the controlling grappler breaking down his opponent and securing a finishing hold of some type. In many situations, a sambo grappler will control his opponent with a ride, break him down, and put the opponent into a hold-down or, if that is not possible, into another controlling position before securing a submission technique or finishing hold.

Okay, let's now examine some common and effective breakdowns used in sambo.

BREAKDOWNS WHEN ONE ATHLETE IS ON ALL FOURS OR LYING FLAT ON HIS FRONT

A large number of effective breakdowns can be applied when the defensive grappler is positioned on all fours or lying flat on his front in a defensive position. Some of these breakdown are presented here.

FAR ARM–NEAR LEG BREAKDOWN

This breakdown has a high rate of success at all levels of sambo.

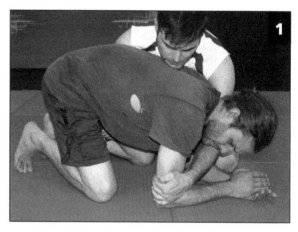

The attacker uses his left hand and arm to reach under his opponent's head and grab the bottom grappler's right elbow low to the mat.

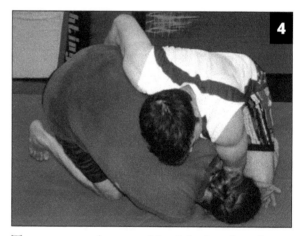

The top grappler uses his right hand and arm to lift his opponent's left leg as the attacker continues to use his left hand and arm to pull in on his opponent's right elbow. Doing this forces the bottom grappler to roll as shown.

FAR ARM-NEAR LEG BREAKDOWN

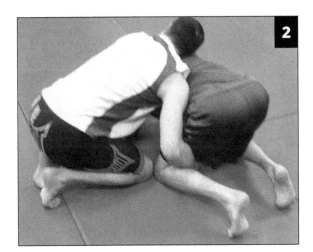

The attacker uses his right hand and arm to reach around his opponent's right upper leg and grab it firmly just above the left knee.

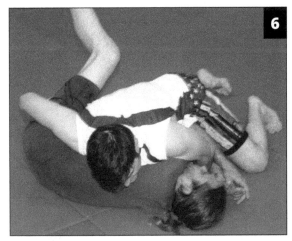

The attacker uses his left hand and arm to pull in on the bottom grappler's right elbow.

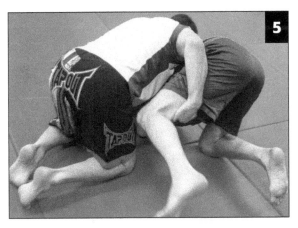

This view shows how the attacker uses his right hand and arm to lift his opponent's left leg.

The attacker rolls the bottom grappler over onto his back. As he does this, the top grappler makes sure to use his chest and upper body to drive his opponent over and to have good body contact.

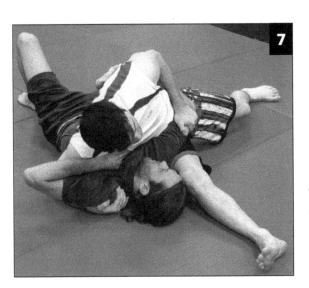

The attacker rolls his opponent over and applies a hold-down.

BOTH ELBOWS BREAKDOWN

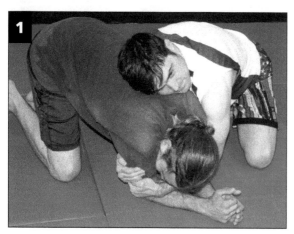

The top grappler is positioned at the left side of his opponent as shown. The top grappler uses both hands and arms to reach under his opponent and grab the bottom grappler's right arm. Look at how the attacker uses his hands to grab low to the mat on his opponent's right elbow.

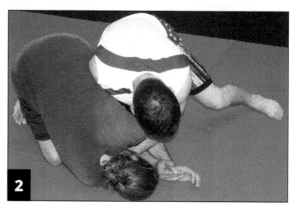

The attacker uses his right shoulder to drive into his opponent's left upper torso as he uses both hands and arms to pull in on his opponent's right elbow.

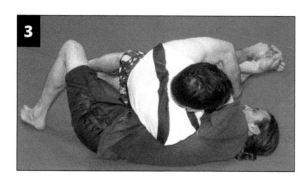

The attacker drives hard into his opponent and rolls the bottom grappler over onto his back.

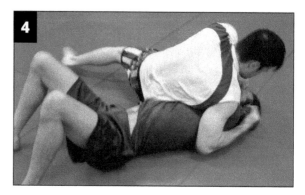

The attacker drives his opponent onto his back and applies a hold-down.

BOTH KNEES BREAKDOWN

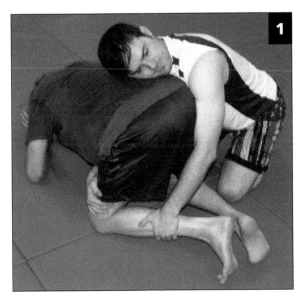

The attacker uses his right hand and arm to reach under his opponent's torso and grabs the bottom grappler's left leg just above the knee. The attacker uses his left hand to grab his opponent's left lower leg near or at the ankle.

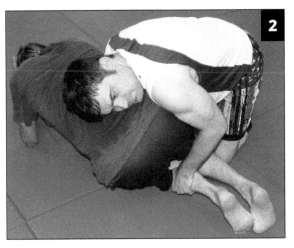

The attacker uses his upper body to drive against his opponent's right torso as the attacker uses both of his hands and arms to pull in on his opponent's knees. Doing this collapses the bottom grappler as shown.

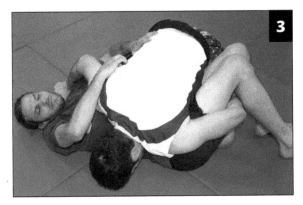

The attacker breaks his opponent down and rolls him onto his back.

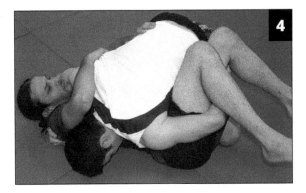

The attacker immediately secures a hold-down.

NEAR WRIST TO NELSON BREAKDOWN

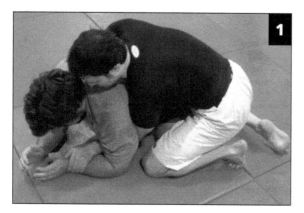

The attacker uses his left hand to grab and control his opponent's left wrist. This near wrist control prevents the bottom grappler from escaping. The attacker's right hand and arm are placed at the bottom grappler's right hip in a spiral ride.

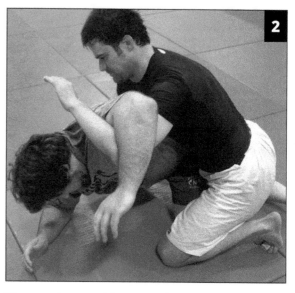

The attacker quickly moves his left hand and arm under his opponent's left shoulder as shown.

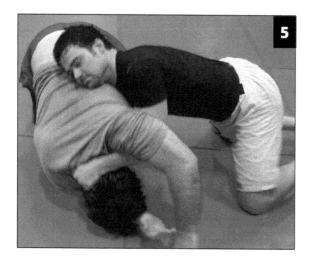

The attacker uses his right hand to pull in on his opponent's right elbow as he continues to pry his opponent's head as shown. Doing this forces his opponent to roll over.

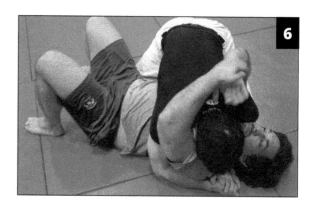

The attacker rolls his opponent onto his back and secures a hold-down

NEAR WRIST TO NELSON BREAKDOWN

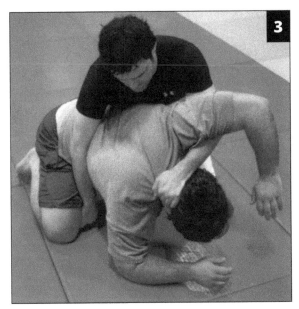

The attacker places his left hand and arm under the bottom grappler's left shoulder and on the back of his head as shown. The attacker uses his left hand and arm to pry his opponent's head down.

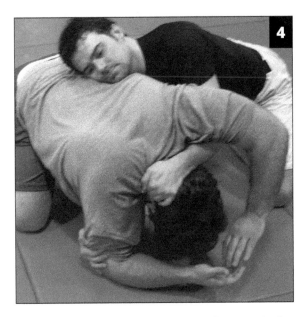

The attacker uses his right hand to grab his opponent's right elbow low to the mat as shown. As he does this, the top grappler continues to use his left hand and arm to pry his opponent's head down.

GUT WRENCH

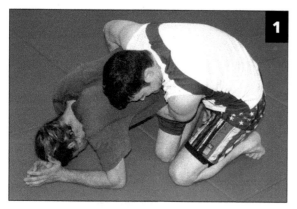

The attacker rides his opponent from the side as shown. As he does this, the attacker uses both hands and arms to grab around his opponent's stomach and to squeeze forcefully on his opponent's gut.

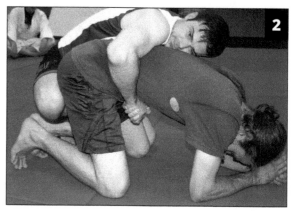

This view from the opposite side shows how the attacker uses his hands and arms to trap, control, and squeeze his opponent's torso. The top grappler squeezes hard and makes it uncomfortable for his opponent.

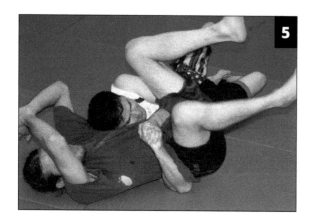

The attacker continues to roll and apply pressure with the gut wrench as he rolls his opponent over onto his back.

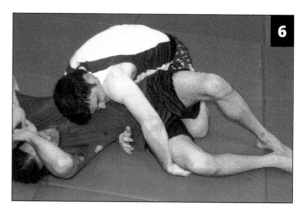

The attacker completes the gut wrench roll and rolls his opponent onto his back as shown.

GUT WRENCH

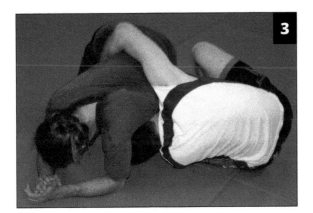

The attacker forcefully dips low under his opponent and drives his head under his opponent's body as shown. The attacker does this quickly and with explosive power.

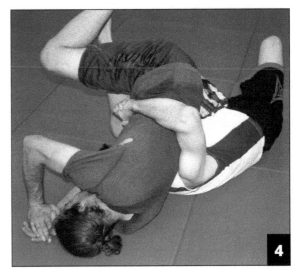

The attacker rolls hard and forces his opponent to roll over as shown.

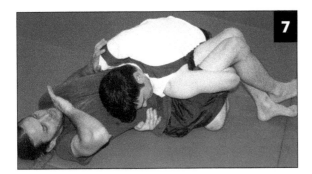

The attacker immediately secures a hip hold.

TWO-ON-ONE WRIST TRAP BREAKDOWN

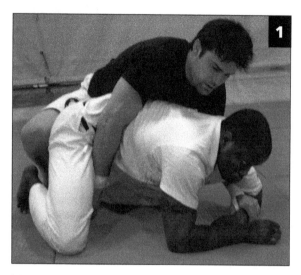

The top grappler uses his left hand to grab and control his opponent's left wrist. The top grappler uses his right hand and arm to reach around his opponent's lower back and hip and place his right hand on the inside of his opponent's right thigh.

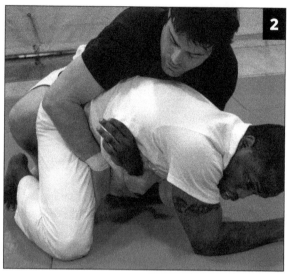

The attacker uses his left hand to pull his opponent's left wrist and arm under the bottom grappler's torso as shown.

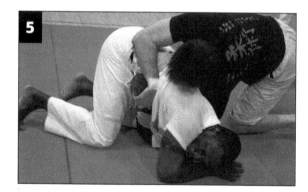

The attacker continues to move to his left and pull upward on his opponent's left wrist. Doing this forces the bottom grappler to roll over his left shoulder as shown.

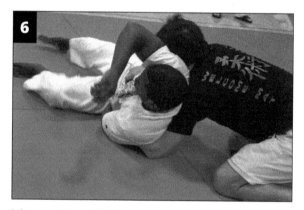

The attacker rolls his opponent onto his back.

TWO-ON-ONE WRIST TRAP BREAKDOWN

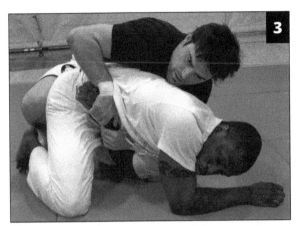

The top grappler uses both hands to grab and control his opponent's left wrist and arm as shown. The attacker uses his hands and arms to pull upward on his opponent's left wrist.

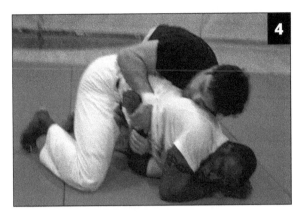

The attacker moves to his left (in the direction of the bottom grappler's head), and as he does this, the top grappler continues to pull upward on the bottom grappler's left arm as shown.

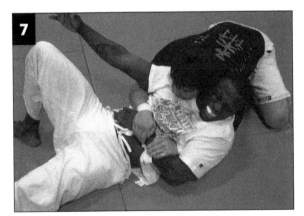

The attacker pulls his opponent onto his back and continues to use both hands to grab and trap his opponent's left wrist, pinning it to his torso as shown. The attacker uses his chin to drive downward on his opponent's right shoulder and upper pectoral area to force the bottom grappler onto the mat.

BELT-AND-NELSON BREAKDOWN

This is an effective, yet simple, breakdown with a high rate of success at all levels of sambo.

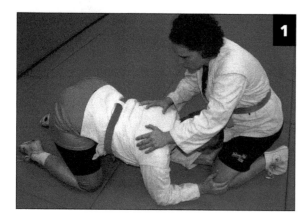

The top grappler is on her knees at the front of her opponent who is on all fours as shown.

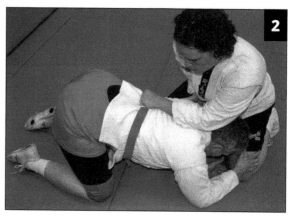

The top grappler uses her left hand and arm to reach down the middle of the bottom grappler's back. The top grappler uses her left hand (palm down) to grab her opponent's belt. Look at the position of the top grappler's body relative to her opponent. The top grappler is positioned at the left side of the bottom grappler, near her left shoulder.

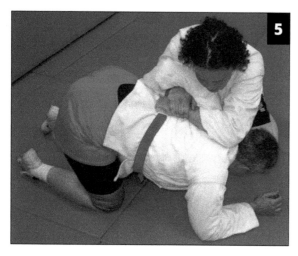

The top grappler uses her upper body to drive into her opponent at the bottom grappler's left side as shown.

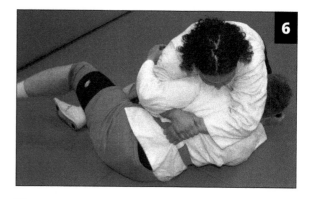

The top grappler forces her opponent over onto her back.

BELT-AND-NELSON BREAKDOWN

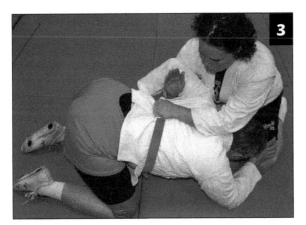

The top grappler uses her right hand to move under her opponent's left upper arm and shoulder. The top grappler's right hand is positioned as shown in the photo.

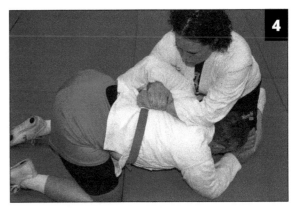

The top grappler uses her right hand to grab her left wrist and form a "nelson" hold, trapping her opponent's left arm and shoulder.

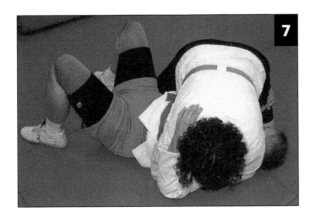

The top grappler breaks her opponent down and applies a chest hold.

BELT-AND-NELSON BREAKDOWN WHEN OPPONENT IS FLAT

As mentioned above, when your opponent flattens out on his or her front and waits for the mat official to call a halt to the action, say thank you and go to work.

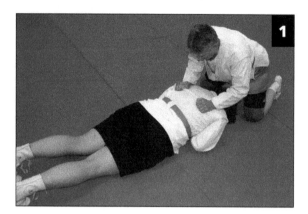

The attacker is at the top of her opponent who is lying flat on her front in an extreme defensive posture.

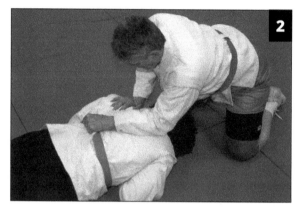

The top grappler uses her left hand and arm to reach down the middle of the bottom grappler's back. The attacker uses her left hand (palm down) to grab her opponent's belt.

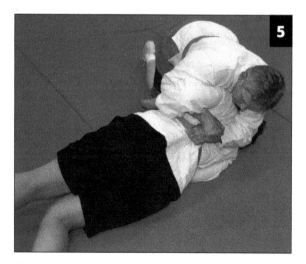

The attacker drives her opponent over and onto her back.

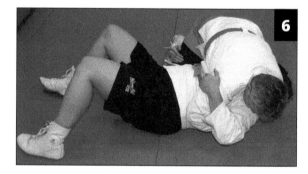

The attacker breaks her opponent down onto her back and secures a chest hold.

BELT-AND-NELSON BREAKDOWN WHEN OPPONENT IS FLAT

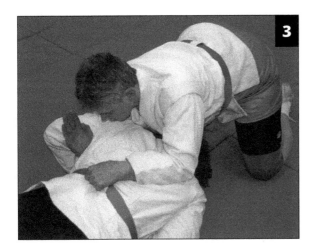

The top grappler uses her right hand to move under her opponent's left upper arm and shoulder. The fingers of the top grappler's right hand are pointed upward as shown.

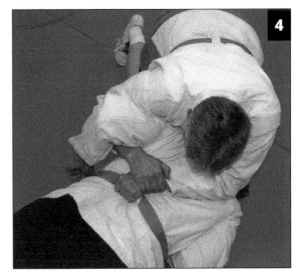

The attacker uses her right hand to grab her left wrist. The attacker moves to her right so that she is positioned over her opponent's left shoulder. The attacker uses her upper body to drive under her opponent's left shoulder as she levers her opponent onto her back.

BREAKDOWNS WHEN BOTH ATHLETES ARE IN A NEUTRAL POSITION

Sometimes, the sambo wrestlers are positioned facing each other and in a kneeling position, either on both knees or on one knee. Here are a few breakdowns that are done from this position.

HEAD-AND-ARM HIP THROW BREAKDOWN

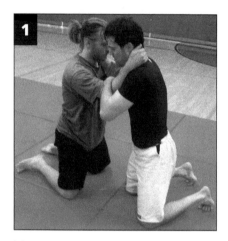

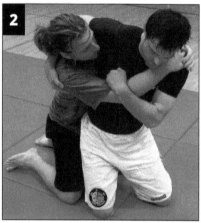

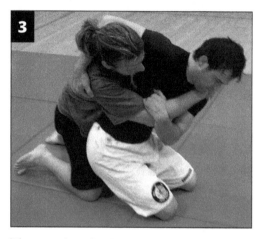

The athletes are in a neutral position on their knees as shown and holding onto each other with a head-and-arm grip.

The attacker uses his left hand to pull on his opponent's right elbow and his right hand and arm to reach around his opponent's head. As he does this, the attacker turns to his left so that he will roll his opponent over his right hip.

The attacker fits his body in place so that he rolls his opponent over his right hip.

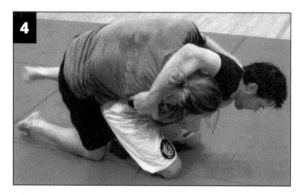

The attacker rolls his opponent over his hip.

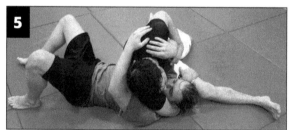

The attacker rolls his opponent over his right hip and directly into a head-and-arm side chest hold.

FRONT BOTH LEGS BREAKDOWN

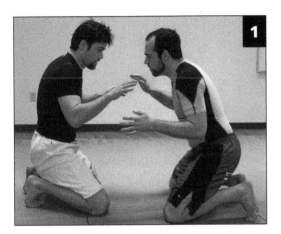

The athletes are positioned on their knees and facing each other in a neutral situation.

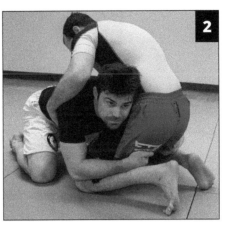

The attacker drops low and drives his left shoulder into his opponent's midsection. As he does this, the attacker places the left side of his head on his opponent's left hip. The attacker uses both of his hands and arms to grab his opponent's legs as shown.

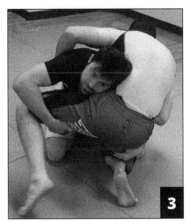

The attacker uses his head to drive his opponent to the attacker's left. As he does this, he uses his hands and arms to scoop his opponent's legs to the attacker's right. Look at the angle that the attacker is taking his opponent to at this point.

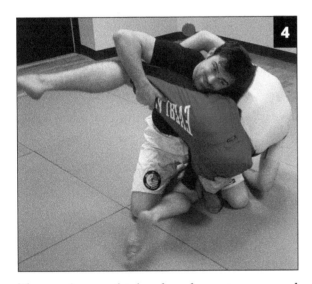

The attacker uses his hands and arms to scoop and lift his opponent off the mat, driving the defender to the attacker's right side.

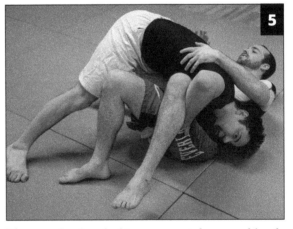

The attacker breaks his opponent down and lands on top of him as shown.

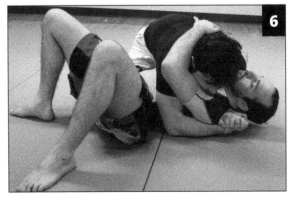

The attacker immediately secures a chest hold.

KNEE TAP BREAKDOWN

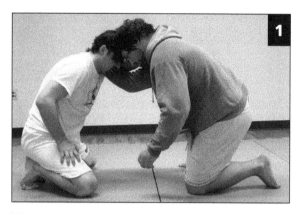

The attacker (on the left) faces his opponent, who is positioned with his left knee on the mat and his right foot on the mat.

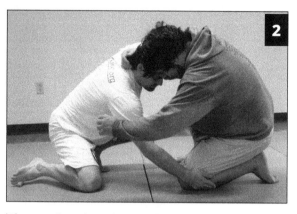

The attacker places his right hand on his opponent's left knee. As he does this, the attacker uses his left hand to grab and control his opponent's head.

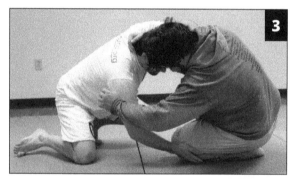

The attacker drives his opponent to the attacker's right side with his body movement and, pushing with his left hand, as he uses it to block the outside of his opponent's left knee.

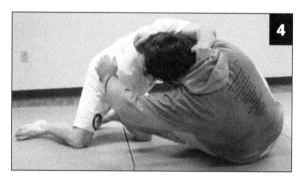

The attacker drives his opponent over onto the defender's left side.

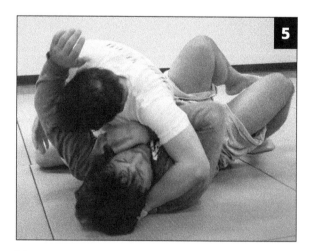

The attacker drives his opponent to his back and applies a hold-down.

ANKLE PICK BREAKDOWN

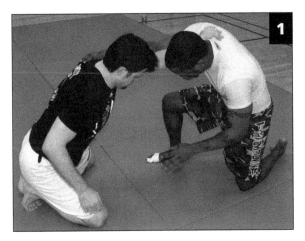

The attacker (left) faces his opponent, who is positioned on his left knee and right foot. The attacker uses his left hand to grab his opponent's left shoulder.

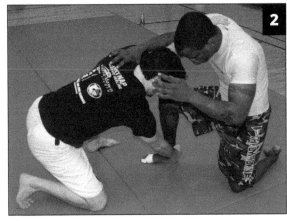

The attacker steps up on his left foot and reaches with his left hand and arm and grabs his opponent's right ankle.

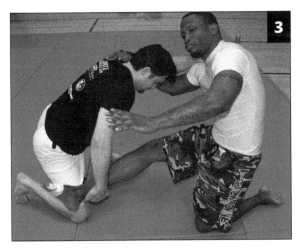

The attacker uses his left hand to pull his opponent's ankle and leg to the attacker's right hip, which extends the defender's right leg straight. As he does this, the attacker uses his left hand to pull his opponent's right shoulder to the mat.

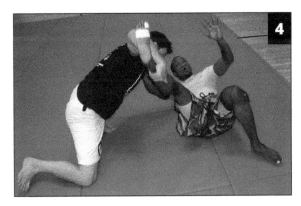

The attacker pulls his opponent's right leg out and forces him onto his back.

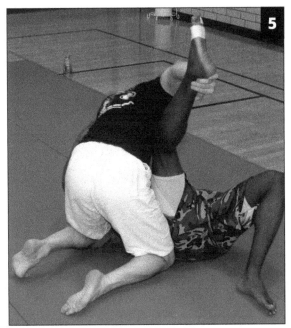

The attacker breaks his opponent down and flat onto his back.

HAND SWEEP BREAKDOWN

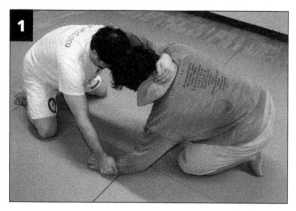

The attacker (left) controls his opponent with his left hand on the defender's head. The attacker uses his right hand to grab his opponent's left wrist.

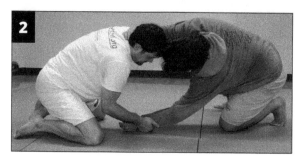

The attacker uses his right hand to pull his opponent's left wrist to the attacker's left. This action starts to break the defender's balance and topple him to his left.

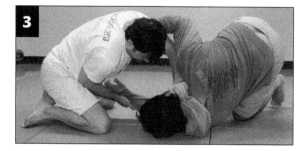

The attacker continues to pull with his right hand on his opponent's left wrist and push with his left hand on his opponent's head. Doing this forces the defender onto his left side as shown.

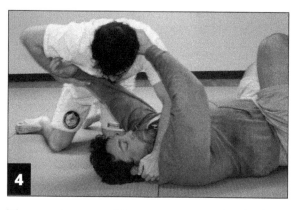

The attacker turns his opponent onto his back.

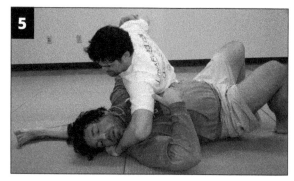

The attacker follows through and applies a head-and-arm side chest hold.

BREAKDOWNS FROM THE BOTTOM POSITION

No sambo wrestler dominates his opponent from the top position all the time. Every grappler has been on the bottom, and the better he knows how to handle the situation, the better he will succeed in getting out of trouble and gaining the dominant position.

TECHNICAL TIP: When on the bottom, get out from there! There are few things worse in sambo or any fighting sport than being the guy on the bottom. If you do get caught on the bottom, think logically and take things step by step so that you first get out of trouble, and then work to take back control of the situation. If you can't take back control initially, you may have to get into a "scramble" with your opponent. A scramble takes place when neither sambo wrestler has the advantage in groundfighting. A scramble may not be the ideal situation, but it's better than being controlled by your opponent.

SAMBO SWITCH TO BOTH LEGS BREAKDOWN

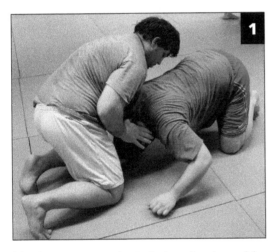

The bottom grappler is being dominated by his opponent as shown.

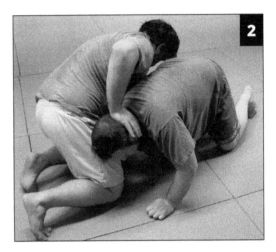

The bottom grappler immediately gets his head from out of the middle under his opponent and places the right side of his head on the right hip of his opponent. It is vital that the bottom grappler get his head out from the bottom. Otherwise, the top grappler will continue to dominate the position and gain more control.

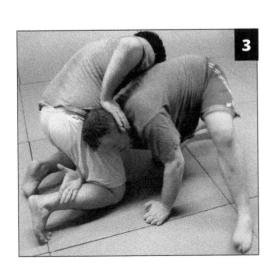

The bottom grappler immediately steps up and onto his left foot. As he does this, the bottom grappler uses his right hand to hook on the inside of his opponent's right leg just above the knee. The bottom grappler's right hand is positioned as shown. The bottom grappler uses his head to drive into his opponent's right hip.

SAMBO SWITCH TO BOTH LEGS BREAKDOWN

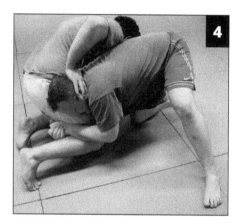

The bottom grappler grasps both hands together in a square grip and forcefully traps his opponent's right upper leg. Doing this traps the top grappler's right leg and prevents him from sitting out or moving to a better position. As he does this, the bottom grappler starts to move to his left.

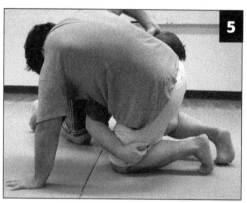

The bottom grappler uses his right hand to grab his opponent's left leg just above the knee.

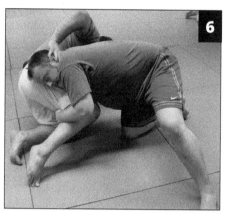

The attacker uses his left hand and arm to hook and lift his opponent's right leg just above the top grappler's knee. Look at how the bottom grappler drives to his right and starts to topple his opponent.

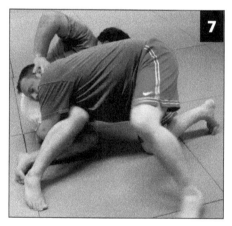

The bottom grappler continues to drive his opponent to the bottom grappler's right and breaks his opponent down onto his left side.

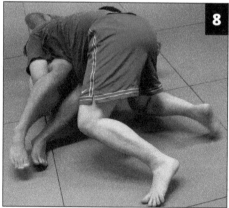

The bottom grappler breaks his opponent down and onto his back.

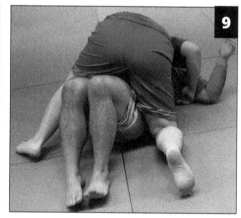

The bottom grappler isn't the bottom grappler anymore and immediately applies a hold-down.

SODEN ROLL

This is an effective breakdown from the bottom position when the top grappler uses his hands and arms to reach around the bottom grappler's body.

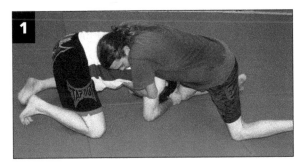

The bottom grappler is being controlled by his opponent who is positioned on his knees near the bottom grappler's head.

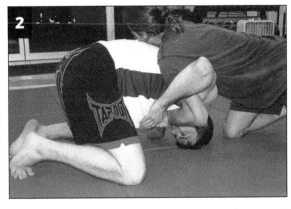

The bottom grappler posts on the top of his head for stability as he uses both of his arms to hook and trap the top grappler's arms. Look at how the bottom grappler hooks his opponent's arms between the elbow and shoulder for maximum control.

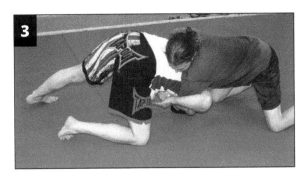

The bottom grappler (making sure that he has trapped his opponent's arms firmly to the bottom grappler's body) quickly turns to his left. Look at how the bottom grappler posts his left foot and leg to his left for stability as he initiates his roll.

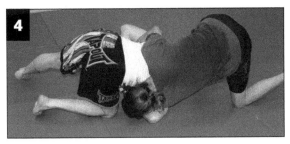

The bottom grappler continues to roll his opponent as shown. A fast, explosive rolling movement is necessary.

SODEN ROLL

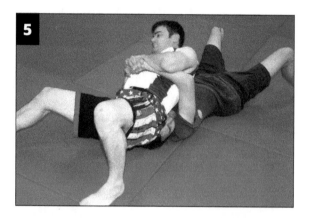

The bottom grappler completes his roll (still using both hands and arms to trap both of his opponent's arms firmly to the bottom grappler's body).

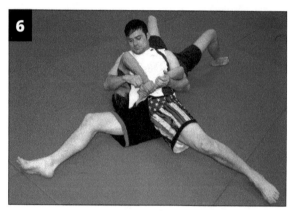

As part of the rolling movement, the attacker ends up with his right hip positioned at the right side of his opponent's head. Look at how the attacker continues to use his hands and arms to trap his opponent's arms to the attacker's body. Immediately after completing the roll, the attacker positions his legs as shown in the photograph. Doing all of these actions allows the attacker to be positioned on his right hip, holding his opponent.

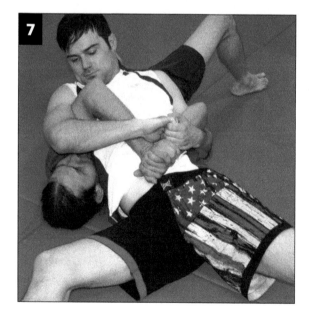

If necessary, the top grappler can grip his hands together as shown, trapping his opponent's arms against the attacker's torso for more control.

PETERSON ROLL

Named for Olympic Champion Ben Peterson, this is a common but effective breakdown for the bottom grappler.

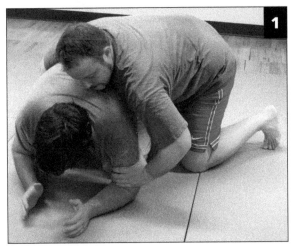

The bottom grappler is being controlled by his opponent.

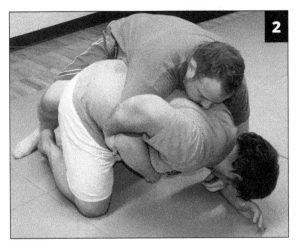

The bottom grappler uses his right hand and arm to grab and hook his opponent's right arm just above the top grappler's right elbow. The bottom grappler pulls tightly, trapping the top grappler's right arm firmly to the bottom grappler's body.

TECHNICAL TIP: The Peterson Roll is a good example of a "get out of trouble move" where, if the bottom grappler can't break his opponent down, the bottom grappler can at least get out of a bad positon and get into a neutral situation. Sometimes it's not possible to break an opponent down or immediately move into a scoring technique, and it's important to know how to get out of trouble.

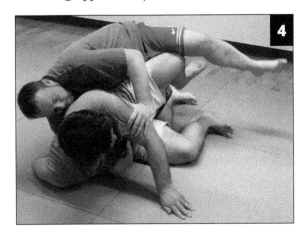

The bottom grappler rolls over his right shoulder using his right hand and arm to firmly trap and control his opponent's right arm, forcing the top grappler to roll over the bottom grappler's back as shown. An important part of this roll is how the bottom grappler uses his left bent leg to help lift his opponent's left upper leg. The power of the bottom grappler's leg lift along with the momentum of the rolling action forces the top grappler to roll.

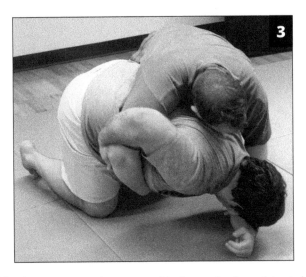

The bottom grappler moves his lower body to his right so that the top grappler's right arm is trapped against the bottom grappler's upper back. Doing this gives the bottom grappler a better angle to roll his opponent over his back.

PETERSON ROLL

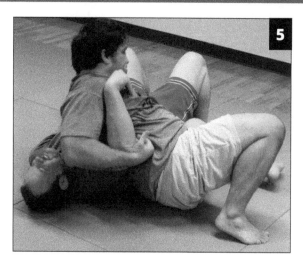

The attacker rolls his opponent over his back and hip and immediately completes the rolling action to turn and face his opponent's legs as shown.

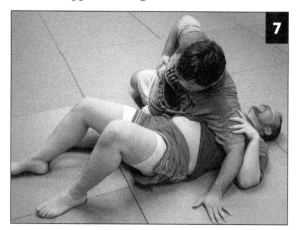

If this hold is precarious, the attacker can switch to another hold. The attacker uses his left hand and arm to post on the mat as shown.

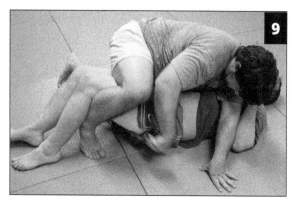

The attacker moves his right foot and leg over his opponent's lower body as the attacker starts to position his body on top of his opponent.

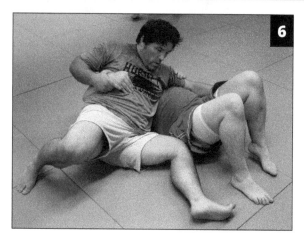

The attacker completes his roll and ends up in this holding position. Look at how the attacker continues to use his right hand and arm to hold and trap his opponent's right arm firmly to the attacker's body. Doing this gives the attacker strong control in this holding position.

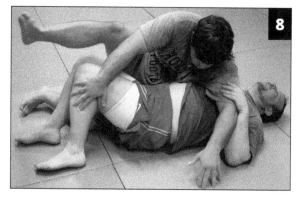

The attacker places his right hand on his opponent's left leg just below the knee and pushes inward. This action gets the opponent's left leg out of the way for the attacker to move his right foot and leg over his opponent's legs as shown.

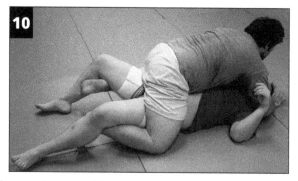

The attacker transitions to a stronger position and holds his opponent with a vertical chest hold.

BREAKDOWNS WHEN THE TOP SAMBO WRESTLER IS ON TOP AGAINST AN OPPONENT DEFENDING OFF OF HIS BACK

Sometimes, the bottom sambo wrestler is skilled at fighting out of the "guard" position used in judo, jujitsu, and MMA. If the top grappler is not able to directly apply a front chest hold from this position and the bottom grappler is skillful at using his feet and legs to make space, the top grappler can use an ankle or leglock. But in some situations this may not be possible, and the top grappler can use the following move (or other breakdowns similar to it).

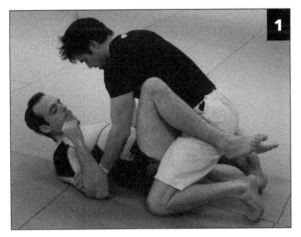

The top grappler is situated between his opponent's legs and in the bottom grappler's guard. The top grappler uses both of his hands and arms to pin the bottom grappler's uppers arms to the mat.

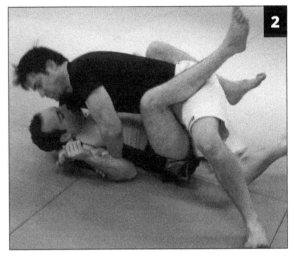

The top grappler turns to his left as he places his left foot and leg out to his left as shown. By doing this, the top grappler turns his hips so that his right hip is now facing the middle of the bottom grappler's body.

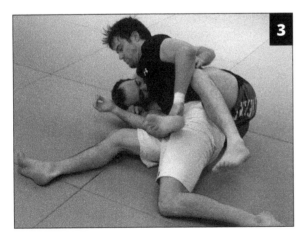

The top grappler moves his right foot and leg forward and sits through so that his right hip is now positioned on the bottom grappler's right upper leg. As he does this, the top grappler wraps his right hand and arm around his opponent's head for upper body control. The attacker starts to move his left hand and arm under the bottom grappler's right lower leg.

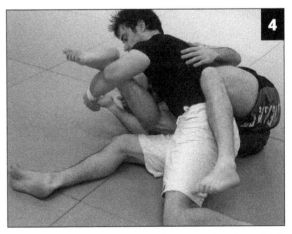

The top grappler uses his left arm to hook and lift forward on the bottom grappler's right lower leg or ankle. This is painful and weakens the bottom grappler.

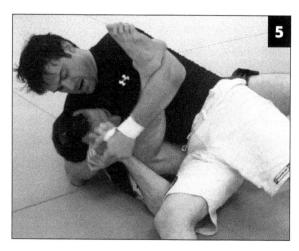

The top grappler's right hand and arm are hooked around the bottom grappler's head and neck. The top grappler's left hand and arm are hooked under the bottom grappler's right leg. The top grappler grasps his hands together and forms a strong square grip and squeezes tightly. Doing this creates a nasty and painful hold, bending the bottom grappler in half.

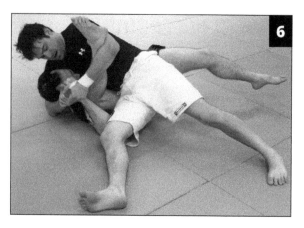

The top grappler controls his opponent as shown. If the bottom grappler doesn't tap out from the pain of the hold-down, the top grappler will hold him for time.

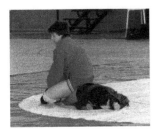

Chapter Six: Epilogue
"World-class skills are simply fundamentals performed to their full potential."

SOME CLOSING THOUGHTS

As mentioned in this book's introduction, sambo is an eclectic, open-ended fighting sport with a tradition of pragmatic innovation.

It's been my purpose to give you a book that will serve as a foundation to build on. Whether you are an elite sambo wrestler, coach, mat official, or a novice to the sport, this book can be a reliable resource for many years to come. The information contained in this book can be used by hard-core sambo exponents as well as athletes, fighters, and coaches in other combat sports such as MMA or submission grappling.

Another purpose of this book has been to provide an organized and systematic approach to the theory and technique of the sport of sambo. To my knowledge, this is the largest and most comprehensive book yet published in the United States on the subject of sambo. It's my sincere hope that anyone, regardless of nationality or language, can benefit from what has been presented in this book.

This book is titled *Sambo Encyclopedia: Comprehensive Throws, Holds, and Submission Techniques* for two reasons. First, sambo is an eclectic, open-ended, and dynamic sport with a tradition of innovation as well as a future of innovative development. Second, the vital and essential skills of sambo are at the forefront of this book. No claims are being made that this is the final word or ultimate authority on sambo, but a comprehensive book like this can serve as a solid source of information on sambo. Hopefully, the work that is being presented here will impel others to produce books or other media that will enhance and improve the theoretical and technical principles of sambo.

On a personal level, this book was a joy to write and I sincerely hope that it will be a positive addition to the world of sambo. It's always been my belief that, in any book and on any topic, the author has a discussion with the reader. If I'm successful as a writer, the words and photographs in this book will elicit thought on your part and compel you to explore new areas of thought and technical exploration and innovation. Books are marvelous tools that you can come back to at a later date and gain another insight or perspective that you didn't have before. This is certainly the case for me. There are books that I have read and reread for many years, learning something new or gaining a different insight every time. Books make us think and, of course, the purpose of this book is to make you think. Hopefully, you will come back time and again to think about and reflect on what is written in these pages and we can continue our discussion for many years in the future.

Steve Scott
Kansas City, Missouri

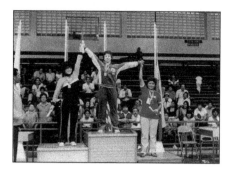

Special thanks to my wife Becky Scott. Her contribution to this book has been immense; from discussions on every phase of technical skill when this book was in the planning stage to the editing of the final proofs, her input has been both welcome and substantial. Becky is a World and Pan American Sambo Champion as well as a six-time U.S. National Sambo Champion. She is the first woman from the United States to win a World Sambo Championship. Becky also won national and international titles in judo as an athlete and served as a coach for official U.S. judo teams to a variety of international tournaments, including the World (Under 21) Judo Championships. We have been married since 1975 after having met at a judo tournament in 1973. After having travelled the world, we continue to be happiest when we are together at home with the cats.

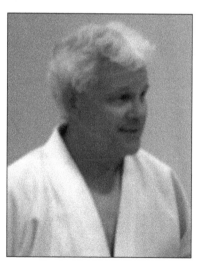

Special thanks to my friend Jim Schneweis. Jim is one of the best coaches I've ever met, in any sport. Jim is a U.S. National Sambo Champion, World Team Alternate, U.S. Olympic Festival Coach, and coach of over 150 national and international sambo champions. He was also instrumental in the success of the first women's teams at the Pan American Games and World Championships. Jim is a pioneer and unsung hero in sambo in the United States.

In February of 1977, I organized the first sambo tournament in the Kansas City area, and it was then and there that I met Jim Schneweis, a local high school wrestling coach. This was Jim's first exposure to sambo and he was immediately hooked. Since that time, Jim and I have worked closely on many sambo tournaments, training camps, demonstrations, and anything else we could think of. He is a skilled sambo man, and we've spent many hours on the mat training and learning from each other. Jim's insight into both the technical and coaching aspects of sambo have been a positive influence on this book.

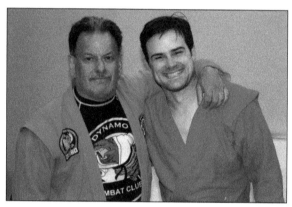

Special thanks to Gregg Humphreys (left) and Derrick Darling (right). Gregg proved to be a good sounding board for a variety of ideas and subjects during the writing of this book. Gregg has travelled and trained in Russia, Belarus, and Ukraine fifteen times (more than any other American) and is one of the most knowledgeable and skillful sambo men in the United States. He is also the editor for the DVD series by Igor Kurinnoy titled *Sambo for Professionals* and is Coach Kurinnoy's North American representative for his organization. Derrick appeared in over 75 percent of the photographs in this book. His technical expertise is of the highest quality as is his understanding of sambo's theoretical foundation. His suggestions and input during the photo shoots as well as during the many workouts when we took photos provided a positive contribution. Derrick is a U.S. National Sambo Champion and World Sambo Championships Team Member. He has also won numerous National AAU Judo Championships and Freestyle Judo Championships as well as the Pan American Judo Union Championship and many international medals in judo, submission grappling, and sport jujitsu. At the time of this writing, Derrick is a young man and will be a positive influence on sambo and other fighting sports for years to come.

ABOUT THE AUTHOR

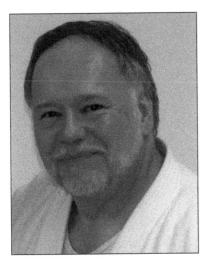

This is the sixteenth published book by Steve Scott on the subject of sambo, judo, jujitsu, fitness and martial arts. Steve is a professional coach and CPR instructor and is a graduate of the University of Missouri–Kansas City. Starting his judo career in 1965 and his sambo career in 1976, he has trained, competed and coached in over a dozen countries. He has personally coached four World Sambo Champions and several other world-class medal winners and members of world and international teams. He is considered a pioneer in sambo in the United States and is a member of the U.S. Sombo Association Hall of Fame. As a coach, he has developed over 350 national and international champions and medal winners in sambo, judo, submission grappling and sport jujitsu. He is the innovator of women's sambo in the United States and hosted the first women's U.S. National Sambo Championships in 1980. He was the coach of the U.S. women's sambo team at the Pan American Games where the U.S. won the women's team championship with four gold and six silver medals. As an athlete, Steve won two gold medals and a bronze medal at the National AAU Sambo Championships and was an alternate to the World and Pan American teams in different years. He also won numerous smaller national sambo tournaments in the 1970s and 1980s as well as being an active judo athlete and athlete in the Scottish Highland Games for many years. As a mat official, Steve was a national and international sambo mat official for many years. As an administrator, Steve introduced sambo to the Kansas City area in 1977 and served as a member of the National AAU Sambo Committee for many years and was one of the three founders of the U.S. Sombo Association in 1985. Steve is the founder of the Welcome Mat Judo Club in 1969 and continues to coach Shingitai Jujitsu, sambo, judo and submission grappling at the Welcome Mat Training Center in the Kansas City area.

BOOKS FROM YMAA

AND MANY MORE . . .

VIDEOS FROM YMAA

AND MANY MORE . . .

more products available from . . .
YMAA Publication Center, Inc.   楊氏東方文化出版中心

1-800-669-8892 • info@ymaa.com • www.ymaa.com